Denise:

Thanks for all the help –

It's the little things that count

Don Hunt

SHAPE Shift

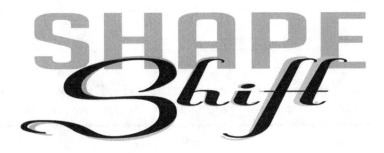

SHAPE *Shift*

The Shape Intelligence Solution
Getting Healthy While Creating Your Ideal Shape

DR. GREGORY KELLY
DR. MARK PERCIVAL

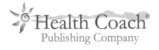

Health Coach®
Publishing Company

Health Coach Publishing Co.
3225 McLeod Dr., Suite 110
Las Vegas, NV 89121
1.888.888.8565

ISBN 978-0-9845374-0-2

Printed in the United States of America.
First Edition
10 9 8 7 6 5 4 3 2 1

Printed on recycled paper

Book Design by Cheri Percival
Cover Design by Eric Blais

Neither the publisher nor the authors are engaged in rendering professional advice or services to the individual reader. The ideas, assessments, and suggestions in this book are not intended as a substitute for consulting with your physician. All matters regarding your health require appropriate medical supervision. Neither the publisher nor the authors shall be liable or responsible for any loss or damage allegedly arising from any information or suggestion in this book.

While the authors have made every effort to provide accurate telephone numbers and Internet addresses at the time of publication, neither the publisher nor the authors assume any responsibility for errors or for changes that occur after publication.

This book is dedicated to our two wonderful mothers, Joanne Kelly and Betty Percival.

Acknowledgements

More than a decade ago, we became frustrated with the conventional wisdom of weight sciences. This boiled to a head when a prominent health expert wrote on their website words to the effect of; if you want to lose weight, I'll give you the advice I give all my patients, eat less and exercise more. In our work with people with shape challenges, we knew it wasn't this easy. We wanted to find out why, and we wanted to find ways to make it easier. This book is the end result of our investigation. Along the way, there have been many people who have helped directly and indirectly. We want to thank them all.

First, we owe a considerable debt to those authors and experts whose research and ideas were used as elements of this book. Without the efforts of these individuals, whose specific works are mentioned in the notes and references section, this book would not have been possible. As the saying goes, we are standing on the shoulders of giants.

We want to thank all of our patients, clients and students, past and present: Without you to work with, teach, and learn from, we would never have seen what did and didn't work, especially over long periods of time. You have also been instrumental in helping us find new ways to convey important points with a simplicity and directness that you readily understand (which is often very different from the ways we, as doctors, communicate with each other).

We want to acknowledge all of the health professionals who have taken our courses on shape. One of the biggest leaps forward we had in our investigation was when we committed to teaching a course on shape improvement to other doctors. Our thanks go out to all of you who were willing to take a course that diverged substantially from the conventional wisdom around weight gain and loss. We especially want to acknowledge those of you who stuck with this work and became core members of the health scene investigation team. In alphabetical order these persons are: Katherine Ackland, N.D., Shannon Bell, Stephen Bircher, D.C., Kim Clarke, Mark deDubovay, D.C., Kenneth Gilman, D.C., David H. Haase, M.D., Janet Haase, Timothy Houlton, D.C., Donald Huml, D.C., Debbie Martin Belleville, N.D., Todd Norton, D.C., Richard Perryman, D.C., Richard Powers, D.C., Russel Sher, D.C. and Daniel Therrien, D.C.

We want to acknowledge and thank Eric Blais for designing our cover. We want to thank Janet and David Haase, Richard Powers, and Natasha Efross for reading rough drafts of this book. Your feedback and editorial assistance are tremendously appreciated. We want to acknowledge the support, enthusiasm, and occasional expertise of our family and friends, among them Sepi Day, William Fenton, Betty Percival, Joanne Kelly (and all the Kelly clan). Thanks for your encouragement and patience. We want to specifically mention Aspen and Lexi Percival (Mark's daughters). Thanks for helping with our HSI team events, for being willing guinea pigs for some of our efforts into self-experimentation, and for helping us to see some of this information through your eyes. And, lastly, and most importantly, we want to acknowledge and thank Cheri Percival. Thank you for hosting our HSI events, for preparing nutritious food and showing the doctors and their staff that healthy eating can be fun and easy, for all of your assistance with the different teaching aids we have used over the past decade, and lastly, for all your efforts on this manuscript and in the publishing process.

Contents

PART 1: EVIDENCE

PART 2: ANALYSIS

PART 3: SOLUTIONS

Foreword

The aim of medicine is to prevent disease and prolong life; the ideal of medicine is to eliminate the need of a physician.
William J. Mayo

What three year old has not played the "Why" game? "Why do I have to go to bed?" "Because you need your sleep." "Why do I need my sleep?" "So that your body can grow big and strong." "Why does my body need to grow big and strong?" "So that you can play with your friends and have fun." "Why should I play with my friends and have fun?" and on and on and on. Parents usually surrender with "Just because," or "Everybody knows that." As a physician, even though I am over forty years old, I still find myself playing this game and asking lots of "Why" questions. And in the same way it caused frustration to my parents, I and other "Why" gamers (maybe you) are frustrating the health care experts with simple questions leading to answers that usually lead to more questions. "Why can't I lose weight anymore?" "Why does disease occur?" "Why can two people with nearly identical lifestyles have such different shape and weight results?" "Why is our healthcare system focused on treating disease rather than creating health?" "Why do we see some people get fatter after a diet?" and so on.

"Why" is a powerful question. It is the essence of root-cause analysis, and the best route to find meaningful solutions to the most persistent problems of today. Sadly, the cop-out answers heard too often in reply to "Why?" questions, often borne more out of frustration than understanding, are "Because I said so," or "It just does," or "Everybody knows that". Those kinds of answers will not provide the results we desire for our health. You will not find any such cop-out answers in this book. Doctors Kelly and Percival have created a very thoughtful and exceedingly well referenced work that gives us context for understanding the issue of shape and weight in a way never presented before. They boldly ask "Why", and, by examining the scientific literature with careful eyes, come up with answers that are not only surprising, but as I have found in my clinical practice, notably effective when it comes to improving shape and weight.

I have personally struggled with my shape and weight. So, with deep empathy for the pain of being overweight, I studied "weight loss" diligently over the years, determined to help others who, like me, struggled with their shape and weight. I put what I learned into practice, and operated a standard weight loss program within my medical practice—complete with the use of appetite suppressing drugs and strict, very low-calorie diets. But about the time I passed the board exam for the specialty of Bariatric (obesity) Medicine, two things happened in my life that shifted my perspective on shape and weight. The first of these was that patients who had appeared to be "successful", having lost large amounts of weight by severely restricting calories and in many cases taking weight loss drugs, started to come back. They weren't coming back because they wanted to fine-tune their results or show me how great they were doing. They were returning because, they had not only regained the twenty to one hundred pounds they had lost under my previous care but, in some cases, they had surpassed their previous all-time-high weight. The rebound effect, of this conventional approach to weight loss, was leaving many of them fatter than ever. While repeat customers are the foundation of every great business model, I found this outcome wholly unsatisfying. It ran counter to my deeply held passion for improving the long-term (lasting) health and well-being of my patients. I began to question what I had learned, and had been practicing. Without better answers, and disillusioned with these results, I shut down this part of my practice.

The second event, the one that ultimately got me re-excited, and changed my approach to shape and weight, was being introduced to Dr. Kelly and Dr. Percival. Within a very short period of time of working together, I came to realize I had been approaching the problem of obesity in a way that was contrary to how the body functions and heals. As I was learning this new way of viewing shape, I found one thing truly remarkable. I had been using many of these concepts, or similar ones, in my efforts to find and treat the underlying causes of other disease states. But I had a huge blind spot when it came to the subject of fat. If someone came to me with auto-immune disease, allergy, heart disease, chronic fatigue syndrome, depression, or anything else for that matter, I would always seek to find the cause(s), and focus treatment in that direction to bring about healing. But with obesity, I (like much of society at the present time) was blinded by what I thought I knew: I had been convinced that weight was an issue of controlling how many calories we take in and how many we use. Eating less, exercising more, and using medications to do things like suppress appetite and boost metabolism, were the sensible solutions to this issue. While these approaches will produce temporary weight loss, they generally don't produce the kinds of sustained results we want, and are more akin to trying to manage a problem, than actually solving it. In other areas of my practice, I had been dedicated to solving health issues. What you will learn in this book is this solution-based approach to shape and weight. You won't be told how to manage shape issues, or given tips on how to make quick, but temporary changes. Instead, you will be given something even better. You will be given answers to "Why"; answers that will help you find and make changes in the underlying, and often hidden, areas that really make a difference when it comes to producing lasting changes in shape and weight.

Please allow me tell you about Susan (not her real name), and how this approach affected her. She had been through three other weight loss programs during the last five years, and had gained and lost as much as forty pounds in between each of these weight loss adventures. She was tired, discouraged, depressed, and said she felt like a "failure." Susan came to me shortly after my "Great Shape Awakening", so when she asked me to help her to lose weight, we had a very different discussion than she had previously experienced. We dove into what could be the cause(s) of her increased fat mass, why she gained weight when she did, why her body could actually want to hold on to fat given her current and past circumstances, and why changing her approach could change her results. We worked together for six months, doing what we call at the MaxWell Clinic for Proactive Medicine "Peeling the Onion," which is systematically finding and addressing the many layered barriers to health creation—be that removal of excess stressors of body, mind, or biology, or the replenishment of the ingredients needed for healing. What were Susan's results? Over six months time, she shed sixteen pounds of fat and gained four lbs of muscle mass. This was a significant shape change. The rest of the story is even better. Her depression cleared, her energy went through the roof, her sex drive returned, she started the business she had dreamt of for years, she slept through the night without the use of sleeping aids: All that and a change of two dress sizes! But Susan's story continued to get even better. Susan left my practice because her husband was transferred to another city. Five years after our last meeting, she appeared on my schedule once again. When she walked in, I didn't recognize her. It wasn't because of the passing years; it was because she was now fifty-two pounds lighter than when I had first met her. The overall shift in her shape was even bigger than this loss in pounds. She had added an additional ten pounds of muscle since our last meeting, making her shape change even more dramatic, healthy, and transformative. She was once again wearing a size 4; a dress size she hadn't been able to wear since she was a teenager. Her business was thriving, as was her marriage. When I asked her how she had accomplished what she had, she replied, "I just kept asking 'why?' and running better experiments on myself." It brought tears to my eyes, because it confirmed, in such a beautiful way, the truth that health creation is a process that comes from the inside out. It is not something that some doctor can do to you from outside in. It is something we each do for ourselves. The quote by Dr. Mayo, at the beginning of this forward, is one of my favorite takeaways from my time practicing at the Mayo Clinic. It is my hope that approaches based upon it become the standard for whatever comes next in the realm of health-care delivery. Excellence in health-care is not defined by more medical treatment, it is defined by producing better and lasting results; results which provide greater quality and quantity of life.

You're probably curious what Susan did. I will refrain from giving you her recipe, because I fear it would only distract you from finding your own. Every person is unique because of their genetics, the environment in which they live, and more. This being the case, everything we do in the realm of medical treatment or health creation must be individualized; it is, in other words, an experiment of one. My goal is to help my patients produce exceptional and lasting results, by guiding them to find the biggest opportunities for improvement in their lives, and then to run increasingly wholesome experiments in these areas of opportunity. This is the miracle of the Health Scene Investigation approach; an approach founded on helping you investigate your own Health Scene, and which intimately involves *you* in the process of both discovering these areas of opportunity, and changing them.

Our medical system is technologically more advanced than at any point in human history. We also spend more on healthcare than at any previous time. And, while the current medical system does a tremendous job in many areas, it has arrived at a crossroads of sorts. We are in the midst of epidemics of obesity, cancer, heart disease, and the list goes on and on. Just to pay for our current obligations to fund Medicaid and Medicare, each family in the United States would need to pay $400,000.00 into the United States Treasury *today*. By the year 2030, the cost to pay the interest on the money borrowed to fund health care in the United States will exceed our entire nation's Gross Domestic Product, effectively making us financially insolvent due to medical treatment costs alone. Treatment of preventable chronic illness accounts for 70 to 85 percent of our total yearly health care expenditures. Please, read that last sentence again and let it sink in. Obesity is related to many of the preventable chronic illnesses that are producing this runaway train when it comes to both the downward health of our society, and funding its treatment. Obesity is often blamed as the cause in this relationship. It's more complicated than that: You'll find out why in this book. Improving shape, both our individual shape and our society's shape, is imperative for our personal and national well-being. How do we do this; how do we get in shape?

We have to make a shift in how we view things and in what we do about them. There is really no other choice. We can wait until an issue with health is so advanced that it becomes a medically recognized problem, or we can take pro-active steps to change the direction our health is taking. We can hope that someday medicine will be able to fix people in spite of themselves (which, trust me, is unlikely), or we can strive to turn the hope of Dr. Mayo into a reality—we can, because of our individual choices, help prevent disease and prolong our own lives, drastically reducing the current and future role medicine will need to play for us. This will shift our personal well-being, and if enough of us do this, it will make a shift in corporate well-being, and even our societal-well-being. At LifeStrive (a company Dr. Greg, Dr. Mark, and I helped co-found), we refer to this shift in how we look at things, and what we do about them, as "Health Response-Ability". The greatest opportunity most of us will ever have when it comes to our own health, and our shape, won't come from what medicine will do for us; it will come from our ability to choose to do things differently. We have the ability to respond differently; we also have the responsibility to do so.

By becoming an effective Health Scene Investigator, you will be practicing Health Response-Ability. You will be solving your health scene in ways that improve the shape and health results you produce today, but also improving them in ways that offer a form of insurance for tomorrow.

Many health challenges seem to occur suddenly. We don't notice they are a problem, until they are already a big problem. We are noticing things late in the game. The causes have often been ongoing for years, or in some instances decades. In most of the patients I work with, there are ongoing opportunities to make changes that will alter the outcome of the health game much earlier, long before a big problem has occurred. Shape is a clue to this opportunity. Shape doesn't occur in a vacuum. It has causes. It's also a clue to the direction our health is traveling. A slowly increasing waistline is a trend that predicts catastrophic long-term outcomes. Paying attention to this trend, and altering the course as early as possible, will take you to an entirely different destination in the long-term. If coming to grips with the idea, that a small change early in the course of life would make a big long-term change in outcome, is difficult for you, I ask you to ponder how a very small change in course early in the voyage of the Titanic would have changed the outcome of that tragic story. No matter what your current shape, or whether it's early, in the middle, or late in your own personal health game, what you do starting today can alter the direction you are trending.

While very enjoyable, this book is not fluffy. Serious topics deserve a respectful and thorough investigation. Shape is one of these topics. It is time the world has access to a book of this caliber. I do my best to answer the question of "Why?" when my children ask it, and when my patients ask it. I am certain that this book, and the approach to shape and health it offers, will help you to answer this and other questions for yourself.

Be Well.

David H. Haase, M.D.
Founder, MaxWell Clinic for Proactive Medicine
Chief Medical Officer, LifeStrive®

Introduction

Definitions:

Shape (*noun*): The contour of a person's body; the figure.
Shape (*verb*): To give a particular form to; create
Shift (*noun*): A change (in direction or appearance)
Shift (*verb*): to (cause something or someone to) move or change
from one position or direction to another

Shape provides information that can be missed when the only detail
we focus upon is weight. Weight can also lead us into thinking one
thing when the truth is something quite different, or at the very least,
more complicated. My own shape story highlights these points. I
gained 55 pounds during my four years of college. In our weight-
obsessed culture, the tendency would be to look at this number—55
pounds—and think, oh my, that's a lot of weight: You must have
gotten really fat. The truth is more nuanced. I started college short
and skinny. I grew a few inches and put weight on my chest, back,
arms, and legs. At the time, I considered gaining this weight as a
positive thing. I still do. I also gained about 4 inches around my
waist. I wasn't as thrilled with this weight. My shape had shifted
through my college years. Some of the shifts were for the better;
others were for the worse. Soon after graduation, my shape would
shift again.

I graduated from college in 1984 and was commissioned as an
officer in the United States Navy. Prior to commissioning, I was
fitted for uniforms. My waist measured slightly more than 33 inches.
The tailor recommended getting size 34-inch pants. His opinion was
that it was far more likely that I would gain more weight around
my waist than lose it, so it made sense to build in a little cushion.
I agreed. We were both wrong: My waist size never expanded to
reach 34 inches. In fact, during my first few months in the Navy, it
went significantly in the other direction: I dropped about 3 inches
from my waist and about 20 pounds of weight. My uniform pants

were too loose around the waist and remained that way for the five and one half years I stayed in the Navy. It is two and one half decades later and they would still be too loose for me.

In our culture we tend to overemphasize weight loss and underemphasize more important changes. Weight didn't really tell an accurate story in either of these two shifts in shape. I wasn't trying to lose weight during my first few months in the Navy. I was trying to get in better shape. That some weight was lost as I got in better shape was more of a side effect. And the loss of 20 pounds I experienced failed to accurately capture the totality of the shape change I experienced. My muscles became bigger and better toned. Put another way, I gained weight in some areas of my body. At the same time my stomach became flatter and more defined. I didn't just lose weight; my overall shape changed. Sometimes this happens when we lose weight, but many times it doesn't. Paying attention to shape, in all its subtleties, is a better barometer.

Shape is changeable. It shifts based on our habits and circumstances. Mine shifted when I went to college and lived a very different life than the one I had lived in high school. It shifted again when I went into the Navy. It has continued to evolve since. This is what shape does. It adapts to our habits and circumstances in what might best be described as evolutionarily sensible ways. Our shape is a reflection of our genes interacting with the lives we have led and are leading. I didn't experience the big change in my shape during my first few months in the Navy because of restricting calories or going on some fad diet. My shape changed because my habits and circumstances changed. What I ate, when I ate it, my exercise routines, my sleep-wake cycles, and more, radically changed during my first few months in the Navy. I went from being a night-person—going to bed most nights at 2 to 3 in the morning and waking around noon—to being an early to bed, early to rise person. I stopped eating late at night and started eating breakfast, lunch, and earlier dinners. I became more serious about training with weights. I walked more. I decided to learn about what constitutes healthy food and took more responsibility for what I would, and conversely wouldn't (at least not regularly) eat. I swapped soft drinks for water. I started to associate more regularly with people who cared about their shapes, and I asked them for advice. My diet, lifestyle and environment shifted, and, not surprisingly, my shape did as well.

I arrived at my first ship in the beginning of 1985 lean and fit. This did not go unnoticed. The Navy had a problem with overweight sailors in the mid 1980s. My understanding is that they still do. On my first ship, it wasn't long before this became my problem. Before going to a ship, an officer receives official orders. The orders include the ship you will be assigned to, where and when to report, and your job assignment. My ship was the USS Ouellete. I was to report at the beginning of February of 1985 to Pearl Harbor, Hawaii. My job was going to be working in the ship's engineering department. This would be my primary job; it wouldn't be my only one. Officers often have one or more collateral duties. I was no exception. I had a handful of collateral duties, one of which, since I looked to be in shape, cared about what I was eating, and exercised regularly, was to be in charge of the shipboard fitness program, including all of the sailors who were having trouble meeting Navy weight standards. This was a relatively fruitless job. Most of the sailors who had difficulty meeting the Navy's weight standards didn't want to be in this program: Adherence was a constant issue. Navy menus, at least at the time, were cafeteria style, all-you-can-eat, with many tempting and fattening food choices. Snack food—soft drinks, cookies, crackers, chips, and candy—were one of the few things you could purchase on a ship. Navy personnel, especially at sea, are chronically sleep-deprived. Body clock disruption is an ongoing stress that becomes even more exaggerated when the ship pulls out to sea because of watch schedules and the availability of midnight meals. Dedicating time to exercise while at sea typically meant taking time away from sleeping. And, as a last ditch effort to pass the weight standards, overweight sailors would typically go on a crash diet; restricting calories to lose enough weight to meet Navy weight standards for one moment in time (their weigh in). Not uncommonly a sailor would "succeed", only to regain the lost weight in time to fail the next fitness test. These factors all acted to stack the deck against producing a sustainable shape improvement. In fact, they were contributing to the problem in the first place. Many of the circumstances that life in the Navy entails are fattening. Most sailors don't arrive onboard their first ship over-fat. Their shape shifts in a fattening direction after they arrive. In this book you will learn to identify the factors that contribute to this shift. Some, perhaps many, of these same factors are likely contributing to your shape.

My understanding of shape has evolved in the more than two decades since I left the Navy. The biggest leap forward in this evolution came when my paradigm around shape, the metaphor I used to think about this subject, shifted. Suddenly information that hadn't made sense did. Results that had been puzzling came into focus. Cases that couldn't be solved were. With this shift in paradigm some of what I once considered sensible now seemed nonsensical, and some things I had viewed as unrelated to shape now took on big roles. This book is the product of these shifts in understanding and perspective.

The most important shift I had was in realizing that I am in a *cooperative* relationship with my body. In nature there are many relationships that are characterized by mutual benefit to both parties. Each party advances their individual interests, but this plays out in a way that allows both parties to gain, trading favors so to speak. A bee pollinates a tree, but the tree provides food (pollen) for the bee. This is a reciprocal relationship. The bee does its part; the tree does its; and both benefit. Health and shape are a lot like this reciprocal relationship. There are many things your body does for you without any need for your conscious mind to be involved, and there are other things it is dependent upon you to do for it.

When most of us think of our body, and more specifically our shape (or weight), we tend to think about it as if we are in charge or control. This control metaphor is reflected in the most common strategy followed to alter shape—dieting. The theory behind dieting postulates that we can control our weight by eating less food. This control metaphor misses a key point: Our body behaves as if it has a mind of its own. We might want one shape, but if our body wants a different one, guess who usually gets what they want. What we want doesn't occur in a vacuum. Our body wants what it wants and needs what it needs. We have a much better chance of getting what we want if we help it get what it needs. We observe this with sleep. The body wants and needs sufficient sleep to be healthy and to stay lean. It is our job to help it get enough. If we do our part, it does its, and we're both better off. If we resist doing our part, sleeping far less than we need, we suffer, it suffers, and shape usually suffers. If your goal is to improve your shape, there are absolutely things you can do that will all but guarantee this outcome. You will need to do your part when it comes to these things. You will also need to trust that your body can do its part.

The body is capable of tremendous feats of intelligent adaptation, but the way it adapts when its needs are met, in contrast to when they are unmet, can be extremely different. It takes intelligence to survive in a constantly changing world. It also takes flexibility, a willingness to alter strategies to adapt to new circumstances. The human body is an expert when it comes to intelligent adaptation.

The human body is capable of adapting to all manner of real world challenges. Many of the adaptations it makes, including shape, are evolutionarily sensible. What you do and don't do will influence shape significantly, because your habits and circumstances will cause your body to adapt in ways that make sense to it. Shape is a dynamic thing. It is adjustable, but it adjusts itself based on its rules, not ours. Understanding these rules can be the difference between succeeding in co-creating a sustainable shape you will be satisfied with, or failing over and over again. The most important rule of this game is that your body will do its best to adapt intelligently to the circumstances and situations it faces. Your shape is a reflection of these adaptations, and all of the past and present factors that have contributed to them. If you want a different shape, something will need to shift in one or more areas of your diet, lifestyle habits, or environment. If you want to sustain the improvement, the factor you shifted will need to remain shifted. Temporary changes in weight or shape can be obtained by temporarily changing something about your life. Lasting change in shape requires more than temporary changes in habits. Because of this, the focus of this book is to point you in the direction of habits and circumstances that can be changed in ways that are sustainable.

It's our hope that the information contained in this book will help you shift your shape. It's also our hope that this book will shift your perspective—point of view and understandings—when it comes to shape. We believe that our bodies are trying to do their best to take care of themselves and us. This is an incredibly important job; one our conscious mind could never do entirely on its own. Many of the adaptations the body makes are intended to protect us against a perceived threat or to better prepare us to face situations the body thinks we might face again. Shape is one of these intelligent adaptations. It is protective in nature, intended to better prepare us for things we might encounter again, and is, at its most fundamental level, a survival mechanism. We might not always agree with how the body goes about protecting us or altering our shape, but it is our hope that this book will help foster an appreciation that your body will be trying to do its best given what it knows how to do, and what it has available to do it.

Over the past decade, Dr. Mark and I have coached clients on the principles in this book. We have also taught classes to health professionals and helped them work with their patients on shape issues. Arising from our work in this area was an appreciation that improving shape often involved what amounted to detective work. We needed to investigate areas of a person's diet, lifestyle, habits, environment and beliefs about shape, gathering clues as we went. This process of investigation required help from our clients. In a sense, we helped them become better detectives when it came to their own personal health scenes. With their help, once we had gathered the right clues, the mystery often solved itself. Mark and I eventually came to call this investigational approach to shape (and in a bigger sense health) Health Scene Investigation (HSI). In this book we will be sharing this approach with you.

Before we can solve a health scene, we must be able to properly investigate it. But how do we do this? *CSI: Crime Scene Investigation* (commonly referred to simply as CSI) is one of the most popular TV shows. It is about a team of criminal investigators who solve difficult crime cases. *House* (formerly titled *House, M.D.*) is about a team of physicians who go to extraordinary lengths to find the real answers behind unusual ailments. The characters in these shows are investigation specialists. They are experts in looking for clues and gathering evidence. They use the latest technology and techniques to analyze the clues they find. And, only after all of this is done, do they solve the case. *CSI* and *House* are modern day versions of Sherlock Holmes.

Sherlock Holmes has been an enduring literary figure for more than 100 years. His cases usually have an official inspector, who represents a conventional point of view that causes them to miss clues and go about solving cases incorrectly. In many ways, they are analogous to the conventional approach to shape cases. The other key character is Dr. Watson; the trusted sidekick and narrator of the stories. At the beginning of a case he is in the dark (uninformed) just like us. The case either looks completely unsolvable or very obvious from his initial vantage point. It is usually neither. He is given access and insight into Holmes' method of investigation. While he might not have had the genius of Sherlock Holmes, he was able to become a better investigator by learning his methods. The goal of this book is to help you become like Watson, to improve your ability to investigate your shape and to, in a phrase, solve it. This book is intended to help you shift the way you solve problems, shift your point of view, shift your actions, and ultimately shift your shape and health. As you proceed with this investigation you may find that what you've thought is important might not be, and other things you had previously overlooked, might be the critical clues when it comes to producing a sustainable new shape. With these things in mind, I want to welcome you to the HSI team.

Dr. Greg

Chapter 1

The Sherlock Holmes Way
and the Mystery of Shape

It is a capital mistake to theorize before one has data. Insensibly one begins to twist facts to suit theories, instead of theories to suit facts.

Sherlock Holmes

Opening Dialogue

Health Scene Investigator: Tell me, why does a person become overweight or obese?

Apprentice: It's because people eat too much and don't get enough exercise.

Health Scene Investigator: That's possible.

Apprentice: What do you mean possible? It seems obvious to me that this is the cause.

Health Scene Investigator: I think you will find that when it comes to health scenes in general, and shape specifically, what appears "obvious" often hinders investigation. It has the potential to mislead. Let me ask you an important question. How do you know this is the cause? What evidence do you have that supports what seems so obvious to you? Are there any facts that are exceptions?

Apprentice: I don't have specific answers to your questions.
I assumed...

Health Scene Investigator: Please forgive me for interrupting you. Never trust to general impressions and assumptions. Learn to concentrate on details in advance of theorizing. It is a common error to theorize before we have looked at the totality of evidence. When you look at any health scene, a shape case being one such scene, there are many possible ways to explain how it arrived at its current situation. However if you enter the case with a theory that you believe already explains the case, you are apt to overlook or misinterpret important details. Investigating a health scene is, or ought to be, an exact science. Allow me to introduce you to my method.

Shifting Our Shape Paradigms

Thomas Kuhn, author of the book *The Structure of Scientific Revolutions*, wrote, "You don't see something until you have the right metaphor to perceive it." He argued that science does not evolve gradually toward truth, but instead undergoes periodic upheavals during which the prevailing scientific theories radically change. He called these upheavals *paradigm shifts*; a time when existing theories got replaced with new theories that better explain the facts. A paradigm shift is in many ways identical to Dr. Watson's moment of insight in one of Holmes's cases; where his previous way of looking at a problem shifted.

Kuhn argued that up until a paradigm shift occurs scientists can be guilty of twisting facts to fit the prevailing theory, ignoring facts that don't fit, or both. What is the result? It is an unsolvable case, a mystery that persists, not because of a lack of facts or evidence, but despite their existence. In this scenario, science is guilty of the mistake Sherlock Holmes cautioned Watson against. Facts are twisted in ways that suit the existing theory. Is it possible we have been guilty of making this mistake with weight? To answer this it is important to understand that science and medicine already has a theory of weight. They have had it for more than 100 years.

The conventional theory has been, and continues to be in most of society, a theory we could best describe as *controlling energy balance*. According to this theory, if a person is overweight it is because they did a bad job controlling their weight: They took in more energy than they used in metabolic processes and activity. In other words, they ate too much, exercised too little, have a slow metabolism, or have some combination of all three of these. The solution to this problem is simple: Create a negative energy balance. This is accomplished by reducing the amount of calories we consume (energy in), by using more energy in activity or metabolism (energy out), or both. It is a very appealing theory. Weight sciences have fit facts to this theory for more than 100 years now. Why shouldn't they? No theory could be more obvious. No case could possibly be easier to solve. But as Sherlock Holmes might have warned us, the obvious is often wrong.

The theory of controlling weight by creating a negative energy balance has guided the way experts have approached real life shape cases— your cases. It is argued that virtually anybody can, with a reasonable amount of conscious effort and willpower, control how fat or thin he or she becomes. All we need to do is eat less. Unfortunately the best scientific evidence, and real world experience, indicates that this approach doesn't work. With rare exceptions, a person who tries to directly control their weight by eating less food than their appetite dictates loses weight temporarily, and then, despite great determination, gradually regains all of it. Eating less works until it doesn't. Application of the theory fails the one test that really matters, the real world test. Based on the real world results, maybe we should be asking whether we made the capital mistake of theorizing before having the data. Are we being misled by obvious facts? Is there evidence being ignored that might cause us to look at weight differently? Has the metaphor of controlling our weight been the correct metaphor? Are we in need of a paradigm shift?

> **HSI CLUE**
>
> The controlling energy balance theory implies that we can have, and will get to keep, whatever shape and weight we desire by eating less. Does evidence support this theory? In the real world what happens when a person eats less for a few days, weeks, or months? Does it get easier? Does it get harder? Is the body comfortable at a reduced weight that is arrived at by dieting?

The Mystery

In December 2001, the United States Surgeon General issued a health warning. Americans are experiencing an epidemic of overweight and obesity, it's out of control, and it's getting worse. Estimates suggest that 65 percent of adults are overweight, as are one out of every five American children. The latest government statistics indicate that obese Americans outnumber overweight Americans, and the group that has been expanding at the fastest rate during the past decade is the severely obese group, persons who are 100 pounds or more overweight. If the epidemic is allowed to continue on its current path, by the year 2025, 40 to 45 percent of us will be medically obese and the amount of people either overweight or obese might well be upwards of 75 percent. What is causing this epidemic?

H S I   C L U E

The "logical" approach to weight loss for the past century has largely focused on eating less. This approach matches our intuitions about how things should be. Yet, as any dieter can attest, dieting works right up until it doesn't. It requires greater and greater feats of abstinence to lose incrementally smaller and smaller amounts of weight. The struggle does not end when weight is lost. It's far easier to regain lost weight then it was to lose it. Fat appears to be resisting our efforts to lose it. Why?

The conventional theory is that we, as a society, as well as many individuals within our society, do a poor job of controlling our weight. We eat too much and exercise too little. If we want to reverse this epidemic, if we want to be leaner as a society and as individuals, we have been told the solution is simple: We need to eat less and exercise more. The problem and its solutions are theorized to be this simple. Are they? Let's look at one piece of statistical evidence that doesn't quite fit. In 2006 scientists from the Harvard School of Public Health reported that there had been a 73 percent increase in the prevalence of obesity in young infants (less than 6 months of age) since 1980. In a 2009 Newsweek article (*Born to Be Big* by Sharon Begley) endocrinologist Robert Lustig points out "Since they're eating only formula or breast milk, and never exactly got a lot of exercise, the obvious explanations for obesity don't work for babies. You have to look beyond the obvious." Babies are not an isolated case. There are many other examples, some of which we'll investigate in subsequent chapters, where the conventional explanation does not fit the facts. If we hope to solve the mystery, we'll need to learn to look beyond the obvious.

Despite considerable money and 70 years of research, more people are fat now than at any time in human history. Even after repeated efforts to control weight, the average person will be as dissatisfied with the shape of their body today as they were last year. Often times, they will be more dissatisfied. If it is really as simple as eating less, why is the epidemic worsening? And, if it isn't really this simple, why do we continue to act as if it is?

A prerequisite to solving any problem is having an understanding of the nature of the problem. Is the problem weight? Or is it something else? We must seek to uncover the real causes. How do we do this? Is there a formula we can use to help us in our investigations? Is there a way to approach seemingly "unsolvable" problems? The answer is yes. We can follow in the footsteps of a master in the art of detection. In order to solve a mystery, we can approach the case the way Sherlock Holmes would.

The Sherlock Holmes Way

Sherlock Holmes was a master at making the mysterious less mysterious. He described himself as a consulting detective, an expert who was brought into cases that had proven too difficult for other, typically official, investigators. The following six principles were central to his method:

Extraordinary powers of observation: As Sherlock Holmes explained to Watson, on more than one occasion, his method was founded on the observation of trifles. By trifles Sherlock Holmes did not mean unimportant facts or evidence; he meant the finer details that other observers either ignored because they did not fit their existing theory, or escaped their detection because they were not trained to see them. Holmes understood that there might be nothing as important as a trifle when solving a case. Could it be that seemingly insignificant details of our lives and environment play an important role in determining our shape?

HSI CLUE

What has changed since 1975; the time when the epidemic of overweight really took off? Is it possible that some of these changes might be contributing to our expanding waistlines? Are there any trifles, smaller details of our lives and environment that are less obvious than how much we eat, that better explain our shape and weight?

A deep understanding of advances in science and technology: As an expert in the advances of science and technology of his time, Sherlock Holmes had tremendous knowledge of chemistry, botany, medicine, and what we now call forensic sciences. If Holmes were alive today, it is certain that he would be adept in the new sciences: Complexity theory, Chronobiology, and Network theory. And he would find these new understandings critical to solving the mystery of shape.

A commitment to gather and analyze all evidence before drawing conclusions: Sherlock Holmes repeatedly cautioned Watson against approaching a case with a preconceived theory. Having a theory before gathering evidence greatly increases the risk that one might twist facts to support that theory and ignore other facts that do not fit. In other words, we will likely find what we expect to find, and may fail to observe other more important clues. Holmes thought it better to approach a problem without any pre-formed theories, with a blank mind. Gather all of the evidence, analyze it, and then, and only then, come up with a theory (or theories) that explains the facts.

The ability to look past obvious facts: Obvious facts, according to Sherlock Holmes, could mislead the most astute investigator. By obvious facts he meant common knowledge, things so seemingly obvious that they simply did not warrant questioning, much less a search for a competing explanation. Being able to avoid obvious facts is an essential part of investigation.

A willingness to examine all competing explanations for a body of evidence: After gathering and analyzing evidence with the technology at his disposal, Sherlock Holmes used his understanding of what was scientifically possible and impossible. He was only able to do this because he was an expert in the science of his day. He was willing, initially, to consider competing theories and then let the evidence disprove these one by one until only the possible remained. Many of his most famous sayings have to do with this process of eliminating the impossible and being left with, however improbable, an explanation that solved the case.

A logical reasoning process to uncover the hidden solution: The last part of the Sherlock Holmes way was a process of logical reasoning. The British have an adjective that describes this process: Holmesian. A Holmesian approach involves using a logical process after amassing a large body of evidence, to produce a number of possible explanations of that evidence. The goal is to find one explanation that best explains the totality of the evidence.

Become Your Own Detective

When it comes to our shape and weight we could use a Sherlock Holmes. Unfortunately he won't be walking through our doors any time soon. That's the bad news. The good news is that he won't have to. We can each learn to solve our own cases. The next six chapters of this book will arm you with tools of investigation. Mastery of these concepts will prove invaluable to you as you tackle your own *shape case* as well as other "mysteries" you may encounter in your lifelong quest for health. Subsequent chapters of this book will continue our investigation into other areas of shape, and aspects of diet, lifestyle, and the environment. You will learn about new clues to gather with your extraordinary powers of observation and will be introduced to circumstances and situations that have big impacts on shape. You will enter *health scenes* that may even look like your own and learn to apply investigative principles within specific areas related to your life and shape. You will learn why shape, not weight, is what really matters. And, most importantly, you will discover how you can, starting today, improve your shape in healthy and sustainable manners.

Ending Dialogue

Health Scene Investigator: Now that you are more familiar with my methods, let us return to my original question. You told me that the reason a person becomes overweight is because they eat too much and don't exercise enough. Do you know of any other events that could cause a person to get fat?

Apprentice: That's a good question. To be perfectly honest I haven't the slightest idea.

Health Scene Investigator: When investigating a new case it is critical to know what type of events might lead to the current situation, to remain open to the possibility that there will be further events discovered that could have led to this situation, and lastly to discount an event only when it can be proven to not apply.

Apprentice: You mean there might be other things that could make a person gain weight besides how much they eat and exercise?

Health Scene Investigator: Yes. It is precisely what I mean. We must remain open to that as a possibility. The initial inspection of the health scene, generally speaking, gives the impression that...

Apprentice: Generally speaking? What are you saying?

Health Scene Investigator: I am trying to tell you the facts. There are certain details of the case, details I would prefer not to go into quite yet, which give rise to some perplexity, to certain, let us say, reasonable doubts.

Apprentice: This is incredible. It is like something out of a detective novel.

Health Scene Investigator: That is exactly what it is.

Chapter 2

Extraordinary
Powers of Observation

It has been an axiom of mine that the little things are infinitely the most important.

Sherlock Holmes

Opening Dialogue

Health Scene Investigator: When Holmes made statements such as "little things are infinitely the most important," what do you think he really meant?

Apprentice: I must admit that I have no idea. Little things seem to me, well, little. I would have thought the big things would be the most important.

Health Scene Investigator: Big things, by which I mean the obvious, can be important. But less obvious clues, so called little things, can be as well. Allow me to explain.

The Importance of "Little Things"
Sherlock Holmes had extraordinary powers of observation. But what exactly was he observing with these powers? In many of his conversations with Watson he mentioned that his method was founded on the observation of trifles. By trifles Sherlock Holmes did not mean unimportant facts or evidence; he meant the finer details,

little things that other observers ignored or for some reason were incapable of seeing. The power of seemingly little things can be seen in the concept of *tipping points*.

The term tipping points was coined by Sociologist Morton Grodzins to describe the flight of Caucasians from the urbanized areas of the Northeast into the suburbs. Grodzins looked at all types of factors to try to identify the reasons for this flight to the suburbs; school systems, crime, and other big, obvious factors, but nothing provided a good explanation. Finally, he discovered that when a city neighborhood reached a certain threshold of minority residents, about 20 percent, the majority of the remaining Caucasian residents would spontaneously move away: The neighborhood tipped. An epidemic of flight to the suburbs had broken out and the force most responsible for this was the percent of residents of different ethnic backgrounds, which when compared to crime or school systems, seems like a little thing.

Malcolm Gladwell, in a book called *The Tipping Point: How Little Things Can Make a Big Difference*, further elaborated the concept of tipping points. This book is about transitions and how things spread. And, most importantly, it is about how and why things really happen in the world that surrounds us. As the title suggests, his book teaches us that little things, seemingly unrelated or overlooked minor details, can and do make big differences. They can make big differences in the way information, behaviors, or even infections spread through a group of people. They can make big differences in the way an individual responds and behaves. Could little things make a big difference when it comes to our shape?

We are conditioned to believe in scale. To get a big effect we need a big cause. This is called *proportionality* and is a central tenant of a scientific theory called *Reductionism* (Reductionism will be discussed in chapter 3). For most of the 20th century science believed only big causes could cause big changes. We see this tendency in how weight changes are typically explained. If a person gains a large amount of weight, the knee-jerk reaction is to usually blame in on a big thing— overeating. How much food is being eaten gets the blame whether or not it is actually the problem. Let's look at a real world example, the *Case of Neutering a Pet*, to highlight this point.

It's not unusual for a neutered pet to get fatter after the procedure. How do we react when this occurs? Many pet owners reduce the amount of food they feed their pets. But in the *Case of Neutering a Pet* is eating more food the tipping point? Is it the force that causes the fat gain? Because if it isn't, and something else is, is feeding the pet less really going to solve the case? Evidence indicates that for pets that gain weight easily after neutering, most of the weight gain will be fat. This means that shape or body composition, even more so than weight, is changing. Scientific studies also inform us that this gain in fat can occur even if the animals are fed the same amounts and types of food as before the procedure. In fact, some neutered animals will get fatter even when fed less food. In this latter instance, they aren't getting fatter because they are eating more food; they are getting fatter despite the fact that they are being fed less.

In this case the big and obvious, the amount of food, is not the tipping point. More food is not causing the fat accumulation. The procedure of neutering is the point at which the pet's shape shifts. It was the tipping point. What the animal eats after this procedure is an effect. Something about neutering causes the animal's body to shift in a way that makes getting fat easier. While neutering is not a little thing in terms of the effects it can have on our pets, it is a little thing in the sense that we often over look the effects it has on shape, and, instead, mistakenly blame food and eating as the cause of the changes we are observing in our pets.

Most of us have had a tipping point experience, when it comes to shape, at one point in time. We might have had a very stable weight, sometimes for years, and then suddenly gained a few pounds (or far more). Or, our weight might have stayed the same but its distribution suddenly shifted leaving an extra inch or so in unwanted areas. Shape tipped but what was the tipping point? Was it because after months or years we suddenly started to eat so much more or exercise so much less? In our experience, while this can be the case, it often is not. There are one or more hidden causes. It is the job of a health scene

HSI CLUE

The dominant metaphor, when it comes to weight, seeks to explain the nature of the problem in terms of big things like overeating. A tipping point metaphor would shift our perspective, and introduce the notion that one or more seeming trifles might be more important. It would also clue us in to both focus our powers of observation into detecting these things, and to be aware for shape tipping points.

investigator to identify the real causes, the differences that really made the difference.

As mentioned in the last chapter, Kuhn was of the opinion that, until one had the correct metaphor to perceive something, one wouldn't. When it comes to many real world issues and problems, the concept of tipping points is this more correct metaphor. To get a big effect, we don't necessarily need a big cause. Sometimes, a little thing will cause a big change. Things can have geometric progressions; they can cascade. And things can have effects far out of proportion to their size. Adding a tiny amount of weight to a perfectly balanced heavy object can cause it to topple. A slight drop in temperature can make the difference between water being a liquid or solid (ice). The smallest of changes can shatter a potential epidemic's equilibrium and cause it to affect many more people. It might take only a slight change in a product or idea for its popularity to spread suddenly to the masses. This same principle applies to our shape and health. It might take just a few changes in the finer details of diet, lifestyle, or environment to shatter the balance point that had previously been a stable shape or state of health, changing it for the better or worse. Identifying these finer details that are acting as individual tipping points, and, taking steps to address these details is the secret to producing sustainable improvements.

HSI CLUE

When you look back at your life, from a time period around when your body shape seemed to change suddenly, what was really going on? What details, seemingly little things, were occurring in your health scene during those time periods?

The tipping point metaphor teaches us to prepare ourselves for the possibility that big results can occur from seemingly small causes. Things that look stable or seem to resist all efforts at change might be just a small push in the right place away from a large shift. Sometimes it only takes the smallest of actions to produce large results. It also informs us that the real forces behind the unwanted shifts in our shape are likely to be things most of us do not notice, seemingly little things or trifles hidden in the periphery of our lives.

To solve a real life health scene an investigator must, like Sherlock Holmes, be able to observe trifles. When it comes to shape, in our experience, the typically overlooked little things are infinitely the most important. To solve a Health Scene it is these several, sometimes many, seemingly unimportant "little things", factors that often lie at the margins of our lives and awareness, that we must put our efforts into discovering, understanding, and changing.

Avoiding the Fundamental Attribution Error

Imagine seeing an overweight person eating a large bowl of ice cream. How would you rate their willpower? Is it low, medium, or high? Are you likely to blame the ice cream as part of the reason they are overweight? If you rated their willpower as low and judged the ice cream as a problem, you are not alone. Most people would see this scene and assume low willpower and ice cream are a significant cause of the person's weight challenge. Very few people would look at this same image and wonder things like (1) how much sleep the person had the night before, (2) whether they have been dieting, and, if so, for how long, or (3) whether they just had a very stressful day. We look at the person eating ice cream and the tendency is to blame the behavior on a character attribute like willpower. But the truth is that situational influences are much more likely to be the real reasons for the observed behavior. The same is true for shape changes and weight gain. It might seem inconceivable that a behavior like eating a bowl of ice cream is not a statement about willpower, and, instead, could be a result of some more arbitrary and seemingly insignificant aspect of lifestyle or the environment, such as the quality or duration of last night's sleep, this morning's breakfast, or a stressful situation. But the truth is that context is powerful. In fact, it is a far more powerful influence on our behavior than we realize. Getting fewer hours of sleep than we need causes many of us to increase snack food consumption, especially in the evening hours. People who have lost weight by dieting tend to crave fattening foods. Some people are exceptionally prone to stress eating. Having a bowl of ice cream, or some other comfort food, is not an unusual occurrence in these situations; it is a common response.

Scientific experiments have shown that humans have a strong tendency to come up with explanations of behavior that over emphasize character and disposition traits. We see a person do something and we tend to explain the behavior in terms of the kind of person he or she might be. In the case above, the result is we explain the eating ice cream behavior in terms of a character trait— willpower. Coupled with this, is an equal and opposite tendency.

We usually underestimate the significant role context—circumstances and situations—has on behavior. Because of this, we are prone to underestimate the influence that things like sleep, stress, dieting habits, or the amount of time since a person last ate, have on a person's food choices at any moment in time. This tendency is called the *fundamental attribution error*. It is a fancy way of saying that when it comes to interpreting people's behaviors, human beings invariably make the mistake of overestimating the importance of fundamental character traits and underestimating what is going on in a person's life.

HSI CLUE

The average adult has about 40 hours a week of free time. In 1965 about 10 of these 40 hours were spent watching televisions. By 1995 this had increased to about 15 hours a week. Could this increase be a shape tipping point?
In 1975, the average American slept 7.5 hours, down from 9 hours in 1910. Today, adults sleep about 7 hours a night. Do you think this might be a tipping point for shape?

Let's use the TV show *Survivor* to highlight the fundamental attribution error. What types of food do the Survivors crave after 10, 15, 20, or more days as castaways? Anyone who has watched this show can answer this question. They crave foods like chocolate, desserts, burgers and fries, pizza, etc. They talk about these foods, think about these foods, and, if the opportunity arises, they will eat them. If we were to stumble into this Health Scene and were unaware of the context of *Survivor*, we might conclude that these people have no willpower, don't care about their shapes, and have unhealthy eating habits. And if some of the Survivors are overweight, we might blame their weight on this aspect of their character. But is lack of willpower or a character disposition towards eating these foods why the Survivors behave this way? Or are they behaving this way because of the context created by *Survivor*? In *Survivor* the participants have insufficient food to maintain their body fat reserves. They lose weight, usually rapidly. As they lose this weight, seemingly out of nowhere, high degrees of hunger emerge, as do cravings for what most of us would consider fattening foods. Why? Since the behaviors were not there before the *Survivor* experience, it seems a poor explanation to blame it on some fundamental aspect of the character of the participants. Maybe there is a better explanation.

The better explanation is that as fat reserves get depleted, hunger accumulates, especially for foods that allow the body to rapidly replenish the lost body fat (we will discuss why this occurs in more detail in later chapters). What foods allow for this? The answer is fattening foods. No matter how disciplined a person might be in the context of their usual life, if placed into a *Survivor* experience long enough, they would behave in the same manner. They would crave similar foods. Character flaws do not cause the cravings. They emerge because of a context that would cause them to emerge for all of us.

The tendency to overestimate fundamental character attributes and to underestimate the importance of the circumstances surrounding our lives is one of the reasons most of us have a difficult time spotting the little things that are the real reasons for behaviors. It is part of the reason we miss the clues hidden at Health Scenes. Since most of us will have this tendency, it is important to question causes that seem big and obvious; we might be overestimating their importance. It is also important to search the Health Scene for little things; factors whose importance we would be likely to underestimate or completely miss. Focusing on what the person is doing and generalizing this behavior to be about some character defect (like lack of willpower) will not help us solve cases. But if we are able to use our powers of observation to find the context around the behavior, we just might.

> **HSI CLUE**
>
> Per capita fructose consumption (excluding that which occurs naturally in fruits and vegetables) increased from less than 0.5 g/day in 1970 to more than 40 g/day in 1997 (more than an 80-fold increase). Is it possible that the addition of this one little thing to the diet can be having a big effect on shape?

Develop and Use Your Powers of Observation

Most of us want to believe that the key to making a big impact in someone's life lies with making some large dramatic change. With shape this often manifests in going on a crash diet or severely restricting entire types of foods like fats or carbohydrates. These "big change" approaches tend to work until they don't. Given the advice of Holmes and the power of tipping points might we be better served taking a different approach?

We are far more susceptible and sensitive to the smallest details of everyday life than we are conditioned to believe. We are not programmed to use extraordinary powers of observation to find hidden clues. Even worse, when it comes to shape issues, we have been educated to miss them. We have been taught to focus on things that usually are, at most, minor clues.

Watson learned to see hidden clues. You'll learn to spot them as well, and when this happens, little things will no longer seem to be trifles. You will understand the power they have on shape. The lessons from tipping points match what Sherlock Holmes knew: It can be the smallest details of the immediate environment that really matter. Minor seemingly insignificant factors can cause shape to tip in an unwanted direction. The good news is that they can also cause a tip in the other direction, to a more desirable shape.

Our shape can seem impossible to budge. We go on a diet and several months later find that all the lost weight has returned. But with the slightest push in the correct place, our shape can be tipped. It is not the big things like radically changing diet to something a person will never be able to sustain that will create the results we desire. The solution lies in modifying smaller and sustainable details of our life. We would never be able to live the rest of our life on a low calorie diet—semi-starvation—like the participants on *Survivor* endure throughout their contest. In fact, just like the Survivors, we will rebound to our old weight once the constraints on food intake are lifted. But if we can identify the right little things and make changes in smaller details of our life, details we can readily live with, we won't have to.

Closing Dialogue

Health Scene Investigator: When Holmes made statements such as "little things are infinitely the most important", what do you think he really meant?

Apprentice: I think what he was trying to say was that when investigating a health scene one must be able to detect the things other people are missing. These things are little in the sense that they are being missed, but not little in their importance.

Health Scene Investigator: Very good. Now how might we apply this lesson to shape?

Apprentice: I imagine it means that to solve shape cases we would need to look at things differently. We would need to look for the things that are being missed because we either (1) don't think of them as being big enough to cause the problem, or, (2) have no idea that some of these little things can cause shape changes.

Health Scene Investigator: That is it exactly. And how might we start to identify some of these hidden clues?

Apprentice: I would start by creating a list of the things that have changed just before and since the tipping point for obesity in America was reached. Experts pinpoint the mid 1970s as the time of this tipping point, so I would look at what things, even if they are seemingly trivial, changed significantly in diet, lifestyle, and the environment from then to now.

Health Scene Investigator: I think that would be an excellent start.

The Apprentice's List

Diet:
Increased reliance on commodity vegetable oils
Addition of trans fats and hydrogenated oils to many foods
Increased consumption of corn-derived sweeteners
Increased consumption of artificial sweeteners
Increased use of flavor ingredients and other food additives
Increase in snacking
Rise of the fast food industry and super-sizing of meals and beverages

Lifestyle:
Decreased sunlight exposure
Less time spent sleeping
Increased air travel across time zones
Increased TV and computer use
Increase in sedentary lifestyles
More meals eaten out of the home and fewer family meals

Environment:
More Stress
Increased pollution
Increased electro-magnetic exposure
Increased use of fluorescent lights

Can you think of anything to add to the Apprentice's list?

_____

_____

_____

_____

_____

_____

_____

_____

_____

_____

Chapter 3

Understanding Advances in Science

Detection is, or ought to be, an exact science and should be treated in the same cold and unemotional manner.

Sherlock Holmes

Opening Dialogue

Health Scene Investigator: Can you tell me what the scientific process includes?

Apprentice: Yes, it includes making observations, creating hypotheses that might explain these observations, and then testing these hypotheses. If exceptions are found, the hypothesis can be assumed to be falsified or untrue.

Health Scene Investigator: Excellent. In your opinion, should we be scientific in our approach to shape cases?

Apprentice: Of course we should. If we are not, how can we possibly hope to accurately solve them?

Health Scene Investigator: Very well then, which scientific model should we use to guide our efforts?

Apprentice: To be perfectly honest I haven't the slightest idea. I didn't realize that there were different models we could choose from.

Health Scene Investigator: Yes, there are very different models and these models disagree on a number of important points. I think that you will find that our choice of a scientific model will make a big difference in the way we understand shape cases. Let me explain.

An Exact Science

Readers originally met Sherlock Holmes, as did Watson, in the short story titled *A Study in Scarlet*. Dr. Watson had a competent background in applied sciences because of his medical training. Yet he was confounded by what he observed of his new flatmate's interests and knowledge base. While it was apparent that Holmes was endeavoring to be an expert in something, he was at a loss as to what this something might be. To help answer this question, Watson compiled a list of things he observed. His list included:

- Knowledge of Botany: Variable. Well up on belladonna, opium, and poisons. Knows nothing of practical gardening.
- Knowledge of Geology: Practical, but limited. Tells at a glance different soils from each other.
- Knowledge of Chemistry: Profound.
- Knowledge of Anatomy: Accurate, but unsystematic.
- Knowledge of Sensational Literature: Immense. He appears to know every detail of every horror perpetrated in the century.

While Watson had a difficult time understanding how these different interests could fit together in any profession he knew of, Holmes was practicing something similar to what we now call forensic science or crime scene investigation; the use of science to answer questions related to the criminal and legal system. However, it would be limiting to think of Holmes as only a forensic scientist. Holmes was applying knowledge derived from a broad spectrum of sciences to answer questions that were of particular interest to him. Many of these pertained to criminal or legal matters; some did not. If Holmes lived today and was determined to solve cases involving shape what might a list of his interests look like? Perhaps the list would include interests and specialized knowledge like:

- Knowledge of the Stock Market: Impractical. Knowledgeable about trends and cycles. Seems to know nothing of actually investing in or buying stocks.
- Knowledge of Weather: Variable. Well up on the science of predicting weather. Seems to care little for what the weather might be on any given day.

- Knowledge of Insects: Practical but limited. Keenly interested in ant colonies and beehives. Little interest in *entomology*—study of individual insects.
- Knowledge of Health Diagnostics: Accurate but unorthodox. Fixated on how things change and measuring things at different times of the day, month, and year.
- Knowledge of *Bariatrics* (weight sciences): Immense. He appears to know details from studies on weight that date back decades.

Looking at this list might leave you feeling equally as perplexed as Watson had been. You might have a difficult time understanding how these diverse things might fit together. What could the weather, the stock market, or an ant colony possibly have to do with shape? The answer is that these real world phenomena are examples of things that can be best understood by a new kind of science called *Complexity Science*, the science of complex adaptive systems—systems that show an ability to adapt and learn. As Holmes might have said, an *exact science*; just a very different type of exact science than most of us learned in our high school or college science courses.

Life Finds a Way

Science is a process used to acquire knowledge. It consists of making observations, creating hypotheses that might explain these observations, and testing these hypotheses. If a number of related hypotheses appear to be accurate, they are grouped together to form general *theories* or *models* that are used for describing and predicting the behavior of a category of natural phenomena. The acid test for the utility of a scientific model isn't how well it explains past observations; while this is important, it is even more important that the model be able to accurately predict *future behavior*. It is this ability to predict what will happen next that separates out things that look scientific from things that are scientific.

Science isn't made up of just one model; it's comprised of a collection of models, with different models existing for different categories of natural phenomenon. A model might excel in one area but might be extremely limited, or even unusable, in another area. It is vitally important that the right model be used for the natural phenomenon being investigated if we hope to make accurate scientific predictions. As examples, *Newton's theory* of physics allows us to accurately predict the behavior of many physical interactions like balls moving on a pool table. *Quantum theory*, on the other hand, is not very useful for describing movement on a pool table, but it is a far better model for describing and predicting the behavior of subatomic particles. Both Newtonian and Quantum theory are extremely useful models in some scientific areas but not in all scientific areas. This is a critical point.

HSI CLUE

The purpose of science is the accumulation of knowledge, which can be used to produce useful models of reality. These models are used to make accurate predictions about how (and why) things behave the way they do. What does it tell us about our model when it fails to make accurate predictions? It tells us that this model is not useful for this data. In no uncertain terms, it informs us that we need a better model.

Scientific models are useful where they are useful and where they aren't, as the saying goes, *Houston, we have a problem*. If we attempt to use a scientific model to understand, explain, and make predictions in a category of phenomena where it is a poor fit, the model won't help us to better understand things. More often than not, it will be an obstacle in the path of understanding. We learn this lesson from Holmes. An incorrect theory can cause an investigator to see clues where none exist and to miss clues that are present. This is only part of the problem. When our theory is incorrect most of us are quite capable of fitting a square peg into a round hole while being convinced that the fit is perfect. In many of Holmes' cases, the official investigator, usually a police detective, has a pet theory; an explanation of the facts that they are supremely confident is correct. As they uncover more clues, it further cements this false sense of confidence. The confidence is unshakeable right up until Holmes proves them wrong. How is it that they could have been so spectacularly wrong yet have been so confident that they were right? The short answer is that it is in most of our natures to use a theory as a way to filter information. We do the opposite of what Holmes advises. One would think that if our theory were incorrect, we would readily notice this and abandon the theory. We don't. Instead our biases lead us to ignore, distort, or misinterpret clues that don't quite fit. As Holmes informs us, "Insensibly one begins to twist facts to suit theories…" Misapplying a scientific model is, in a practical sense, no different from the errors these official investigators make. It causes a scientist to miss important clues, see clues where none exist, and misinterpret clues that are collected. It allows one to be magnificently wrong while feeling unshakably certain of being correct. This is a recipe for disaster when it comes to understanding issues and coming up with solutions to problems. Using a scientific model that would be perfectly valid in one area, in an area where it is a poor fit, can lead to what amounts to scientific gibberish; nonsense, but nonsense that looks and feels scientific. One of the big problems, when it comes to making sense of shape, has been this wrong model problem. This problem is in the process of being corrected.

Over the past few decades, a silent revolution has occurred within many scientific fields of inquiry—a *second scientific revolution*. The first scientific revolution occurred in Europe's Renaissance period. During a relatively brief time period in European history, centering about the year 1600, there were dramatic changes in the ways in which *natural philosophers*, what we today would call scientists, thought about and investigated the physical world. They saw the world in a new light. This fundamentally transformed astronomy, biology, chemistry, and physics. The widely held model of the universe, a largely theological model that existed prior to this first scientific revolution, became obsolete. It was replaced with a new model, the universe being akin to a big machine, that has influenced scientific thought ever since. Today we are in the midst of a second scientific revolution; a revolution in thought that promises to radically change the way we think about and explore our world. This revolution is being fueled by what we'll call the *Jurassic Park* metaphor.

> **H S I   C L U E**
>
> What if, rather than thinking we can control our weight, we believed that there was some intelligent system operating in the background learning and adapting; how might this change the way we approach and solve shape cases? How might this color our behaviors?

In the book and movie *Jurassic Park*, written by the late Michael Crichton, the InGen scientists were convinced they could build, what amounted to, a safe dinosaur zoo. They were wrong. It turns out that controlling dinosaurs is easier said than done. Dinosaurs, like all living things, learn and adapt. They have minds of their own. Trying to control them wasn't possible. It also had disastrous unintended consequences. The reason that these scientists were so spectacularly wrong boiled down to a simple pivot point. They used the wrong scientific model. The InGen scientists were using a scientific model called *Reductionism*. They assumed that dinosaurs were little different than balls on a pool table, an assumption that proved to be catastrophic. One character in the book, Dr. Malcolm, looked at this same situation using a different scientific model, one that assumes complexity. What did he conclude? He assures us, "There is a problem with that island. It is an accident waiting to happen." Here we have what amounts to two groups of scientists both looking at the same situation, yet, because they are using different scientific models to inform their interpretations of facts, they give us what amount to diametrically opposed predictions about what is likely to occur. Who was correct? Dr. Malcolm was: It was an accident waiting to happen. Dinosaurs are an example of a complex adaptive system. They don't play by reductionist rules. The thing that seemed so simple, controlling dinosaurs, ended up being incredibly complex in the real world; complicated in ways the InGen scientists hadn't imagined and didn't anticipate, but that Dr. Malcolm, and his scientific model, had.

Living things don't play by pool table rules. They learn, adapt, store information for later use, and change the rules of the game as they go. They don't like being controlled and they tend to push back. They have a way of coming up with creative solutions to get what they want. In a phrase, *life finds a way*. This idea that life adapts and finds a way is the *Jurassic Park* metaphor. If our goal is to understand a system as complex, and as capable of learning and adapting, as the human body, we need to use a scientific model that takes into account this metaphor. This scientific model is called *Complexity Science*. It is far better suited for investigating, understanding, and predicting the behaviors of complex adaptive systems of all types. Up until recently, the dominant scientific model used for understanding health and shape has been the same one used to understand movement of balls on a pool table. This has been a mistake. Our bodies and their shapes are far more than just balls on a pool table. Like dinosaurs, the human body learns and adapts. It finds ways to get what it needs or wants. We have been using the wrong scientific model. It's time to use a better one. This point of choosing the correct scientific model can't be overemphasized. While something might be a valid and useful scientific theory, if it is used as a model to predict the behaviors of a category of natural phenomenon for which it is a poor fit, we end up misunderstanding the phenomenon and making bad predictions. There is in fact, nothing less scientific.

Old Models, Old Assumptions

Different scientific models tend to have very different assumptions about the nature of the phenomenon they are attempting to understand. From the time of Newton until recently, the dominant scientific model has been Reductionism. This theory has as its fundamental assumption that the nature of complex things can be understood by reducing them to simpler things. If we want to understand shape, we might study a fat cell. To understand a fat cell we might study its chemical reactions, receptors, and messenger molecules. It's assumed that if we eventually know enough details about an individual fat cell, we will be able to figure out how shape works. And, if we are smart enough, we might be able to eventually design drugs targeted at fat cells that block or inhibit chemical reactions, receptors, or messenger molecules; ultimately enabling us to pharmacologically control shape and make it behave the way we want it to. The implied promise is that with enough time, money and computational power, we will be able to figure everything out, fix all problems, and control anything we want—the environment, economy, disease, and even our shape. Unfortunately, entire categories of real world phenomenon have proven resistant to these assumptions and to this promise. In the real world there are, quite simply, events and organisms that can't be completely figured out by taking them apart and putting them back together again. Reductionist informed predictions in these areas often prove to be inaccurate. Put another way, actual behavior indicates that these systems don't follow the rules of Reductionism.

> **HSI CLUE**
>
> Reductionism tells us that the *gas mileage* our body gets will be constant. Complexity Science tells us that our body might act intelligently; conserving or wasting fuel as it adapts and learns. In the upcoming chapters notice what happens to metabolism after dieting and after overeating. Is it constant or does it adapt?

New Models, New Assumptions

Complexity Science is the preferred scientific model for describing how *complex adaptive systems* behave. These systems may be insects in a hive or colony, the Internet, stock market trends, the immune system, or fat cells. What do these systems have in common? Each of these systems is made up of a great number of individual agents (individual insects, computer users, investors, immune or fat cells, respectively) that are somehow connected together. As a group these agents display a collective type of intelligent behavior that is far richer than could be guessed by studying any of the individual agents in isolation. As an example, we could study an individual computer user for the next year; yet find ourselves no closer to predicting the behavior of the Internet. We could study individual ants, and be left with little to no idea how an ant colony behaves and adapts to real world challenges. Paraphrasing a metaphor used within Complexity sciences, we could study a snowflake for the rest of our life, but get no closer to understanding avalanches. This same principle applies to all complex adaptive systems. To truly understand them we need to study how the entire system, not isolated agents, responds. We need to pay attention to the behaviors that emerge at the level of the whole, which might hardly have been guessed at when we were studying the individual agents in isolation. What does this mean for shape? It means that if we want to truly understand shape we need to focus on how the body learns from, responds to, and adapts over time as it encounters different real world situations. It means that we need to stop thinking of our body as uncaring and passive and start to appreciate it for what it really is, an intelligent organism with its own objectives, an organism that uses *collective intelligence*.

HSI CLUE

What if instead of thinking about fat cells in isolation, we viewed body fat as an intelligent superorganism? What if we thought about muscle in the same way? What if our shape were the result of an intelligent superorganism adapting to the world around it? How might this influence how we think about our shape? How might it change what we do in our efforts to improve how we look?

An ant is a living thing. It matches our intuitions about what a living thing should look like and how it should behave. But what about an ant colony, is it "living", does it behave "intelligently"? The answer to both of these questions is yes. An ant colony is an example of collective intelligence. It is a living *superorganism* consisting of many organisms. It learns from and adapts to its environment; with the entire colony being a problem-solving unit. An ant on its own is actually not very bright. Removed from a colony, it will wander without purpose, directionless, until it dies of exhaustion or starvation. Yet put it in a colony with other ants and a collective intelligence emerges that is capable of remarkable things. A colony will find new sources of food or a new place to live if needed. It will adapt to all manner of real world challenges in ways that an isolated ant can't.

What if body fat was akin to an ant colony? Is it possible that all of our fat cells might be working together? Could body fat be a single superorganism capable of collective intelligence? Like the dinosaurs in *Jurassic Park*, when it comes to shape, the body seems to find a way to get what it wants. The science of complex adaptive systems, and the collective intelligence these systems are capable of, offers a new perspective for understanding why this is the case.

Complex Adaptive Intelligence

Complex adaptive systems have the ability to learn from experience; they also tend to have *decentralized intelligence*. This intelligence is different than the centralized intelligence of a brain. Instead of being located in one particular place, it is spread through the entire system of interacting agents. The immune system is an example of this decentralized type of intelligence. There is no one single location for which we can say, "this is where immune system intelligence resides". Immune intelligence is everywhere and nowhere. Yet this immune system intelligence will remember lessons it received from when a person was vaccinated years, or even decades, ago. It will learn from and adapt to emergent threats such as a new bacteria or virus. It will store this information

> **HSI CLUE**
>
> What might an intelligent system learn from a couple of episodes of dieting? How might this experience affect its predictions about the future? Hint: What would you learn if you ran out of gas a few times? Is it likely to convince you to keep less or more gas in your tank?

in case it needs it again. And if the same bacteria or virus threatens it in the future, it will recall the needed information and respond quickly and decisively. After immune system intelligence has solved a problem once, and it is great at solving bacterial or viral problems or we would have been wiped out long ago, responding to the same problem in the future is an exercise in recall, a matter of immune system memory, and our immune system has a tremendous memory and is exquisitely designed to perform this exercise.

An ant colony uses this same type of decentralized collective intelligence. Individual ants aren't very bright, but, as mentioned, an ant colony is capable of remarkable things and shows extremely intelligent behavior. Where does this intelligence come from and who's in charge? The answer is the same as it is for immune system intelligence. There's no one in charge. The intelligence is diffused throughout the entire ant colony; it's everywhere and it's nowhere. It arises from the group of ants interacting. The colony—

superorganism—is what adapts to its environment, and it can and will adapt to all manner of stimuli and then remember these solutions if similar situations arise again.

Complexity science informs us to expect that a complex adaptive system, like our body, will rely on decentralized intelligence for some important jobs. Immunity is one of these jobs. Could shape be another? Might we have a complex adaptive *Shape Intelligence*? Complexity science teaches us that, if we do, this Shape Intelligence would be spread diffusely through the network of interacting fat cells, muscle cells, and other cells and systems that collectively are adapting and learning from the experiences we give them. It teaches us that if we try and take direct control of our shape, we will be taking on this collective, decentralized intelligence, and it might have far different plans than we do. We would find ourselves up against an intelligence that learns quickly, adapts to whatever new things come its way, has the memory of an elephant, so to speak, never gives up, and has access to internal processes that we can't see or even hope to control.

The Human Body:
An Unintelligent Machine or Does Life Find a Way?

Reductionism promises that everything can be figured out and controlled. Complexity Science tells a different story; living systems are complex, intelligent, and adapt. Using an analogy, Reductionism tries to tell us that the human body is a lot like a car, just a very complicated car. Complexity Science informs us that, if this were true we would be more like Herbie the Love Bug; the human-like fictional Volkswagen Beetle featured in several Disney films, than the car we have in our driveway or garage. Which do you think we are more like? You will be introduced to a variety of cases—to evidence and data—in the next few chapters. Your task is to notice the behaviors and the real world responses. As an example, when you review cases concerning underfeeding, notice what happens initially, short-term over weeks or a few months, and long-term over many months. Do we respond like the car in our driveway might or more like Herbie would? Both Reductionism and Complexity Science predict that restricting calories will result in weight loss, but they disagree on how the body will respond over time. The assumptions within Reductionism predict that as long as a calorie deficit remains constant, the rate of weight loss will continue unabated and indefinitely. Complexity Science predicts that the body will adapt: Even if the calorie deficit is kept constant, weight loss might not continue, it could plateau and given enough time to figure things out, the body might find a way to get back what it lost. Reductionism assumes that it is equally as easy to be at any weight: The body does not care how much it weighs any more than a car cares about how much gas it has in its tank. Complexity Science assumes that the body is intelligent: Not only is it likely to care, it just might actively defend its shape. Reductionism tells us that if we want to lose weight, it is easy: Just eat less. Complexity informs us that eating less isn't going to be easy and it's likely to get harder the longer we diet and the further below the body's defended weight we move. Reductionism assumes that it doesn't matter what we have done in the past. The key thing is what we are doing now. Complexity tells us the body has a memory. It keeps track of the kind of person it houses and remembers the things the person has done in the past. Reductionism essentially concerns itself with what we do. The critical variable is creating an energy deficit. Complexity is concerned about what we do, but it is more concerned with how the body might adapt to what we do and what might be learned in the process. Reductionism informs us that calorie restriction is the solution. Complexity offers a different perspective: Dieting is an experience, one that might be difficult and fail to permanently alter shape, and that just might cause the body to learn things and adapt in unintended ways.

The purpose of a scientific model is to make accurate predictions about how things behave. Do its predictions match what really occurs? If it does a poor job, it is a poor theory, at least for describing that type of real world phenomenon. If it makes accurate predictions, it is a useful model. As you move through the next few chapters, reviewing the evidence and paying attention to what really occurs, not what some theory says should occur, ask yourself a question: When it comes to shape, is the body acting like an unintelligent machine or is life finding a way?

Closing Dialogue

Health Scene Investigator: What is your answer now? Which model should we use?

Apprentice: Shouldn't we observe the evidence first and after that determine whether one of the models explains the evidence?

Health Scene Investigator: Excellent answer. I see you have taken to heart our earlier lessons. Let us proceed to investigate the evidence.

Chapter 4

Gathering and Analyzing Evidence

We approached the case, you remember, with an absolutely blank mind, which is always an advantage. We had formed no theories. We were simply there to observe and to draw inferences from our observations.

Sherlock Holmes

Opening Dialogue

Health Scene Investigator: Are you familiar with the TV show *Survivor*?

Apprentice: Yes. It is a show about people placed into a castaway experience, who attempt to win a million dollars by, as the show's tag line states, trying to *Outplay, Outwit, and Outlast* each other.

Health Scene Investigator: Since you are very familiar with the show, please be so kind as to answer a few questions for me. Do the Survivors get enough food to eat?

Apprentice: No. Between what they can gather and what they are given, they never seem to get enough to eat.

Health Scene Investigator: And what does this lead to?

Apprentice: They all lose weight.

Health Scene Investigator: Yes, we would expect that. What else happens?

Apprentice: I am not so sure I know what you are asking.

Health Scene Investigator: Allow me to explain.

A Blank Mind

Sherlock Holmes was committed to gathering and analyzing evidence *in advance of theorizing*. He believed it was a disadvantage to approach a case with a pre-conceived theory because we might view the evidence in a way that distorts certain facts to support our theory. We might ignore facts that don't fit. And we might be incapable of seeing some facts because our theory does not allow for their existence. Sherlock Holmes thought the better way to approach a problem was to enter a case without any formed theories, with what he called a blank mind. With this mindset, an investigator should gather evidence, analyze it, and only then, come up with a theory that explains the facts. Why is this important to shape? It is important because there is already a theory about why people are overweight. The generally held theory, a theory of *energy balance*, argues that a person can, by exerting a reasonable degree of conscious effort, get to and stay at a desired weight. This theory gives rise to behaviors aimed at creating a negative energy balance. If we want to lose weight we reduce the energy we take in (calories), increase the energy we are using (exercise and metabolism), or both. The three options for energy balance are listed in the box. Losing weight is theoretically a matter of taking control in a manner that creates the third situation, an energy deficit.

Energy Balance and Weight Gain or Loss

(1) Calories In = Energy Used in Activity + Metabolism: Weight Stays the Same

(2) Calories In > Energy Used in Activity + Metabolism: Surplus of Energy Resulting in Storage of the Surplus → Fat Gain (and, Hence Weight Increase)

(3) Calories In < Energy Used in Activity + Metabolism: Deficit of Energy Resulting in Use of Stored Surplus → Fat Loss (and, Hence Weight Loss)

If we have failed to do a good job controlling our weight, one or more of three things must be occurring. We must be eating too much, taking in too much energy. We must be exercising too little, using too little energy in exercise and activity. Or we must have a slow metabolism, needing less energy to run our body processes than a normal person would. It follows that solutions for improving shape would be consistent with addressing these issues. We would attempt to eat less and exercise more. We might even consider a medication or supplement to boost our metabolism. Case solved.

The energy balance theory predicts that after we lose weight by following one of these approaches, our body should be as comfortable at this reduced weight, and as willing to stay there, as it was at our previous higher weight. Since each of us is ultimately the one in control of our weight, it should be as easy for us to be at a new reduced weight as it was for us to be at our old heavier weight. Is it? Is there any evidence that contradicts this theory? As you review the evidence we are about to share with you below, it is important to remember one of Holmes' famous axioms; "an exception disproves the rule." If we uncover clues that indicate the body is not content to remain at a reduced weight or that it is adapting against approaches designed to create a negative energy balance, we can conclude that a theory predicated on controlling energy balance is logically flawed.

The energy balance theory has been the dominant way of thinking about shape for more than one hundred years. Weight gain and loss have been approached with anything but a blank mind. Has this approach been helping or hindering when it comes to solving the mystery of shape? Does it help individuals attain and keep the shapes or weights they desire? Are any facts being twisted, ignored, or missed completely? Is the theory biasing our investigations? What would we observe if we had a blank mind? For the energy balance theory to be correct, we must assume that the body doesn't really care how much fat it has or where this fat is stored. What if it did care?

Cases of Underfeeding

Three cases of underfeeding will be investigated in this section. In each case, a negative energy balance was created and sustained. Weight was lost. Reductionism predicts this will occur. Complexity science does as well. Where they differ is in predicting what else occurs. As you explore the next three cases—the *Case of Army Rangers, the Minnesota Experiment, and Starving in the Desert*—pay attention to *what else* occurs.

Each year more than 1,000 soldiers in the United States Army will be picked to enter the elite Special Forces training programs to become a Ranger. This training program lasts nine weeks and is characterized by high amounts of strenuous physical activity. Throughout much of this time period soldiers are deliberately underfed and are held to an average of less than four hours of sleep per night. These stressors are produced intentionally to mirror potential real world conditions that Rangers might encounter on a future mission. The *Case of the Army Rangers* is a study of this training program and the effects its multiple stressors produce on shape. A negative energy balance, or energy deficit, was created by the combination of eating less and exercising more, so, naturally, the soldiers lost weight. The average soldier lost about nine pounds of body fat during the first nine weeks of training. This finding is consistent with the energy balance theory. But are there other important clues in this case worthy of consideration?

HSI CLUE

Did the Rangers get fat because of being big eaters or having a lazy body or slow metabolisms?

Or were these possibly effects caused by the manner that they went about depleting fat? Based upon what occurred, both short-term and long-term, when they lost weight by what amounted to a restricted calorie diet, what can we infer will happen to us if we attempt to change our shape by dieting?

In this same study, stress hormones went up, thyroid hormones went down, and testosterone levels plummeted during the nine weeks of Ranger school. These changes mirrored fat depletion. Stress hormones reached their maximum, and thyroid and testosterone levels their minimum, when body fat reached its lowest amount. In no uncertain terms, fat depletion appears to be treated as stress, and elicits both a classic stress response and a slowing of metabolism. Coinciding with the fat loss, the soldiers became hungrier and hungrier. Even after training, when they were allowed to eat as much as they desired, this hunger did not go away by eating a few big meals. None of these changes are predicted by the energy balance theory. We have all heard them, the reasons for why people get fatter: being a big eater, having a lazy body or a slow metabolism. Yet, in this case, the evidence is clear, two of these things occurred during Ranger training only after body fat was lost. They appear to be effects of fat loss. Who or what is causing them? Could a possible explanation be that we are observing adaptations by some form of intelligence that is dissatisfied with the fat lost in this fashion? So what happened next in this study?

As mentioned, soldiers lose body fat during Ranger training. In this case, on average, a soldier began Ranger training with 21 pounds of body fat. When they finished nine weeks later, body fat had decreased by an average of nine pounds; they now had twelve pounds of body fat. If this is the only time interval we focus our powers of observation upon, we would probably come away feeling certain that if we want to get rid of body fat, Ranger training is the way to go. But in this case there is a rest of the story.

Soldiers frequently complain that, after Ranger training has ended, they end up fatter than they have ever been before. To test this, the soldiers were reassessed five weeks after the end of Ranger training. On average a soldier now had 30 pounds of body fat. This represents a 40 percent increase in body fat when compared to the 21 pounds of fat they had before they began the training program and a whopping 250 percent increase compared to the 12 pounds of fat they had at the completion of training. The soldiers' complaints were justified. But how do we explain such rapid fat gain? Even more importantly, what was it about Ranger training that caused them to be so much fatter five weeks after it ended than they were prior to it beginning?

HSI CLUE

Hunger does accumulate; there is really no question of that. Dieters demonstrate it. Participants in *Survivor* experience it. So do the Army Rangers and the men in the Minnesota Experiment. What is really accumulating under these instances? What is causing the hunger?

The energy balance theory tells us that post training fat accumulation must be the result of the over-eating, laziness, and slow metabolism. But what does the actual evidence tells us? In the case of the stress and metabolism hormones, post-training fat super accumulation resulted in a prompt return to normal values of both. The same was true for hunger. It decreased after these soldiers gained the extra fat. If the causes were truly over-eating, laziness or slow metabolism, why did these issues only appear with fat loss and vanish with fat gain? Why did these shift with the changing circumstances? Could these things, which many people blame as the cause of being overweight, be something entirely different? Might they be evidence of the body adapting by intentionally slowing its metabolism, increasing its appetite and decreasing activity levels, in response to the way these soldiers went about losing body fat?

The next investigation is the *Case of the Minnesota Experiment.* On November 19, 1944, 36 healthy young men entered the Laboratory of Physiological Hygiene at the University of Minnesota for a long-term study in underfeeding that would later be called the Minnesota Starvation Experiment (or simply the Minnesota Experiment). The study had three phases. Phase One was a three-month observation period during which the men were fed enough food to maintain their normal weight. Phase Two was a six-month underfeeding period: Participants were expected to walk daily and were fed about 1800 calories a day. The goal was a weekly weight loss of approximately 2.5 lbs, and ultimately a loss of 25 percent of starting weight. Phase Three was a three-month nutritional rehabilitation period during which time participants were allowed to eat about 4000 calories a day. What was observed?

Shortly into the underfeeding period the men became preoccupied with food; they thought about food, talked about food, read about food, and even dreamed about food. This preoccupation increased as the study progressed. And it did not go away when they were allowed to eat more food during Phase Three: It persisted until the men had regained almost all of the body fat they had lost. In addition to this preoccupation with food, the men experienced persistent hunger that did not go away with eating. Because of this hunger there were times when the men failed to adhere to their diets and lost control of what and how much they ate. There were instances when participants ate between 8,000-10,000 calories at a single setting and were still hungry. These splurges were followed by self-reproach or feeling guilty about the inability to stay on the diet. Even after 12 weeks of being allowed to eat more food during Phase Three, the men frequently complained that they were still hungry. The men experienced a dramatic slowing of their metabolism. At the end of Phase Two, the men's metabolism at rest had dropped by about 40 percent from normal despite the fact that weight had only dropped by 25 percent. Metabolism had slowed faster and further than could have been predicted by either the amount of weight they had lost or the amount of metabolically active tissue, like muscle, they still maintained. During Phase Three, as body fat reserves increased, metabolism sped up and eventually normalized. The men found it more difficult to exercise and responded to weight loss by reducing physical activity. They became tired, weak, and lacked energy. Voluntary movements became noticeably slower. Although they continued walking, lethargy led them to avoid as much work, study, or play as possible. While this was the norm, there were occasional instances of men pushing themselves to exercise excessively so that they would be allowed to eat more food. Weight decreased by an average of 25 percent, but the decrease occurred relatively early during the Phase Two underfeeding period and leveled off. Further weight reductions, despite continued underfeeding, did not occur. And, most importantly, eight months after the end of Phase Two, the men had regained the lost weight, but were much fatter—they had 140 percent of their original body fat—at this weight than they were prior to prolonged calorie restriction. In the long-term, underfeeding was fattening. It took nearly two years for these volunteers to recover from the fattening effects of underfeeding, and for body fat to return to the levels it had been at before the Minnesota Experiment.

If the energy balance theory were correct, it should have been as easy for these men to be at a reduced weight as it was for them to be at their original Phase One weight. It wasn't. How can we best explain why after losing weight, by intentionally restricting calories, the men became preoccupied with food and experienced persistent hunger? Or, that their motivation to control the exercise part of energy balance was sapped? Why did their metabolism become unexpectedly slow when fat was depleted, but returned to normal once the lost fat, plus more than a bit of extra reserves, was restored? Yet we observed each of these things. The conventional theory of weight reduction, one based upon notions of creating a negative energy balance, does not predict that controlling energy balance will become more difficult after we lose weight, yet the evidence tells us it became progressively more difficult for these men. What can we learn from these observations?

The third case of prolonged underfeeding is the *Case of Starving in the Desert*. In September 1991, four women and four men were sealed inside Biosphere II, a 3.15-acre enclosed and self-contained ecological system built in the desert near Tucson, Arizona, for two years. They were supposed to be able to grow and raise sufficient food to meet their energy needs, but because of crop problems were unable to. During the first six months, calorie intake averaged 1784 calories a day. During the next 15 months, it ranged from approximately 1750 to 2100 calories. This was sufficient to create a sustained, albeit modest, energy deficit, especially during the first six months. While this had not been intended, Biosphere II had become a long-term study in underfeeding, and, not surprisingly, the men lost an average of 21 percent and the women an average of 14 percent of their initial weight during the first year. After two years they exited Biosphere II and underwent extensive medical testing. Along with the reduced weight, a lazy body and a slow metabolism were detected. Six months later five of the eight participants underwent another series of testing. They had regained the weight they had lost, an average of about 19 pounds. And, similar to the Army Rangers and the volunteers in the Minnesota Experiment, there was a disproportionate gain of fat with an average of 18 of the 19 pounds of the regained weight being fat. With the fat gain, metabolism had sped up and laziness had decreased.

Where There's Smoke, There's Fire

Are people fat because they are big eaters, lazy, or have a slow metabolism? The above evidence indicates the answer might be no in many instances. In each of the above cases, these appeared to be effects not causes. Metabolic slowness and gluttony only showed up at the health scene after weight loss was induced by creating a negative energy balance, by doing the equivalent of going on a long-term diet. And they disappeared from the health scene as soon as weight, and more specifically body fat, had been re-acquired.

We are all familiar with the saying that "where there's smoke, there's fire." Smoke shows up when there is a fire and vanishes after the fire is put out. It doesn't cause a fire. We know this so we look for other clues at the scene of a fire. We look for things like matches or fuel that can actually cause a fire. We do it because we know it is silly to confuse *effects* of a fire with *causes* of a fire.

In the shape Health Scenes described in this chapter we observed consistent findings. We saw that if people take control of energy balance and manage to create and sustain a deficit, they will lose weight, at least temporarily. They will also experience an increase in hunger and think about food a lot. The inference we can draw from this fact is that there is an increased pressure to eat more calories that accompanies losing weight when the weight is lost by means of calorie restriction. From where is this pressure coming? Why does it emerge? And why does it go away once lost fat is regained? We also observed a reduction in daily physical activity and a dramatic slowing of metabolism with fat loss. We can infer from this evidence that at least in these individuals, a lazy body and slow metabolism accompany fat loss produced by dieting and are corrected by fat regain. The prevailing theory tells us that how much we eat, our level of activity, and the speed of our metabolism, are like the match with fire; they are causes. But if this is true, why do they look so much like smoke (effects)? We observed that the people in these cases eventually regained lost weight. If we can really take control of energy balance and the body doesn't care how much we weigh, we should be as comfortable at a reduced weight, after fat loss, as we were at the higher weight. The prevailing theory allows for no other possibilities. Yet the best evidence and real world experience indicate that the body doesn't seem to get comfortable after a period of eating less. It gets very uncomfortable. And the solutions this theory leads to don't work very well. Most dieters, just like the people in these cases, lose weight temporarily, reach a weight loss plateau, and then, despite great determination, gradually regain all of it.

The last finding we observed we might call *body fat over shoot* or *dieting-induced fatness*. Dieting left a scar. This scar was an increase in body fat above and beyond the pre-calorie restriction levels of body fat. Regaining lost weight almost exclusively as body fat was observed in the Army Rangers. It was detected in the volunteers in the Minnesota Experiment. It occurred in Biosphere II. It has been observed in famine victims and in patients with anorexia nervosa, cancer, sepsis, and AIDS. It is so common it was given a name by Ancel Keys and the other researchers responsible for conducting the Minnesota Experiment—*post-starvation obesity*. We can infer from the evidence that there is something about losing weight by creating and sustaining a negative energy balance that results in the body often being much fatter when it returns to its old weight. But what is it about restricting calories that causes this and why? Why does the body appear to resist fat loss with such determination and respond against it so drastically? Nothing like this is predicted by the energy balance theory.

H S I   C L U E

What inference can we draw from the observation of body fat over shoot occurring after a period of dieting? Has *something* decided to be better prepared for the next period of famine; with better prepared being more stored energy (body fat)? Has this *something* learned and adapted? Is it protecting itself against another period of dieting in the future?

Conclusion

The theory that we can consciously control our weight by creating an energy deficit sounds simple and reasonable. If we want to get rid of fat, what could be more sensible than restricting calories to create an energy deficit; forcing our body to use up some of its reserves? If we eat less long enough, of course we can have any weight we desire. Once we are satisfied with our weight loss, all we need to do to keep this improvement is make sure that energy in equals energy out moving forward. The theory's simplicity and apparently logical construct has led to its broad acceptance. But is this how things work in the real world? Is the case really this simple and easy? The evidence reviewed in this chapter teaches us the answer is no.

The cases of *the Army Rangers*, *the Minnesota Experiment*, and *Starving in the Desert* provide compelling evidence against the popular notion that body weight is easily lost or permanently altered by eating less. Yes weight is lost, but new clues emerge—preoccupation with food, persistent hunger, loss of control over what and how much is eaten, lethargy and physical laziness, and an unpredicted slowing of metabolism. These clues don't fit with the existing theory. Neither does the clue that when the lost weight is regained, it is disproportionately as fat. The theory that we can consciously control our weight by choosing to intentionally restricting calories appears to be an elaborate fiction; a belief in a world that, the evidence indicates, does not exist. While this might sound discouraging, please bear with us. The first step in getting somewhere, in this instance to a sustainable improvement in shape, is to face the facts, to confront reality. Once this has been done, the case begins to take on a new outlook, and from this different perspective solutions can be found.

Closing Dialogue

Health Scene Investigator: Now that you have observed the evidence from these cases, can you tell me what else happens to the Survivors?

Apprentice: Yes, they experience many of the same things described in these cases. They become obsessed with food and eating. In fact, they seem to be especially obsessed with foods that are high in fat and starch—junk food. When they first arrive at the island they always have lots of energy. After losing weight they become lazier. It is a struggle to get work done and complete the challenges.

And I have noticed that in the final show, which occurs months after they have left the island, they appear to have regained the weight they lost.

Health Scene Investigator: Excellent. How can we explain these observations?

Apprentice: I have believed that each of us is in control of our weight and chooses how much or little we eat. If we want to be slimmer we simply choose to eat less. I don't know how to explain what occurs to the Survivors when they eat less. None of this seems to make sense.

Health Scene Investigator: You are correct. These responses don't make sense with a theory that predicts weight can be controlled. But if I were to look at this evidence with a blank mind, I would infer that something was opposing their weight loss efforts, adapting, quite successfully. Naturally, that is only a hypothesis at this point.

Chapter 5

Avoiding Obvious Facts

There is nothing more deceptive than an obvious fact.

Sherlock Holmes

Opening Dialogue

Health Scene Investigator: Do you recall my telling you that when it comes to shape and weight, very few things can be termed "obvious".

Apprentice: Yes, I do. We had been discussing why people are overweight and I said it was obviously because they ate too much.

Health Scene Investigator: Exactly so. Do you remember what else I told you at that time?

Apprentice: Yes, you told me there were details that give rise to reasonable doubts as to the accuracy of this notion.

Health Scene Investigator: Your memory is excellent. Let's discuss those details, but first can you tell me whether being overweight is unhealthy?

Apprentice: Yes, everyone knows this.

Health Scene Investigator: I was afraid you might say that.

Obvious Facts

Steven Levitt and Stephen Dubner, authors of the bestselling book *Freakonomics*, wrote, "We have evolved with a tendency to link causes to things we can touch or feel, not to some distant or difficult phenomenon." We are predisposed to see the obvious facts and miss more subtle clues. This is fine when the obvious is the cause, but in the real world there are many instances when the cause is more subtle, distant or difficult to spot. In these situations we can be easily deceived by what might appear at first glance to be obvious.

According to Sherlock Holmes, obvious facts were the superficially apparent clues that distracted the less keen observer from looking for other, potentially more meaningful, evidence. In some instances they are analogous to conventional wisdom; ideas or explanations that are accepted as true by the majority of the public, and hence, escape scrutiny. The world is flat. The earth is the center of the universe. Malaria is caused by bad air. Disease can be cured by mercury. No one will buy a watch that you don't have to wind. These are just some of the historical obvious facts that we now know to be untrue.

Obvious facts can be correct. They can also be incorrect. In either case, once we latch onto one the tendency is to reject everything else. While this is fine when the obvious fact is correct; it presents a problem when it is incorrect. This was evident in many of Holmes's most famous cases, where an official investigator seized upon an obvious fact, and in large part because of this, solved the case incorrectly. Holmes knew that obvious facts could mislead even the most astute investigator. They mislead us by causing us to believe in false theories, to miss important evidence, and to embrace solutions that don't work. By telling us that obvious facts can be deceptive Holmes was reminding us to look beyond the widely accepted, to question conventional wisdom, and to scrutinize even our most cherished beliefs. Is it possible that our shape might benefit if we were to take this advice to heart?

Does Weight Really Kill?

An important distinction, when dealing with obvious facts, is that there is a difference between cause and correlation. Remember from chapter 4 that smoke and fire show up together, but smoke does not cause a fire. This point is critical because with health and with shape, things that occur frequently together are often presented as if their relationship is causal. Here is an example:

- Observation: In many studies a higher incidence of heart disease is observed in obese individuals.
- Conclusion: Being overweight or obese kills 300,000 to 400,000 people in the United States each year and will soon overtake smoking as the leading cause of death.

The above conclusion is common, but is it actually supported by the evidence? While early death and weight have a relationship, is weight the *match* or is it *smoke*? Claims that a cause-effect relationship exists between two factors must be treated with suspicion. We must be willing to explore competing explanations. Let's explore.

For more than one hundred years a statistical correlation between higher weight (especially extremes of higher weight) and early mortality from heart disease, strokes, diabetes, and kidney disease has been reported. This correlation has been used to blame weight for the observed earlier mortality. Weight is portrayed as the *cause*; we are told it is the *match*. To be sure, this is one possibility. Other plausible possibilities include:

- Heart disease, as an example, causes people to be overweight; the direction of causation is reversed. Weight is a direct effect of heart disease not the other way around (heart disease is the *match*).
- Whatever is causing a person to be overweight is also causing the earlier mortality and the extra weight is a *byproduct* (weight is like *smoke* at a fire).
- Whatever is causing them to be overweight is also causing the earlier mortality and weight is protecting them; if they did not gain weight they would die even earlier (weight is a bit like a *fireman*; while it might be on the scene, it is there to prevent damage).
- Weight has nothing to do with the early mortality and it is a coincidence that it is on the same health scene fairly

HSI CLUE

Data from 7767 patients with previous heart failure enrolled in the Digitalis Investigation Group trial indicated that all-cause mortality rates decreased in an almost perfect line as weight increased. The highest risk of death, 45 percent, was in the people who weighed the least and the lowest risk of death, even lower than that found in persons who were theoretically at a "healthy" weight', was observed among obese participants. How do we rationalize evidence like this if weight really kills?

frequently (weight is like an innocent *bystander* attracted to a fire).

What does the actual evidence indicate? After all, a Health Scene Investigator is in the business of gathering evidence in advance of theorizing. Let's list some of the more consistent observations.

- For a given height, there is a wide range of weights, a range of 80 pounds or more, where health risk is essentially the same.

- In some studies, a modest correlation between being above an "ideal" weight and early death from some health conditions has been reported. In many other studies this correlation hasn't been detected. And, in still other studies, the correlation flip-flops: "Ideal" weight people are more likely to die than overweight ones from these same health conditions.

- The strongest and most consistent correlation between weight and premature death exists for lower weights; being considered underweight is far riskier than being classified as overweight.

- It isn't until extremes of obesity are reached that the health risks of higher weight approaches the risks of lower weight.

- Many studies have observed what is sometimes called the *obesity paradox*. Among people with established heart disease—high blood pressure, heart failure, coronary artery disease, and some other forms of chronic heart disease— being overweight or obese is correlated with a higher likelihood of survival and being at a theoretically "ideal" weight is correlated with increased risk of dying.

- The obesity paradox has been observed in other areas. Higher weight, even extremes of higher weight, has a protective correlation with death from suicide, among dialysis patients, in several surgical procedures, with some cancers, and more.

- Compared to persons whose weight remains stable, people who have intentionally lost weight, or whose weight has cycled up and down several times or more, are at a statistically higher risk of death. In fact, a thin person who has experienced several cycles of weight loss and regain can be at a higher risk than an obese person whose weight has remained stable.

- A thin person with one or more risk factors for heart disease, such as high blood pressure, is at a greater risk for death than an overweight person without these risk factors.
- A physically active overweight or obese person has a lower risk for disease and early death than a sedentary thin or ideal weight person.
- Correlations between weight and health become even more complex when age, race, poverty, and other factors are considered.
- Our shape, as well as the amounts and distribution of body fat and muscle, has a stronger and more consistent correlation with early death than weight does.

The links between weight and health are complicated, far less certain than we are typically led to believe, and there is currently a lack of proof that weight is the cause in the relationship. Does weight really kill; is it the match? We could make just as strong of an argument that weight change or dieting kills. We could make an argument that under some circumstances a higher weight appears to be protective. But we would still be misinterpreting evidence. These things are correlated with early death. Proof of cause requires a higher standard of evidence. There is currently no proof that weight is the cause in this relationship. Nor is there any proof that weight loss, in and of itself, is any benefit to long-term health. In other words, there is no evidence that weight loss puts out the fire. In fact, there is abundant evidence that contradicts the theory of weight as cause and weight loss as solution. What the early investigations done by the insurance industry, and all subsequent research really found was that some heavier Americans appear to be dying a bit earlier than anticipated from *something(s)*. We have been so distracted by the seemingly obvious—weight is to blame—we have failed to search for other clues. Have we been letting the real culprits go undetected and uncorrected?

HSI CLUE

Over a 24-year observation period overweight people whose weight remained stable were at the lowest risk of dying. Overweight persons who lost or gained weight had a 40 percent higher risk of dying. And overweight people who had made deliberate attempts at weight loss were 87 percent more likely to die. Evidence like this leads to a question: Is weight the important variable or is *change* in weight what matters? Is weight the issue or is the real issue dieting?

What are these potential culprits? Evidence suggests they are variables like poor nutrition, lack of exercise, work and relationship stress, inadequate sleep, poverty, and more. These and other aspects of diet, lifestyle, and the environment appear to be interacting in complex ways with individual genetic predispositions to contribute to, not cause, health outcomes. Perhaps it's time we stopped blaming weight or body fat for being the cause. Evidence points to shape as being a reflection of our body's attempts to do its best to match us to our diet, lifestyle, and environment. It might be a symptom of a problem; it is not the problem.

HSI CLUE

In many areas, shape and health included, what might be best described, as the consensus view, seems to be rock solid. But when it is investigated thoughtfully, all of the evidence is viewed and data is analyzed without bias, the consensus view suddenly looks far more fragile. It's not necessarily wrong, it might be, but it is far more uncertain than we have been led to believe.

We expect you to be a bit confused, and perhaps even a bit skeptical, when we tell you that the evidence about being overweight causing early death is not so clear-cut. After all, if you are like most people, you have probably been led to believe that weight is such a well-established cause of disease that it's hardly worth discussing. We assure you that it is worth discussing, but we also understand and appreciate your confusion. The *Case of the News Media* sheds some light on why this obvious fact persists and how scientific findings can be distorted to support it.

A 2007 study conducted by the Center for Disease Control (CDC) found that being overweight, having a body mass index (BMI) between 25 and 30, was associated with a lower risk of dying from heart disease, cancer, and all other causes. In other words, after gathering and analyzing evidence, they concluded that being about 10 to 25 pounds over a "normal" or "healthy" weight appeared to be, go figure, even healthier. But this is not what we want to draw your attention to. There are many findings like this in medical research. We want to draw your attention to how three different news media outlets decided to title their news releases about this research. This CDC research was variously titled as *"Extra weight may have health benefits"* by the Voice of America, *"Extra weight said won't raise death risk"* by the Associated Press and *"Being fat is still unhealthy, experts warn"* by Reuters. If the only thing we read were the titles, we would think they were referring to three different research studies. They weren't.

No wonder so many people get confused about shape. The titles of the three press releases tell us three essentially different things even though they are all reporting on the same scientific information. Sadly, this is not a one-time exception. And even more sadly, the title of a news release is often what draws our attention and gets remembered. The actual evidence is ignored or forgotten in its wake. The result is that conventional wisdom, the obvious fact, persists despite evidence to the contrary. Holmes warned us of the tendency to twist facts to suit our theories. He also warned us against the deceptive nature of obvious facts. If nothing else, the *Case of the News Media* illustrates that Holmes' concerns were justified and that pre-existing bias can color how we interpret evidence.

It is a virtual certainty that you will hear that weight kills on the news, in print media, in conversations among friends and acquaintances, and likely even from health professionals. It is also a virtual certainty that evidence will be distorted, exaggerated, and twisted in all manners of ways to support what amounts to a theory that has as much evidence against it as in its favor. Expect that this will occur, and, when it does, be happy that you know something these people don't. You understand that correlation does not prove cause. You know the difference between an obvious fact and actual evidence; and you know that there is a tendency to "twist facts to suit theories."

In many areas, the consensus viewpoint is far more fragile than we have been led to believe. Reality tends to be nuanced and complicated. Health is a complex subject. Making individual predictions about how healthy someone is or isn't, or even generalizations about a group of people, based on weight has little to do with science and lots to do with falling victim to a pervasive obvious fact. This point was made in a book by Paul Campos called *The Diet Myth: Why America's Obsession with Weight is Hazardous to Your Health*. After investigating this issue he writes, "The absurd notion that something as complex as an individual human being's health can be adequately gauged, or even generalized about, by determining where he or she fits on a body mass index scale is a remnant of a level of medical knowledge (or rather ignorance) that had very little to do with science in any useful sense of that much-abused word."

Are We Fat Because We Eat Too Much?

Another obvious fact is that if we eat more food we will get fat. With this established, the reason an overweight person is overweight is clear; they eat too much. The reciprocal part of this obvious fact is that they could become lean and remain lean if they would only eat *normal* amounts of food. Does actual evidence support these consensus views?

The relationship between how much someone eats and how heavy he or she is, is a weak and inconsistent relationship. Some overweight people eat more than average, but others eat considerably less than average. And many lean individuals eat as much, and even more than the heaviest individuals and do not get fat. We have all observed these patterns. The patterns become even more confusing and inconsistent when we look at shape and amounts and distributions of muscle and fat. We will also discuss many cases in this book, and have already mentioned one, the *Case of Neutering a Pet* in chapter two, where fattening can occur despite there being no increase in calories consumed. The one thing that can be stated with certainty is that the relationship between our shape and how much we eat is anything but simple, obvious and linear. This can be inferred from the three cases described below.

The first of these is the *Case of Overfeeding Identical Twins*. Twin studies highlight the inconsistencies of our individual responses to eating large quantities of food. They also reveal the strong influence genetics has on how readily fat is gained and where it is accumulated. When pairs of identical twins have been overfed by 84,000 calories over a period of 100 days, all pairs gained some weight. We would expect this to occur but we don't necessarily anticipate the wide variety of responses we get. In theory, if a person were to eat 3,500 calories in excess of what their body needs, they would be expected to gain about one pound. Since these individuals ate an excess of 84,000 calories, they would be expected to gain about 24 pounds. In this case, however, some people gained far more, and others far less, than anticipated: Individual weight gain responses ranged from as little as 9 pounds to as much as 30 pounds. A difference of 21 pounds in weight gain represents a significant difference when everyone "over ate" the same amount of calories. Individual shape responses to over-eating were even more varied. Some individuals accumulated much more fat. Others gained muscle more readily. Some individuals stored fat predominantly around the stomach and waist area; others were resistant to fat storage in this area. Despite broad variability in response to excess calories when comparing one pair of twins to another, there was a marked similarity between identical twins. And the similarity among identical twins was particularly striking with respect to how much fat was gained and where it was stored.

Theory informs us that eating 3500 calories in excess of the body's needs should result in about one pound of weight gain. It shouldn't matter if the excess calories are eaten during the first few days or the last few days of an overfeeding experiment. Did it matter? According to the researchers in this case it did. At the beginning almost all the energy surplus resulted in increases in measurable body weight. In an oversimplified sense, a pound of extra calories was adding a pound of weight to the body. By day 100 this proportion had changed. A pound of extra calories was only adding about 6/10ths of a pound of weight; far less of the extra calories were being stored. Instead, they were being used up somehow. We have learned that weight loss by dieting isn't linear and unending; it slows the longer dieting is continued and reaches a plateau. This was evident in the cases of underfeeding from the last chapter. A similar phenomenon in nature, but opposite in direction, was occurring in this case: The body appeared to be resisting more and more as weight deviated further and further from its starting point. It was adapting metabolically and in other ways that were acting to counter continued weight gain. This adaptation was greater in the twins who gained the least amount of weight than it was in the twins who gained the most weight.

Twin studies also point to a third important piece of evidence. Proving that eating more calories results in temporary weight gain is not the same as proving that eating too much causes permanent weight gain. Four months after the overfeeding period ended, virtually all of the added weight was gone, and, on average, upper body fat was actually lower than it had been before consumption of the additional 84,000 calories. While intentionally feeding volunteers an excess amount of calories had caused weight and fat accumulation, it did not cause obesity; at least in a long-term sense.

> **HSI CLUE**
>
> Imagine that two people are over-eating an equal amount of calories. One person is eating in *excess* of what their appetite dictates and the other isn't. Would we expect them to both have an equally "easy" time continuing to overeat? Would we expect both to gain an equal amount of weight? Or to have similar shape changes? Is it, in other words, how much we eat that defines overeating or is it eating more than our appetite dictates?

And the rebound effect from it actually improved shape slightly. The effects of intentionally overfeeding were as transient as the effects of dieting; just in the opposite direction: Weight was gained by using willpower and effort, but then it was easily lost.

HSI CLUE

In one overfeeding study, 16 pounds worth of extra calories were eaten over eight weeks, but no one gained this much weight. There was also a ten-fold difference in fat gain. One person gained almost ten pounds and another less than one pound of fat. How do we account for this difference? Where did the missing calories go? The answer to both questions is *adaptation.* Life found a way. Many of the excess calories were used up in activities akin to fidgeting. This was especially true for the persons most resistant to fat gain.

This case illustrates that genetics influence how much weight is gained in response to overfeeding; and even more importantly, how and where we gain the weight—how much is muscle, how much is fat, and where we store this fat. Some of us appear particularly susceptible to fat accumulation, while others are very resistant. Some of us preferentially deposit fat around our waists; others will distribute fat in areas like arms and legs. Something as seemingly obvious as eating an excess amount of calories for several months produces tremendously varied responses, and these responses appear to be strongly influenced by our genetics. What else can we infer from the *Case of Overfeeding Identical Twins?* Eating more food, even for months, isn't sufficient to make someone permanently fat. There were no persistent negative effects on shape or weight caused by even massive overfeeding. If anything, the persistent effects tended to be shape positive. The rebound effect resulted in a slight reduction of upper body fat.

The next case is the *Case of the Vermont Overfeeding Study.* Ethan Allen Sims conducted the first extensive investigation into long-term intentional excess calorie consumption in the 1960's. He resolved to make a group of thin people fat, so that he could study their metabolism. He began by asking four university students to gain 20 percent over their normally maintained body weight. He theorized that this would be relatively easy and could be accomplished by simply eating more than their habitual food intake. To his surprise, gaining weight wasn't easy. In fact, it was really hard. The students struggled to get 10 percent heavier than their normal weight. We imagine this result must have come as a bit of a surprise to Sims. After all, nothing in the existing theories of weight in the 1960's would have predicted or explained an inability to gain weight *despite* overeating. Not to be discouraged, Sims decided to find people who could make weight gain a full time job. His solution was to use prisoners from the state of Vermont and his subsequent research is sometimes referred to as the *Vermont Overfeeding Study*. The study was straightforward in design and concept: Pay prisoners to overeat until they gained additional weight. The more weight they gained, the more money they were paid. He had, in point of fact, turned gaining weight into a job.

Increasing how much we eat as a means to gain weight seems easy and straightforward; these prisoners found it anything but. It was hard work to gain weight and it got more difficult as they gained larger amounts of weight. Most of the prisoners simply couldn't get 20 percent heavier no matter how much they ate. Once they had gained weight, the hard work did not end. The majority of prisoners had a difficult time staying fatter; they had to force themselves, against the dictates of their appetites, to continue to eat more food than they desired. If they failed to do this, they began to lose weight. And similar to what was observed in the *Case of Identical Twins,* weight gain was not permanent. Within three months after the weight gain period ended, virtually all of the prisoners had rebounded to their starting weights.

HSI CLUE

If we lived in a world that prized being fat over being lean, would we explain the Vermont prisoners' inability to gain weight as a failure to eat enough? Would we criticize them for having too little willpower? Would we say they were cursed with a fast metabolism? We might but none of this would be true. The real issue is that the body has a commitment to a certain shape, and, opposes deviations from this shape.

What can we infer from this evidence? We can infer that consciously deciding to gain weight might be easier said than done. Eating far more food than our appetite dictates can be as much work as dieting, just in the opposite direction. For most people it is virtually impossible to gain lots of weight by consciously over eating alone, no matter how much willpower they might have. As Sims' work shows, people struggle tremendously to even get 10 percent fatter. Most people simply do not have the willpower needed to continue to overeat, day in and day out, to gain and keep even this amount of weight. Lastly, we can infer that, based upon the demonstrated tendency to spontaneously rebound to the initial weight, eating more is simply not a sufficient explanation for permanent weight gain.

The last investigation into eating more is the *Case of Guru Walla*. In Cameroon (Africa) there is a tradition for young men to undergo a fattening ritual called *Guru Walla*. This ritual is accomplished by massive overfeeding, primarily of carbohydrates, for a period lasting four to six months. Observations of one group of young men undergoing this fattening ritual indicated it was "successful". The average weight gain was about 42 pounds, with 26 pounds of this weight being fat. But just as we observed when twins were massively overfed or prisoners were paid to gain weight, the weight gain was not permanent. After cessation of intentional fattening, shape and weight eventually rebounded spontaneously to the initial starting points.

Observations of young men undergoing the Guru Walla fattening ritual have provided an additional piece of important evidence. Everyone does not respond equally to overfeeding, in terms of shape and weight changes. We know this from twin studies. But what was interesting in this case is that fat accumulation had a direct relationship with how difficult it was to continue to eat more. The young Cameroon men who responded to overfeeding by gaining the most weight and fat found it very difficult to continue to consume the excess calories. Those who gained much less weight and fat found it much easier to continue to eat more. What might we infer from this evidence? It seems to be telling us that the observed decrease in appetite that accompanies overfeeding is not caused by the amount of excess food we eat. Calories are not the important variable; a departure from the normally maintained amount of body fat is. Hunger accumulates when people diet and lose body fat. Satiety or fullness accumulates when people add excess body fat by intentionally eating more than their habitual food intake. What is really accumulating under these circumstances? Could it be dissatisfaction; a dissatisfaction that arises when there is a difference between the amount of fat that is on our body and the amount of fat our body apparently considers appropriate or normal for us?

Twins, students, prisoners, and young men from Cameroon found that it was hard work to get significantly fatter by intentionally eating more food. The weight they gained was not permanent. A decreased appetite opposed their conscious efforts at weight gain. The same is true for metabolism; it speeds up to oppose weight gain efforts. In one study, a tremendous increase in the amount of energy spent in maintaining posture and fidgeting occurred. In all these cases, as participants gained more weight, something appeared to be nudging them back in the opposite direction, towards their original weights. In the last chapter, intentionally restricting calories, eating less, as a means to lose weight was very difficult, and ultimately did not produce permanent weight loss. We observed increased hunger, physical laziness, and a slow metabolism. All of which normalized once the lost weight, plus additional body fat, had been regained. Here we observe the exact opposite tendency; hunger vanishes, spontaneous movement increases, and metabolism speeds up when people eat more. Overeaters in these cases, just like dieters, were eventually returned to their original weight.

These cases of overfeeding demonstrate that, even with sustained extreme food overload, it is not easy for many people to get even 10 percent fatter. The weight gain tends to plateau early on. It continues to be hard work to maintain the extra weight. And the weight gain is not permanent. None of this evidence is very supportive of a theory that blames shape and weight challenges exclusively, or mostly, on eating too much. This evidence begs the question, if extreme food overload does not result in permanent weight gain, how could eating a few too many calories here and there possibly be the sole cause?

HSI CLUE

When the men who have gone through Guru Walla lose weight after the fattening ritual ends, we do not observe an increase in hunger like we see with dieters. Why is this? What is the difference between losing weight after Guru Walla and losing weight from our normally maintained weight?

The evidence from underfeeding and overfeeding experiments suggests that *something* appears to be paying very close attention to how much fat we have and where it is located. It also appears to be adjusting appetite, food cravings, activity levels, and metabolism up or down to prevent departures from some pre-determined, actively defended amount of body fat. Shape does not appear to be matters of biological indifference; it's defended. By this, we are not implying that shape doesn't change and can't be improved or worsened. It does and it can. What we do want to communicate is that simply deciding to eat more or less as the path to changing it is unlikely to be as simple and easy as it sounds. More often than not, you will experience a spirited bio-behavioral defense of your "old" shape. This is a clue that the body is resisting the change. Dieting (calorie restriction) serves as an example. When we diet our normally maintained weight, and the weight we are at because of dieting, diverge. We temporarily weigh less than our normal weight. Under these circumstances we usually will experience something very similar to what the people on *Survivor* experience. We feel hungry, crave junk foods, lose motivation to exercise, and feel as if our metabolism is slow. These bio-behavioral changes make losing additional weight progressively more difficult and regaining the lost weight progressively easier. But it would be a mistake to view these bio-behavioral defenses as the *cause* of weight problems in this situation. They are better understood as evidence that *something* is adapting to resist further weight loss and to return us to a shape and weight it feels is appropriate for us.

There are other times when shape changes and the spirited bio-behavioral defenses are absent. We might have gained weight, or we might have lost it, but how we went about doing it make it easy to keep the change. This is not a sign of indifference; it is a clue that what we did caused *something* to change its mind about the shape it is defending. If it is easy to gain or lose weight, there is a reason. *Something* is making it easy. As we will discuss in more detail in the next chapters, this *something* is an intelligent and very powerful shape self-regulating mechanism.

Learning to Recognize Obvious Facts

Economist John Kenneth Galbraith coined the term *conventional wisdom*. He did not think of it as a compliment. He believed, as Holmes did, that conventional wisdom represented simple, convenient, and comfortable explanations; not necessarily true explanations. As he said, "…we adhere, as though to a raft, to those ideas which represent our understanding." But what if our understandings were wrong?

While it would be silly to argue that all obvious facts are wrong—they are not—it is equally as silly to assume that, just because something represents the consensus view and might be considered by most people to be true, that it is actually true. We get in trouble when we cling to an idea or explanation that is simple, convenient, and comfortable but incorrect. How do we avoid this? The answer is that we must learn to recognize and question consensus views and conventional wisdom. How will you recognize these? One clue is that they are often things many people believe to be true; they are, in a phrase, common sense. An example is the idea that artificial sweeteners or fat-free foods help with shape and weight. After all, since they have fewer calories than the foods they are substituted for, it is common sense that they should help. As a Health Scene Investigator we must look beyond this obvious fact and examine the actual evidence.

Another way to recognize obvious facts is by the form they take. They are often appeals to the crowd, to authority, or to tradition. As examples, the statement, "everyone knows eating too much makes you fat" is an appeal to the crowd knowledge: It must be true because everyone thinks it is true. The statement, "all the experts say that if you want to lose weight you must eat less" is an appeal to authority: It must be true since experts say it is true. The statement, "we have prescribed low calorie diets to help people lose weight for decades" is an appeal to tradition: It must be true since we have believed it or done it for so long.

> **HSI CLUE**
>
> If gaining weight is really as obvious as eating too much, how do we explain massively overfeeding twins causing no permanent weight gain, or the difficulty prisoners in Vermont experienced gaining weight despite doubling or tripling their food intake? Could the relationship between how much we eat and whether we gain weight be more complicated?

Obvious facts often arise from self-interested thinking. A clue to detecting when this might be the case is asking a question like; "Who benefits from the perpetuation of this simple, convenient, and comfortable idea or explanation?" Going back to our example of artificial sweeteners, the answer to the "who benefits" question is the companies who produce and sell artificial sweeteners, and experts who work directly or indirectly for them. It is in their financial self-interest for the public to believe that shape is an issue of calories. They are not alone. Estimates suggest that consumers spend $30 billion each year on goods and services that claim to help with weight loss or prevent weight gain. With this much consumer spending, do you think there might be a possibility that self-interest is at least strongly influencing, if not creating and perpetuating obvious facts?

We are told what we should believe. We are sometimes told why we should believe it. But it is a rare occurrence when the process by which a conclusion was reached, and the actual evidence it is based upon, is shared with us. We are given a final product, carefully packaged to appeal to our current understandings or create new ones. We need to be wary when this is the case. While something might seem quite logical and be believed by almost everyone, it still deserves scrutiny and considered investigation.

We have discussed two obvious facts in this chapter; (1) weight kills, and (2) eating too much food is the primary reason people are fat. They match our intuitions of how things should work. They are consistent with what most people believe, experts tell us, and prevailing notions that span decades. Self-interested parties want us to believe these obvious facts. But none of these things make these aspects of conventional wisdom true. Only evidence could do that, but what does the evidence really indicate? The evidence shows us that, in both of these cases, there is much more to the story than the superficially obvious. In fact, there is strong evidence that contradicts both of these theories. These theories are not alone. Much of what we are routinely told, or have come to believe, about how fat is gained or lost is wrong, misleading, or meaningless. The question is not whether obvious facts have prevented us from uncovering important clues; they have. The question is whether we will allow ourselves to continue to be misled.

Closing Dialogue

Health Scene Investigator: You had told me earlier that several things were obvious. Are you as certain now?

Apprentice: Actually, the only thing I am certain about now is that I know much less than I thought I knew. Everything is starting to look, well, quite different.

Health Scene Investigator: You have come a long way then. One of the most important advances in a case is a change in our point of view. Once this occurs, the very thing that we were so convinced was to blame becomes a clue to uncovering the truth.

Chapter 6

Set Points and Self-Regulation

One should always look for a possible alternative and provide against it. It is the first rule of criminal investigation.

Sherlock Holmes

Opening Dialogue

Health Scene Investigator: We have discussed the theory of energy balance. This theory proposes that weight is an issue of calories in and calories out. If a person desires to lose weight the solution is to create an energy deficit by taking in fewer calories than are being used. Yet we have found cases where far more seems to be going on when this approach is put into action. Are you aware of any alternative theories that better explain the evidence?

Apprentice: No I am not. Is there such a theory?

Health Scene Investigator: Yes there is. It has been called *set point* theory. Understanding this theory and its implications is an important element in solving this case. That said we don't want to blindly accept this theory either. The goal is to test theories, making sure they can withstand scrutiny. Allow me to explain.

The Importance of Testing Theories

Many of Sherlock Holmes' most famous sayings have to do with "eliminating the impossible" and being left with an explanation or theory that best explained the evidence, however improbable it might have seemed originally. But before the impossible could be eliminated, Holmes had to do one thing; he had to generate alternative theories and provide against them. Why was this important?

HSI CLUE

Many studies have observed that after losing weight by dieting both humans and animals experience a significant slowing of metabolism. This slowing is *far greater* than what is predicted based upon the amount of weight lost. This slowing represents a metabolic adaptation, a thriftiness that conserves calories. But what is conserving them and why?

Generating alternative theories is important because, by definition, a scientific investigation can never prove that a theory is absolutely true; it can only prove with certainty that other theories are false. The goal of having a theory is not to be correct; it is to be increasingly accurate in one's interpretation of real world observations and ability to make predictions. The confidence we have in any theory's ability to do these things arises from the theory's ability to withstand the process of testing it, of providing against it. This testing process is strengthened immensely when we generate alternative theories. Alternatives cause us to look for new evidence or to re-look at existing evidence in a new light. With each plausible theory we disprove, our confidence in the surviving theory(s) grows stronger. If we fail to look for alternatives, we miss this opportunity.

When we generate alternatives, the goal is not to come up with new theories that will all be correct (how can we know something is correct in advance); it is to generate alternatives that can be tested. Alternatives do not need to be things that fit sensibly with an existing theory. In fact, many advances in science, and no doubt detection, have occurred when the alternative theory started as little more than a hunch, or a flash of insight, that was as different from existing theories as night is from day. As a Health Scene Investigator you are free to use your imagination, experience, and insights from other disciplines in the process of forming alternative theories.

Once we have generated possible alternatives, our next step, as Holmes might say, is "…providing against it"; looking for evidence that doesn't fit the theory. If evidence contradicts a theory, we know in principle that the theory is not a reliable description or predictive model of the phenomenon being observed. As Holmes tells us, "An exception disproves the rule." If we are able to disprove all theories but one, we will be left with something very important, a dependable theory that best explains the evidence.

Exceptions to the Rule

What does the energy balance theory tell us about how we lose weight during exercise? Typically it goes something like this: A pound of fat contains 3500 calories of stored energy. To lose 1 pound of fat, we will need to expend 3500 more calories than we consume (through exercise and metabolism). To help guide our activity behaviors, tables are available that tell us how many calories we should burn during different types of activity. Using walking as the activity, we are told that it takes approximately 100 calories for a 170 pound person to walk a mile. Because it takes more work, and hence energy, to move more mass, theory informs us there is a proportional relationship between weight and calories burned. This means a 160 pound person should burn about 95 calories per mile walked, while a person who weighs 140 pounds, should burn fewer calories—closer to 82 calories per mile walked. So far, so good, everything is straightforward and obvious; if we walk for a certain distance, we will burn a fixed amount of calories and this will be influenced by how much we weigh. We are told that this is how things should work; do they always work this way? Let's answer this question for a real world situation, dieting, and the *Case of Conserved Calories*.

In a study conducted with 11 obese women, researchers determined the energy used—how many calories are burned—while walking before and after losing weight via calorie restriction. Twenty-two weeks into the study, weight had been reduced, on average, by 21 percent. Since weight was now lower, these women should be using less energy to walk; they are moving less mass. And they were: So far, so good. It's predicted that people should burn fewer calories after losing weight by dieting, since they now weigh less, and they do. But in this case, they used *even fewer* calories to walk than was predicted. The energy expended in walking was lower than expected for a person who weighed what these women now weighed. A metabolic adaptation occurred with dieting-induced weight loss and the weight-based estimates of how many calories should have been used to walk were no longer accurate. Calories that, in theory, should have been burned didn't get used: *Something* appeared to be conserving them. The energy balance theory of shape and weight tells us that we should burn a certain amount of calories for a certain amount of exercise. This amount of calories should be consistent for a given amount of weight and it shouldn't matter whether we are at this weight normally or whether we arrived at it by dieting. But the evidence provides an exception and exceptions disprove the rule. What now: Is there an alternative theory that might explain this observation?

HSI CLUE

Rats with damage to the ventromedial region of the hypothalamus act very similar to the people on *Survivor*. They become lethargic. They exhibit a strong preference for fattening foods. They eat more food when given an opportunity to eat. And they become very moody. What do *Survivor* participants and rats with this type of damage have in common?

The next evidence to examine is the *Case of the Damaged Hypothalamus*. Located deep in the brain of all mammals is a tiny region called the hypothalamus. In the early 1940's scientists discovered that if the ventromedial region of the hypothalamus were destroyed, a rat would become lethargic and eat two to three times as much food as normal. It would continue eating tremendous amounts of food and avoid even minimal activity until it was about 70 percent fatter than it had been before the damage was inflicted, at which point, its appetite would decrease and its lethargy would diminish. Scientists later found that damage to this region of the hypothalamus resulted in a preference for high fat rat chow—rat junk food— and an aversion to less *palatable* (less tasty) foods. Scientists also found that if they damaged another area of the hypothalamus, called the lateral region, a very different shape result was produced. Instead of waking post-surgery and eating voraciously, being lethargic, and gaining weight easily, rats who had the lateral region damaged would wake after surgery with no appetite and a strong inclination to exercise. As a result, they lost weight.

In an attempt to make sense of what they were seeing, a theory known as the *dual control hypothesis* of eating was developed. This theory proposed that there were two separate and mutually antagonistic centers that acted as separate on/off controls for eating behaviors. One way to understand this theory is to think of a train with a brake and a gas pedal. Using this analogy, the train is our appetite and the ventromedial region acts like its break; it slows the train or dampens appetite. Once it is damaged, appetite becomes a train without a break, a runaway train so to speak. The animal can't shut off its appetite, so it eats more food and gets fatter. The lateral region acts like the gas pedal; it speeds up the train or increases appetite. Once it is damaged, appetite becomes a train without any gas. Appetite decreases since the animal can't turn it on. The animal eats less and loses weight. This theory seems very logical. It appears to fit what was seen. It is consistent with the energy balance theory about shape and weight, which predicts that weight is about energy balance and is under our control. The animals had failed to control their shape and weight because an important part of the *machine* had been damaged. But as Holmes might have said to Watson, they *saw* but they did not *observe*. The existing theory was preventing them from noticing important clues; clues they would likely have observed had they looked for alternative theories.

Remember Holmes's axiom from chapter one; "It is a capital mistake to theorize before one has data. Insensibly one begins to twist facts to suit theories, instead of theories to suit facts." Now please take a moment to re-read the first paragraph of this section. Three of the things that were *seen* from the very beginning of this case, but apparently not *observed*, are mentioned. None of these three clues were explained by this dual control hypothesis. The *capital mistake* was committed. Facts were made to suit an existing way of looking at weight, instead of coming up with a new theory that fit the facts. The missed clues were that after damaging the ventromedial region, (1) animals became lethargic, (2) the observed changes in appetite and lethargy were not permanent nor was weight gain unending, and (3) appetite was not always like a train without brakes, in fact it was turned down or off for foods that the rats considered less tasty.

If, as the dual control hypothesis contends, damaging the ventromedial region destroys the ability to shut off appetite, how do we explain the emergence of lethargy? Why did damaging the "appetite brake" cause an animal to suddenly get lazy? How does it explain the animal's ability to turn down appetite once the animals are 70 percent fatter? If the appetite brake is damaged, how does it get fixed after this much fat gain? Or how about the observation that the animals avoided less palatable food but had strong preferences for high fat rat chow: Is the appetite brake only for some foods? Again we find that the theory falls short. An alternative theory is clearly needed; one that explains these observations as well as the *Case of the Conserved Calories* and the other cases we have, and will discuss.

Set Point Theory

Decades of research eventually provided against the dual control hypothesis. When the ventromedial or lateral regions of the hypothalamus are damaged, satiety (the brake) or appetite (the gas pedal) is not destroyed, respectively, as originally theorized. In fact, there is no such thing as an appetite brake and gas pedal. Instead something less intuitively obvious occurs. Damage to these areas of the hypothalamus instantly shifts the shape the animal is defending. The behaviors we observe are the means for closing the gap between the old shape *set point* (pre-damage to the region) and the new shape *set point* (post-damage to the region).

A set point implies self-regulation within a physiologically preferred target range. A system with a set point will strive to maintain itself within this range by initiating corrective mechanisms whenever deviations from the range occur. Temperature is an example. The body maintains it within a relatively narrow range. Deviations from this preferred temperature range cause the body to respond in a variety of manners that ultimately act to return temperature to the preferred range. The responses we observe when specific regions of the hypothalamus are damaged make more sense in terms of this notion of a set point. Damaging the ventromedial region increases the set point. Damaging the lateral region lowers it. In both instances, the shape set point is changed and a new biological goal (target range) is now defended.

When the ventromedial region is damaged, there is an extreme upward shift in, very specifically, the amount of fat defended by the animal. The observed increases in appetite, especially for fattening foods, and the extreme lethargy are simply means to an end. They are the corrective mechanisms. The end in this case is arriving at the now higher set point for body fat. Once the animal successfully achieves this 70 percent increase in body fat, reaching its new body fat set point, appetite and lethargy normalize and weight stabilizes. Once body fat amounts stabilize at the new set point level, the corrective mechanisms are no longer needed, and so they disappear. After stabilizing at this now higher body fat set point, opposite corrective mechanisms are initiated if the animal is force-fed and body fat levels rise above the now preferred target range. When this is done, the animal responds with a loss of appetite very similar to that observed in the men in the *Case of the Vermont Overfeeding Study* (discussed in chapter five). Satiety still works perfectly fine, it is just being adjusted, or self-regulated, in defense of a higher amount of body fat.

The same principles are observed at work in animals that have had lateral regions damaged. Lateral hypothalamic damage doesn't actually destroy appetite; it abruptly causes a downward shift in the amount of muscle, and to a lesser extent fat, being defended by the animal. The temporary loss of appetite is usually coupled with increased running behavior. These are corrective mechanisms. Once the animal successfully loses sufficient muscle and fat to stabilize at the now lower set point for these types of tissue, appetite and activity become perfectly normal to allow the animal to stay at a very precise, albeit leaner, shape. They are means to an end. If we attempt to restrict calories after the animal settles into this leaner shape, we observe an increase in appetite similar to that of the people on *Survivor*, or the people in the *Case of the Army Rangers* and the *Case of the Minnesota Experiment* (both discussed in chapter four). Appetite still works perfectly fine. It is dynamically adjusted in defense of the set point.

HSI CLUE

Set point theory predicts that each of us has a specific target zone for how much weight, in general, and body fat and muscle, more specifically, that our individual body views as "normal" or desirable. Our shape *thermostat* is set to a highly individualized amount, with some individuals having a high setting, others a low one. This theory also predicts that when we deviate from our individual shape set point, our body will initiate one or more corrective mechanisms that act to return us to this preferred shape.

Self-regulated processes, including shape, have certain common features. Let's list these features and place them in the context of shape.

1. The variable to be regulated: Body fat would be one of the variables; muscle would be another.
2. A *set point* zone for the variable: There would be a preferred amount of body fat; the same would be true for muscle. This amount would be a target range.

3.   Detector(s). There must be something that monitors the value of the variable and whether we are in the correct zone: The hypothalamus appears to one such detector for both fat and muscle.
4.   Correction mechanisms. There must be some way to restore the variable to the set point zone: Bio-behavioral defenses including adjusting appetite, spontaneous activity, slowing or speeding up of metabolism, fuel conservation, etc., are examples of these correction mechanisms.
5.   Communication or Feedback. There must be some means to inform the detector(s) that the self-regulated variable is above or below the preferred target range. When it comes to body fat, at least a part of this communication feature is done by leptin.

In 1973, a researcher named Douglas Coleman published research that predicted the existence of a substance he referred to as *satiety factor*. This substance, made by the body and under genetic control, presumably influenced appetite, eating habits, and ultimately shape. Before Coleman's work, obesity was largely considered to be an issue of behavior. A person was fat because they ate too much. If they would only behave better, by eating less, they would be fine. His experiments suggested that our appetite, and, hence, how much we eat, might not be something that we choose or control. Instead it appears to be adjusted for us, with satiety factor, as well as an individual's response to it, involved.

The search for the satiety factor would last 21 years and end in 1994 with the discovery of a communication molecule that would be named *leptin*. In the 15 years since this molecule was identified, understanding of its many roles in the body has advanced tremendously. Most leptin is made by individual fat cells. Reproductive organs, skeletal muscle, stomach cells, bone marrow, the pituitary gland and the liver also make small amounts of leptin. Leptin is used as a means of communication between fat cells, as well as other cells and systems in the body. The chief topic in these discussions appears to be the amount of body fat. As body fat increases or decreases, leptin levels rise or fall. With these changes, adjustments in appetite, metabolism, and other bio-behavioral corrective mechanisms are initiated.

When we observe the participants on *Survivor*, read about volunteers in underfeeding studies, or witness the increase in hunger and slowing of metabolism in dieters, we see the effects of the changing leptin levels, and the bio-behavioral corrective mechanisms these changes elicit. In these cases, calorie restriction causes body fat levels to move further and further below the set point range. Increased hunger, the craving for sweet foods and fattening foods, the persistent thoughts about food, the tendency to overeat when food is available, lethargy, and a slowing of metabolism emerge. These are the corrective mechanism. They are the bio-behavioral defenses that both prevent further losses of fat, and help replenish fat levels to the set point range. Once body fat stores are restored to the just right amount for this individual, the corrective mechanisms are no longer needed, and so, just as we see in these cases, they vanish. Leptin plays a key part of this self-regulation. But it also appears to do far, far more.

Leptin is a communication molecule. It is used in the self-regulation of whole body fat stores. It is a way for each fat cell to tell every other fat cell how much fat it contains. It is also the signal that informs some *detector(s)* about the status of whole body fat stores. But leptin is used for more than just socializing between fat cells. It is also used to inform any other cells or systems in the body that care to pay attention about our body fat stores. You might be asking, "What other systems in the body would possibly care about fat stores?" Science has discovered that lots of different systems in the body pay close attention to leptin, and hence, care about body fat stores. These include the cardiovascular, immune, nervous, and reproductive systems. Many tissues, including brain, bones, heart, liver, lungs, and muscle, listen for and respond to leptin. The self-regulation of breathing, sleep, body temperature, and our 24-hour body clock are influenced by leptin. As scientists have continued to investigate leptin, it has shown up in more and more places. The primary topic in all of these discussions appears to be the amount of fat. Based upon all of the tissues and systems

---

HSI CLUE

Shape is changeable, but who is in control of this change? Most of us think we are. We choose to go on a diet. We lose weight initially. But now the weight loss slows, eventually stopping. Great feats of abstinence are needed, in order to keep the lost weight from returning. Our hunger increases; badgering us constantly. Our metabolism slows; we can gain weight while eating almost nothing. We felt in control right up until these adaptations by our body reveal that we aren't.

involved in this discussion, and the bio-behavioral responses leptin initiates, it seems safe to infer that fat stores are not a matter of biological indifference. Not only is the amount of body fat self-regulated, it plays a crucial role in the biological self-regulation of other physiological processes.

Self-Regulation in Action

Self-regulation implies the active physiological *defense* of a particular condition. The hypothalamus is an important center for self-regulating thirst, appetite, metabolism, sleep, activity, temperature regulation, and sex drives. It is also the location of a group of neurons that act as a circadian pacemaker, self-regulating our 24-hour biological clock. As the *Case of the Damaged Hypothalamus* suggests, it is also important when it comes to self-regulating shape. Self-regulated processes are controlled for us. Each of us will have a specific target range for shape as a goal, just as we do for body temperature, and the system in charge will modify internal physiological processes and modify our drives, desires and behaviors to obtain this goal. We don't get to vote on what this size and shape will be, and, we don't get to directly control it. The theory of self-regulation tells us that *something* inside does this for us.

HSI CLUE

Our body operates in a way that might be best described as defending a certain shape. It might "change its mind" and decide to defend a different shape or more or less weight. It will then adjust aspects of our biology and behavior to bring shape into alignment with this new decision. We can do things that influence this decision. We don't get to directly make it.

Humans come in all shapes and sizes. Some of us will be constitutionally leaner. Others will be constitutionally heavier. It will be just as "normal" for a constitutionally lean person to be at a lower scale weight as it would be for a constitutionally heavy person to be at a higher scale weight. In both instances the balance point of self-regulation will be the weight that is normal (or natural) for that person at that point of time in their life. We each have our own set point that is normal for us given our genetics, our environment and the net cumulative influence of our diets and lifestyles. What is normal for us might well be too big or too small for someone else. And this size and shape will not, at least for some of us, always be consistent with some culturally or medically defined idea of "normal". Nor will it necessarily be identical to our dream shape and weight. Our goals, and our body's current goals, might be different.

A hallmark of self-regulated processes is redundancy. Redundancy means that there are several different ways to achieve a goal. In other words, there are multiple corrective mechanisms that can be exploited in order to maintain shape, water balance, body temperature, or any other self-regulated process at a desired amount. Collectively, we refer to these as bio-behavioral defenses. The advantage of this redundancy can be seen from what we have already discussed with shape. If one part of the system is damaged (like in the *Case of the Damaged Hypothalamus*) or over-ridden (by calorie restriction), other parts can kick in and compensate to make sure the system accomplishes its goals. Interfering with one or several correction mechanisms (think *temporary over-ride*) will make the system's shape goals a bit harder to achieve short-term, but there might be little to no long-term benefits, and even perhaps some unwanted consequences, since other corrective mechanisms might now need to be initiated.

An important aspect of redundancy is that the systems responsible for self-regulating, can do so in two ways. These systems can adjust physiological processes. They can also put pressure on us to shift behaviors we typically associate with being under the control of our conscious mind—behaviors like eating, drinking, or sleeping. The first way is easy to accept since all of us know that we can't consciously control the rate of our metabolism or the ease with which fat enters and accumulates in our fat cells, as examples. The second way is a bit harder for most of us to appreciate. So let's take a moment to make this more concrete.

To acquire things needed to make self-regulation within the desired range possible, an organism that is cold must be able to acquire heat, if thirsty then water, or if hungry food. One way to acquire these things is to consciously go out and get them—sit closer to a fire or put on more clothes, drink some fluid, or eat some food. But what if we decide not to do these things? In this case, the intelligence that is self-regulating these areas must have a contingency, a Plan B.

HSI CLUE

Because certain external factors (including availability of food, water, warmth, a reproductive partner, and sleep) are required for survival purposes, our body has developed very complex mechanisms to ensure that these factors are monitored and acquired. Do you think, given the importance of these factors for survival, our conscious mind would be allowed to be in complete charge of their acquisition?

Plan B is to put pressure on us to acquire the things it needs. If our fat stores are below a desired amount (below the set point range being defended), the thing most necessary for achieving shape goals is food. How does, whatever is doing the self-regulating, get more food if we have our mind set on dieting? It ensures this outcome, in part, by pressuring us into obtaining it. This pressure comes in the form of an increase in appetite, persistent thoughts of food, and food cravings. Our sense of taste is also changed. Sweet things taste better longer; we don't get sick of them as quickly. This makes it easier for us to eat more of them. These forms of pressure are precisely what we observe in the contestants on the TV show *Survivor* and what scientists have witnessed in cases of prolonged under-feeding. It is identical to what every dieter eventually experiences. In chapter 4 we mentioned that hunger accumulates. Persistent food thoughts and food cravings also accumulate. We asked, "What is really accumulating in these examples?" The answer is that dissatisfaction is accumulating because of the gap between the quantities of body fat the *something* believes it needs and the amount that is currently in storage. The pressure for us to acquire the thing needed to make the restoration of body fat occur—food—will continue to grow unabated until we eat sufficient food to refill fat reserves.

But what if we resist this increased pressure? What happens if we have lots of willpower and still won't voluntarily eat more food? This might call for the implementation of a Plan C; *a life finds a way* plan. This plan would entail the life intelligence taking more direct control, at least for brief periods of time. What might this look like? It might look like a temporary but complete *loss of control* over eating; binging on amounts and types of food we were consciously avoiding. This is precisely what the volunteers in the *Case of the Minnesota Experiment* experienced. This feeling of complete loss of control is the bane of many dieters. It is what we see in Survivor when participants are given free access to food. They often eat themselves sick. And this is not where Plan C ends; it is only the beginning. In extreme cases, *something* waits until the conscious mind is turned off (sleeping) and then takes control by exploiting eating behaviors for its objectives. The result is *sleep eating*, a person, in a sleep walking state, finds their way to where food is located, typically the kitchen, and eats, with little to no memory of the eating having occurred. Whether with our help or without it, self-regulation implies that *something* will be trying to find a way to acquire what it feels is important.

Who decides whether to sit near or far from a source of heat or to wear a certain amount of clothing? Or whether we drink fluid and how much we drink? Or what, when and how much we eat? All of us were probably pretty clear on the answers to these questions. We do each of these things for ourselves of course. We are in charge. But are we really? The truth is that we are usually *allowed* to be in charge of these areas. This is a *permissive* control; *something* is allowing us to be in control. As long as we are close to the target amount of body temperature, fluid reserves, body fat, or other self-regulated variables, this illusion of control will be allowed to perpetuate. But if we drift away from target amounts, *something* will exploit these typically volitional or conscious behaviors for its own objectives. If we resist, if we don't voluntarily alter our behavior to match its objectives, it will put pressure on us. If we resist this pressure, it will accumulate and build. And if we still are effective in resisting, we just might find ourselves losing control over something we were sure we controlled. Research has shown this over and over again. If our conscious behaviors are interfering with the intelligent system's efforts to acquire what it needs for self-regulation, we will lose the privilege of making the related choices; the choices will eventually be made for us, involuntarily.

> **HSI CLUE**
>
> Eating while sleep walking—sleep eating—occurs in about 1 to 3 percent of the general population, and in 15 to 20 percent of people who have an eating disorder. When a person sleep eats they almost always eat high calorie food, usually a lot of it, and have no memory of eating. How do we account for sleep eating with a theory that tells us we are in control of our weight and our eating? Why is sleep eating so much more common in persons with eating disorders? Could this be Plan C?

The Need for an Alternative Theory

Self-regulation implies that when the supplies of body fat are too low, our behaviors and physiology change to get more. When supplies are excessive, behavior and physiology change to shed the excess. We do not consciously chose the behaviors or set the goals. These are part and parcel of a complicated bio-behavioral shape self-regulatory system that evolved to control shape for us in order to protect us and enhance our ability to survive. Set point theory, and scientific evidence from investigations into self-regulation explain a great deal of the shape evidence; they don't explain all of it. One clue they don't explain is something mentioned in the *Case of the Army Rangers*. The soldiers experienced significant weight and fat loss when they were forced to eat less and exercise more. As predicted by set point theory, bio-behavioral corrective mechanisms were initiated including an increase in appetite and a slowing of metabolism: So far, so good. But one observation from this case wasn't predicted. Five weeks after completion of Ranger training, the soldiers were, on average, 40 percent fatter than before the program. Why did body fat set point increase dramatically? Why did a similar thing occur in the *Case of the Minnesota Experiment?* How do we make sense of this *body fat overshoot* clue?

An alternative theory that explains these, and other clues, would need to consider the following points:

1. *Something* apparently cares how much fat and muscle it has;
2. It appears to precisely monitor their amounts and distributions,
3. It defends these amounts and distributions bio-behaviorally; taking control of appetite, the specific foods craved, motivation for activity, the amount of calories being burned by an activity, and other aspects of metabolism to make sure it arrives, and gets to stay, at its desired shape.
4. It adapts to and appears to *learn* from real world experiences. The amount of muscle and fat being defended are not a fixed attribute; they appear to be dynamically adjusted as needed in an intelligent manner.

This last point is crucial. In the cases of underfeeding, we observed adaptations that countered fat loss and acted to restore it. We also observed what appears to be *learning*. Something seemingly learned that the amount of fat it used to think was sufficient wasn't. As a result, it took *intelligent* precautions, building in a bigger cushion of fat stores just in case it encountered a similar experience in the future. What plausible alternative theory is consistent with these points and can explain all of the findings?

Closing Dialogue

Health Scene Investigator: Do you have any plausible alternative theories at this point in time?

Apprentice: I feel like I am getting closer but I am not there yet.

Health Scene Investigator: Not to worry. There is still one more piece of the puzzle missing, one more key distinction that unlocks the mystery.

Chapter 7

Logical Reasoning

On the contrary, Watson, you can see everything. You fail, however, to reason from what you see. You are too timid in drawing your inferences.

Sherlock Holmes

Opening Dialogue

Health Scene Investigator: Let's assume for a moment that shape is not accidental. It is not a mistake caused by a few caloric indiscretions or mere laziness. How then do we explain a person's shape?

Apprentice: We would need to come up with a new theory that explains the facts we have been discussing.

Health Scene Investigator: Can you surmise this new theory from cases we have discussed?

Apprentice: I am afraid that I can't. I just don't see how things fit together yet.

Health Scene Investigator: You see everything although you may not be able to interpret what you see. It comes down to points of view, imagination, to a special type of reasoning power that allows me to imagine possibilities that you cannot at this time. Let me explain.

Logical Reasoning

Sherlock Holmes is famous for his process of logical reasoning, a logical reasoning process that allowed him to make inferences and solve cases by using elements of *deduction*, *induction*, and *abduction*.

HSI CLUE

Chile peppers adjust the amount of spicy compounds, chemicals that give them their hotness, in response to the world around them. If they are under more threat from insects that spread a fungus that destroys their seeds, they respond by becoming hotter. They adapt to circumstances in what appears to be an intelligent manner. Chile plants are capable of intelligent adaptation. Why wouldn't the system that regulates our shape be equally as capable?

Deduction is a process that allows for one to arrive at a certain conclusion from evidence, the key word in this instance being *certain*. An example of this type of reasoning can be seen with a change in weight. One month ago a person weighed 175 pounds. Today they weigh 170 pounds. We can deduce that they lost five pounds. Presuming our measurements were accurate, we can be certain of this inference.

Despite his fame for deductive reasoning, Holmes often relied as much, if not more, on inductive and abductive reasoning. The British have an adjective—*Holmesian*—that describes these types of logical reasoning processes. A Holmesian approach involves amassing a large body of evidence, producing a number of possible explanations, and then finding one explanation that is the best at explaining the totality of the evidence. Logic refers to this type of reasoning as *argument to the best explanation*. Holmes described it this way: "We balance probabilities and choose the most likely. It is the scientific use of the imagination." This scientific use of the imagination combines reasoning processes— inductive and abductive logic—that allow us to observe evidence and to arrive at conclusions from the evidence that are *supported* by the evidence but not *guaranteed* by it. The critical distinction between deductive reasoning and these types of reasoning is this introduction of doubt or uncertainty.

There is a subtle difference between induction and abduction. Induction implies that we repeatedly observe several pieces of evidence in order to generate a rule that explains the relationship between them. Abduction implies that we know the rule already and use it to reason backwards to one of the pieces of evidence. To place this in practical terms, let's return to our example of a weight change. If we met ten people who had each lost five pounds, and each person tells us they had been dieting during the past month, we might *induce* that people go on diets to lose weight. We create the rule—the reason people go on a diet—from the observed evidence. If we meet a person who informs us they have lost five pounds in the past month, and we already know the above rule, we might use an abductive reasoning process to infer that this person must have been on a diet. While our reasoning would be logical, it might not always be correct. People can choose to go on a diet for reasons other than weight loss. People can temporarily lose weight unrelated to going on a diet, because of reasons like exercise, acute stress or an illness. While the inducted rule and the abducted inference might *usually* be correct, they may not *always* be correct. This distinction is critical. Unlike deduction, abduction and induction introduce an element of doubt or uncertainty.

Deduction is the preferred logical reasoning approach when the relationship between discreet facts is certain. But in the real world many events and circumstances have an inherent degree of uncertainty. When uncertainty is part of the case, inductive and abductive reasoning become essential. Using these logical approaches enables an investigator to draw inferences from many real world events that would not be possible to solve through the strict rules of deduction. These types of logical reasoning also set the stage for new discoveries and advancements; the generation of new theories that better explain the how and why of evidence. They give rise to scientific imagination, which becomes critically important when a piece of evidence doesn't fit within an existing theory. With deduction we would be stuck. With induction and abduction our obstacle becomes an opportunity. This is likely why Holmes said, "When a fact appears to be opposed to a long train of deductions, it invariably proves to be capable of bearing some other interpretation." This "other interpretation" is our opportunity to shift our perspective and arrive at a better understanding of the case.

Our health in general and our shape specifically, are examples of the types of situations and circumstances that have an inherent degree of uncertainty. Shape also demonstrates facts that don't fit neatly within existing theories. If we were limited to deduction we would be stuck. We would never be able to solve the case. Fortunately this is not where things end. We can fall back on our ability to use these other logical reasoning processes, in combination with our scientific imagination, to create new theories that better explain the evidence, with a goal of finding the best explanation for what we are observing. As you explore the cases below, put your scientific imagination to use: What can you come up with that would be an argument to the best explanation?

Adapting to Cold

It is widely theorized that exercise causes shape changes because movement requires energy (calories). To lose one pound of fat a person needs to expend 3500 more calories through exercise (and metabolism) than they consume. For this theory to be correct it shouldn't matter what type of exercise is done as long as 3500 calories are used. Burning the calories is the important thing. Evidence published in the *American Journal of Sports Medicine* calls this assumption into question.

Minimally to moderately obese young women were placed into one of *three different exercise programs* for about six months. Each program began with up to 10 minutes of daily exercise. The length of each workout was gradually increased by five minutes every week until participants were exercising for sixty minutes daily. During the study period participants were allowed to eat as much food as desired. Shape results were as follows:
- Program One: Average of 17 lbs. of weight loss
- Program Two: Average of 19 lbs. of weight loss
- Program Three: Average of 5 lbs of weight gained

Programs one and two also depleted *subcutaneous* body fat, which is the layer of fat under the skin. Program three did not. How do we make sense of what we are observing, of these perplexing discrepancies? Perhaps it will help you to better use your scientific imagination if you know what the types of exercise were in each program. Program one consisted of walking, program two of bicycling, and program three of swimming.

This is not the first piece of perplexing evidence arising from studies of swimming. Competitive swimmers typically have body fat levels that are higher than those of runners or cyclists who expend a similar amount of energy when they train. Endurance swimming is also mildly associated with being fatter. And if swimmers for some reason can't train, they tend to gain significant amounts of weight almost all of which is body fat. How might we go about solving this case? Perhaps we can start by asking, "What is it about swimming that is different than other types of exercise?" Before we answer this question, there is one other important clue. This clue was detected in a study where men exercised for 45 minutes in both cold (68° F) and neutral (86° F) water. The men burned a similar number of calories while exercising in the cold and neutral water conditions, averaging 505 and 517 calories, respectively. But calorie intake after exercising in the cold water was *44 percent greater* than it was after exercising in neutral water. How might we explain this big difference in appetite emerging from something as seemingly unrelated to it as water temperature?

Swimming takes place in water. Walking, bicycling and other types of exercise activity take place in an air environment. Why might this be important? Heat flow from something of higher temperature to something of lower temperature is far greater in water than in air. Because of this, more body heat is lost while exercising in water than while exercising in air and more heat will be lost in cold water than in neutral water. Sea-going mammals protect themselves against this heat loss problem by creating a thicker layer of insulation (blubber). The more fat stored in the layer of blubber under their skin, the better will be the mammal's ability to protect itself against heat loss. This same principle appears to apply to humans as well.

Subcutaneous adipose tissue, the layer of fat underneath the skin, is a depot for energy storage. It also serves an *insulative* role. In the case described above, walking and cycling were effective methods to reduce subcutaneous fat tissue. Swimming wasn't. This makes sense given the importance of preventing heat loss. It also makes sense given other clues from studies of swimmers and divers. Evidence indicates that the thickness of this layer of fat tissue plays a role in how long experienced swimmers will voluntarily remain in very cold water. Evidence also indicates that one of the adaptations made to cold-water exposure is an *insulative* adaptation, with this layer of fat acting

> ## HSI CLUE
> How might it change our notions about shape if we viewed it as an intelligent biological adaptation rather than a "disease"? What might this shift in perspective due to our judgments about our current weight? How might it change what we viewed as "causing" shape changes? How might it alter our perspective when it comes to what we might consider as being sensible strategies for improving shape?

in an analogous manner to blubber in protecting against body heat loss.

HSI CLUE

Sea-going mammals are known for having a thick layer of blubber under the skin. Why is it there? What is its purpose? Like all fat tissue, blubber is a reservoir for energy storage. Blubber is also an intelligent adaptation to living in a cold-water environment. It's protective, preventing heat loss. Can you think of any other situations where specific shape adaptations might be protective?

Insulative adaptation is one mechanism for dealing with cold. Another mechanism can be observed in the *Case of Brown Fat*. Adipose tissue, fat, can be divided into two different functional types based on its color. Most of the fat in our body, including the layer under the skin, looks white when viewed through a microscope; a small amount will look brown. White fat serves as a place for storage of excess calories, and as a means of insulation. Brown fat has an entirely different job. It converts energy into heat. In animals and humans, having more brown fat—greater capability to generate heat from calories—improves the ability to adapt to and survive cold.

When placed in colder environments, brown fat is activated. With this activation, calories, fat in this instance, are converted into heat. This extra heat helps a living thing keep warm and alive. It is a highly intelligent inside out response to what otherwise might be a catastrophic stress—cold stress. This inference is supported by cases where brown fat doesn't work well. All animals of a given type are not genetically equal when it comes to brown fat. In one strain of genetically obese mice, brown fat does not respond to cold to the same degree as it does in lean mice. It's "sluggish." These genetically obese mice sicken and die prematurely if kept in cold environments, despite having a thicker layer of insulation (white fat) under their skin than lean mice. The inability to produce sufficient heat from calories is lethal in this scenario. This is evidence of the incredibly important role of brown fat. Despite this importance, brown fat makes up a tiny proportion of total body fat. Yet this small amount plays a disproportionately large role in overall energy metabolism. Having just one extra ounce of brown fat might make the difference between keeping fat levels the same and gaining ten pounds of fat per year.

Newborns have proportionately more brown fat than humans have at any other point in the life cycle; with brown fat being as much as five percent of their body weight. Why? Newborns can't shiver their muscles to keep warm or chose to put on warmer clothes. They grow into these abilities. While they are waiting for these abilities to develop, they depend on brown fat to keep warm. This is a protective mechanism; an intelligent solution to the problem of "keeping warm" an infant faces. Conventional wisdom has held that little brown fat survives past infancy into adulthood. The theory was that once our shivering mechanism kicked in our body would no longer need brown fat, and we would lose it. Newer research disproves this obvious fact. Recent studies using advanced imaging techniques have provided evidence that brown fat is indeed present and active in a significant percentage of adults. Not only is it present in amounts greater than were anticipated, brown fat activity also increases when a person is taken from a comfortable temperature and placed in a chillier environment. Under the circumstances of cold exposure, adapting in a manner that acts to warm us from the inside out seems like a sensible thing to do; it appears to be intelligent.

In animals the total amount of brown fat is regulated primarily based on the environmental temperatures the animal was consistently exposed to during its life. If an animal is raised in a colder environment, it maintains higher amounts of brown fat into adulthood. If it is raised in a warmer environment, it doesn't. This also appears to be a very sensible adaptation. This same sensible adaptation might also occur in humans. People who work outdoors in Northern climates, in contrast to office workers, have increased activity of brown fat. Brown fat amounts and activity appear to be an intelligent adaptation to circumstances.

When exposed to extreme or prolonged cold, a priority is to maintain body temperature. This priority will influence the amount of food consumed, how much energy is used, how it is used, and ultimately the amount, location, and types of body fat. An animal placed in a cold environment will eat more food and favor metabolic

---

HSI CLUE

Scientist placed mice in a cold room for a week. Brown fat became more active (to warm the animal) and body fat decreased by 47 percent. Did this occur because they were eating less? No. The mice lost weight and depleted body fat despite more than doubling how many calories they ate. A cold stressed mouse eats much more food, but this is an intelligent adaptation. The extra calories are needed as raw materials to be spent in heat generation.

functions that convert energy to heat. If an animal is consistently challenged by cold, it often responds by better insulating itself. It does this by increasing the amount of subcutaneous fat under the skin. It will also activate, and possibly increase amounts of brown fat as a means to generate more heat. These adaptations appear to be both *protective* and *intelligent*. They also indicate that shape isn't only a function of how much we eat and how many calories we burn exercising. We know this because it fails to fit the facts. A better explanation is that shape is integrated with temperature self-regulation. Whatever might be governing shape considers our past and present exposure to cold when making its decision about what types, how much, and where fat is needed, as well as when, at least with brown fat, it should be more or less active.

Body Fat Fingerprints

Most of the fat in our body is white fat. This white fat, whether taken from the hips or the stomach, will superficially look the same under a microscope. Once we get past this superficial level, finer details emerge. White fat is not all the same. It is tremendously complex; with white fat from different parts of the body serving different roles, responding to real world challenges in different ways, and behaving locally in highly unique and self-interested ways.

When faced with the real world problem of energy scarcity, a diet, fat isn't mobilized equally from all areas; it is mobilized preferentially from some areas of the body and not others. As a result, we can, and many of us will, reduce fat stores unevenly when we restrict calories. We might lose a great deal of fat from our face and arms and notice little to no improvement in our hips. The same is true when we eat an excess amount of calories. We won't necessarily gain an even layer of fat everywhere. We each have our own *body fat fingerprint* (unique distribution patterns) when it comes to fat storage and mobilization.

It was once thought that, with something like calorie restriction, fat would be evenly lost in all areas. While this can occur, it doesn't always occur. Many studies have shown that body fat is far from uniform in how it responds to situations like dieting. We can, and quite often do, experience very uneven depletions of fat, with proportionately greater losses in some regions than in others. The same principle applies to the expression of genes within fat cells from different parts of the body. Gene expression can vary considerably from region to region in response to dieting or other experiences. Investigations into this area strongly suggest that our fat is self-regulated *site-specifically*. This implies that, not only does *something* care very much about how much fat is in storage, but it also cares where it is located. This site-specificity is apparent with the fat stored around immune nodes.

Fat stored in immune nodes is relatively insensitive to fasting. This means that when a person goes on a diet, the immune system holds onto its fat much more tightly than do fat cells in other places. When our body is faced with a different type of challenge—an infection—immune cells release and utilize their fat, but the fat cells in our hips do not. Why the difference in response, why the site-specific variations? A possible explanation is that if the immune system gave up its supply of fats when a fasting condition was imposed, it would have less stored energy left to do its job of fending off opportunistic infections. Without this site-specificity, an infection occurring during, or immediately after a period of famine might be catastrophic. With it, fat can be held in reserves especially for immune system use.

The regional behavior of fat cells is not the only site-specific difference. Fat cells from different areas can have different fatty acid profiles. For example, fat cells from our hips tend to have more *monounsaturated fat* and less *saturated fat* than facial fat does. Fat in lymph nodes (immune centers) consistently contains more *polyunsaturated fats* than fat tissue at other sites in the body. These site-specific differences in fatty acid composition—location-specific fingerprints—persist even when the diet is dramatically changed.

HSI CLUE

Because brown fat is found between the shoulder blades in rodents, science looked for brown fat between our shoulder blades. They didn't find it there and concluded that adults don't have any. But in adult humans brown fat isn't located in the same place as in rodents. When scientists eventually searched elsewhere they detected it. The problem wasn't with brown fat; it was with a theory that predicted its location incorrectly.

Once upon a time, the firmly established obvious fact was that fat cells simply stored energy in the form of triglycerides. And, when called upon, they released these stored fat molecules into the bloodstream to be used as energy by muscles and other organs. All fat was thought of as the same. It was a single anatomically and functionally identical tissue that just happened to be widely dispersed in the body. New understandings have led to an appreciation that body fat has highly specific regional behaviors and differences. Something appears to make extremely specific decisions about where to send certain dietary fats and where to send others. It also makes precise decisions when it comes to where to take stored fat from when it is needed. These decisions are contextual; changing based on the circumstances. While most of us think of all fat as the same, nothing could be further from the truth. In a Holmesian sense, what *argument to the best explanation* explains these observed facts?

Complex Adaptive Intelligence

Self-regulation is often thought of as being analogous to a thermostat. Our normally maintained shape is its set point. But this metaphor actually fails to account for some of the clues we have discussed. A better metaphor would be an *intelligent* thermostat; one that not only can resist our efforts to deviate from our shape set point, but which can learn from its experiences; shifting the shape being defended in highly specific ways. The theory that allows for intelligent adaptation is Complexity theory; the theory of complex adaptive systems introduced in chapter 3. This theory of real world living systems is our doorway to understand shape, as well as our health, in a brand new way.

Complexity theory predicts that, to live in an ever-changing world, all living organisms must be able to learn from past and present experiences, store this knowledge, and alter their strategies accordingly. As they gain more experience solving new problems they continue to update their strategies. Of equal importance, survival in a changing world requires an ability to make best guesses about what the future might hold in store. When these understandings are applied to shape the implication is that there must be some form of automatic internal intelligence capable of *adapting* and *learning*. We can also infer that this intelligence will have a good memory, be adept at solving problems related to our diet, lifestyle, and environment, and will have strategies in place to get and defend specific types, amounts and distributions of fat and muscle. And we can infer that this shape will be a best guess about the shape needed to best prepare us for survival in the future. We call this intelligence *Shape Intelligence*.

The most common type of intelligence found in nature is network intelligence. Networks form the basis of living intelligence from the very small to the very large; from a cell to an ecosystem. They are everywhere. They are the backbone of biological sciences and human physiological function. Beehives, ant colonies, and food webs are examples of network intelligence. In our body, the immune system is an example of this type of intelligence.

Networks are decentralized collections of individual agents whose collective interactions act to store data, solve problems, and ultimately produce intelligent behaviors. Ant colonies, a beehive, the worldwide collection of bacteria, the Internet, the stock market, are examples of systems that display some degree of network behavior. In these complex systems there are individual agents—ants, bees, bacteria, personal computers, and individual investors, respectively. These individual agents don't need to be very intelligent because the intelligence at the level of the whole isn't located in any isolated agent; it is produced by the *interactions* of many agents. By interacting in complex ways, often very self-serving ways, a system capable of intelligent behaviors emerges. Immunity is an example of emergent intelligence arising from the complex interactions of individual immune cells. Our shape is another example. In both instances, this intelligence is decentralized.

HSI CLUE

The amount and distribution of muscle and fat is a reflection of the past and present experiences we have had. It is also a reflection of what Shape Intelligence anticipates our needs will be in the future according to those past and present experiences. To change our shape we will need to convince Shape Intelligence to anticipate a different future.

Decentralized intelligence can be observed with ants. There is no single ant "in charge" of the entire colony. An ant colony, while made up of many individual ants, behaves as a unified intelligent *superorganism*. The colony grows, evolves, adapts to its environment, learns, remembers, and responds in intelligent ways when faced with new problems or threats. While an individual ant might never be able to adapt to or solve a novel problem posed by a dynamic environment, the network of interconnected ants can and does.

Ants are an example of a complex adaptive intelligence that emerges from a network. This type of intelligence requires *connectedness*; there must be something that connects otherwise isolated agents, and allows for communication. Investigations into fat cells have revealed that individual fat cells are a far cry from "deaf and dumb." They make, release, and respond to many communication molecules. One of these is Leptin. Leptin, and perhaps other communication molecules, serves this connectedness function with fat cells; allowing for network intelligence to exist and complex behaviors to emerge. Leptin transforms what would otherwise be isolated individual fat cells into an interconnected superorganism, an intelligent network comprised of tens to hundreds of billions of fat cells.

Network intelligence tends to be dispersed throughout the entire system. When it comes to shape this means that it is exceedingly unlikely that there is some master cell hidden somewhere within the brain or anywhere else in the body in complete charge of body fat types, amounts or distribution. Body fat is simply too important to trust to that much centralization. The same is true for muscle. Instead, the intelligence is stored redundantly and diffusely in the entire system of cells. Just like immunity, shape is everywhere and nowhere.

Network intelligence, in living systems, has been naturally selected for optimal survival over millions of years of evolution for several reasons. The first reason is that networks are great problem solvers; they can adapt and learn, and in the real world adaptation and learning are musts. While different networks evolve to solve different kinds of problems, all networks have learning or problem solving as a common strength. How a network goes about solving any given problem will always be a bit unpredictable, but make no mistake, it will find a way to solve it. Because of this, each time we give Shape Intelligence a new experience, a problem to solve so to speak, it will try to come up with a solution.

Dieting is an example of a problem we give Shape Intelligence. As we have discussed in previous chapters, its solution to this *famine problem* is to initially adapt to prevent further fat loss with a longer-term goal of replenishing body fat stores. A slowing of our metabolism, decreasing motivation for exercise, and increasing appetite, especially for fattening foods, are visible clues to the adaptations (emergent behaviors) that might be used to solve the famine problem, a type of problem that our human ancestors encountered and solved in the past. But Shape Intelligence doesn't stop here; it also learns from this experience.

Complexity theory teaches us that networks learn when they encounter novel problems, store this knowledge, and can change their best guesses about the future accordingly. What might an intelligent system learn from a famine? A sensible thing to learn might be that what had appeared to be a sufficient amount of body fat might no longer be enough. It might be smarter to build in a bit of an extra cushion just in case another famine occurs. When this learning is acted upon, we would return to our previous weight, but be fatter at this weight than we would have been had we not experienced a famine problem. This is precisely what occurred in the underfeeding cases. A sensible solution for a period of famine is to be better prepared in case there is a *next* period of famine. The theory of complex adaptive intelligence prepares us to expect that dieting will not convince Shape Intelligence to defend less fat; instead it just might convince it to defend more.

> **HSI CLUE**
>
> How do we go about increasing or decreasing muscle tissue...or bone...or body fat? We will need to give Shape Intelligence experiences, learning opportunities that once solved, will convince it to shift our shape. What types of situations can you imagine that might cause Shape Intelligence to decide that less fat is needed, or that more muscle might be a good idea?

The other big strength of networks is robustness. Since networks always have some, usually a high, degree of decentralization of the intelligence—the intelligence isn't placed solely in one centralized agent and is spread through the entire system—networks are extremely resistant to failure. In a network if one agent fails (a single fat cell, immune node, ant, bee, etc.), the overall performance of the system as a whole is either not compromised or compromised minimally. This is not the case in a more centralized type of intelligence where if one agent fails the whole system can stop functioning. In addition to this resistance to failure, the robustness of networks usually allows it to have many different ways to meet its objectives. There is a great deal of built-in redundancy. If we attempt to prevent a network from achieving its objective by blocking one path, it will find a new way to get there. This is part of the reason that many medications, supplements, and other control strategies fail to permanently alter shape. Given sufficient time, Shape Intelligence finds a way to adapt intelligently. Microorganisms like bacteria are another example of network intelligence. They can adapt intelligently to antibiotics by developing *antibiotic resistance*—the ability to withstand the effects of an antibiotic. In an analogous manner, shape can become resistant to a weight loss medication. The medication works until it doesn't; life finds a way.

The last thing to understand about network intelligence is that its job is not to come up with the *best* solution to a problem; it is to come up with a *good enough* solution. This means the shape we defend is more akin to a *best guess* than to an accurately solved math problem. In a pinch, a guess might be good enough to get the job done. If not, it can be modified later. When determining this best guess, Shape Intelligence works within existing genetic possibilities and takes into consideration our past and present diets, lifestyles, and environmental experiences. Our present shape is a reflection of this complex adaptive intelligence attempting to do its best, given what it knows, what it has to work with right now, and what it has learned in the past.

What we do is important; what Shape Intelligence learns from what we do is even more important. No matter what strategy we might decide to follow in an effort to improve our shape, we want to consider what Shape Intelligence might learn from the experience. The goal is to give complex adaptive intelligence opportunities to learn, that when responded to intelligently, would result in a different shape, one which is more to our liking. We do this by providing it new circumstances and situations—opportunities to learn—that result in it updating its *best guess* in ways that will lead to a shape that is more appealing, a weight that is lower, and health that is more robust. If we don't give Shape Intelligence a reason to modify its best guess, it won't. But if we do give it a reason(s) to believe that a different shape might be wiser, it is, in our experience, completely willing to change its mind. While Shape Intelligence is entirely committed to defending a specific shape today, it is equally as willing to abandon this shape for one it views as a better solution. Before it will do this, it needs to have a reason to update its past *best guess* solution. In our experience it can't be forced into altering best guesses nor is it likely to change its mind about an existing best guess simply because we would prefer to look differently. It will only change its best guesses if there is a good reason. Our job is to give it one or more good reasons.

Many of these good reasons are shared. They are the same for all of us. Some are highly individual. In either instance, when we make a change in a needed area of diet, lifestyle or environment, it can act as a shape tipping point. Each and every change we make is an opportunity for Shape Intelligence to do what it does best, adapt and learn. Shape Intelligence is always open to changing its mind; we just need to give it a reason to do this. The world is our classroom for accomplishing this task. The lessons that will be taught in this classroom will be largely dictated by each of us. If you are dissatisfied with your existing shape, it is time to change the curriculum.

The Shape Intelligence Theory

We are not in conscious control of our shape; a complex adaptive intelligence is. This intelligence adapts to and learns from the world around it. At any given time, it will be defending a preferred shape. We refer to this preferred shape as *natural weight*; the shape and weight each of us normally maintain, give or take a few pounds, when we are not actively trying to control it. We don't get to decide upon our natural weight. It is decided for us based on the way our individual genetics interact with the *learning* our Shape Intelligence has experienced to-date (i.e. our diet, lifestyle and environmental influence). Some of us are constitutionally leaner; others are constitutionally heavier. Some of us will have more muscle; others will have less. No matter what our existing shape might be, if it is a shape that our body naturally gravitates to when we are not interfering, it is normal for us.

A variety of bio-behavioral mechanisms can be employed in defense of natural weight. These might include modifications of internal physiological processes; processes we can neither self-monitor nor control. Our metabolism might be slowed. Entry of fat into fat cells might become ridiculously easy and exit more difficult. We might burn proportionately less fat for energy. Our sense of taste might be changed. These are just some of the things that have been observed to-date.

HSI CLUE

The body appears to keep close track of the kind of person it houses. Is this the kind of person who is likely to diet in the future? Is this person likely to lift heavy weights or move a lot? How does it make decisions about the future? It makes predictions based on what we have done and are doing. Our history matters because it provides information about what might occur in the future and whether or not certain precautions might be needed.

Corrective mechanisms also include the exploitation of behaviors we normally consider as under our conscious control. These are behaviors like how much and what we eat. When we are at our natural weight, Shape Intelligence allows us to believe we are in control of these behaviors. It might be easy to choose a salad. But just like with the *Survivor* participants, if for some reason, like intentional calorie restriction, we find ourselves below our natural weight, we find ourselves being pressured to do what Shape Intelligence wants. It now gets a lot more difficult to choose the salad; junk food is far more appealing. This pressure does not relent with just a few big meals; it persists until depleted body fat stores have been replenished.

Consider the cases we observed in earlier chapters. When supplies of body fat became too low, lower than Shape Intelligence predicted was necessary, behaviors and physiology changed to get more. When supplies were excessive, higher than Shape Intelligence predicted was necessary, behavior and physiology changed to shed the excess. From these observations and other clues, it is apparent that we do not get to consciously choose these corrective shifts in physiology and behaviors that restore us to our defended shape. Nor are we the ones in control of deciding whether our defended weight is too high or too low. Our natural weight is decided for us. This isn't a bad thing; it is a tremendously wise thing. We will present evidence in the upcoming chapters that suggests that, when it comes to our shape, our body, not only has a mind of its own, but its decisions are generally wise *under the circumstances*. While we do not consciously control our Shape Intelligence and the shape it sets for us, we do influence and teach it. New habits and behaviors provide new lessons and the right lessons will lead to improvements in shape.

There are many potential reasons for having Shape Intelligence. One of these reasons is that no animal can afford to run out of nutrients or energy, nor is it always a great idea to carry unnecessary surplus. There must be some reservoir of stored energy on hand, otherwise we would have to be eating 24/7 and would be unable to do anything else an organism needs to do to live. If the reservoir were too large, from an evolutionary perspective, the animal would be at a mobility disadvantage; avoiding predators, securing prey, or even gathering food would be more difficult. If the reservoir is too small, the animal would be at a famine disadvantage; the ability to overcome even short periods of time of reduced nutritional and energy supplies would be severely compromised. Given the relative importance of the need for mobility being balanced against the need for contingency plans against future time periods of low food supply, what types of information and experiences might Shape Intelligence consider when deciding upon a natural weight? Two of the most vital information sources appear to be (1) frequency of movement, or it's opposite, sedentary tendencies, and, (2) stability of food supply (factors like famine, calorie deprivation, skipping meals, and nutrient status).

The primary job of Shape Intelligence is to take into account all of the past and present information stored in terms of genetic determinants, lifestyle habits and choices, and environmental exposures, and then forecast what might be required for the anticipated future. It must determine how much muscle and body fat to defend, and where the most strategic locations are for these. While shape is based on the sum total of all of the information inputs from our past and present, it is also an anticipatory function; a best guess of future need. The result of this best guess is our current natural weight.

When we apply this theory of shape to real world cases, clues and observations take on an entirely new meaning. For example, what is an intelligent system going to learn from a couple of episodes of dieting and how might this influence it's planning for the future? One possibility is that it will view food availability as unpredictable and subject to intervals of insufficient supply. It might then forecast that more of the same is likely in the future. And it might create new contingencies and plan accordingly to ensure it is better prepared for the next time. The end result of dieting, rather than being a body that permanently looks better, would be an unwanted shift in shape to a body that looks worse. Dieting seems like a sensible solution from the perspective of a theory of controlling energy balance. Yet all available evidence indicates it is ineffective and often times counter-productive. With this new theory of Shape Intelligence, we can understand why this might be the case. Even more importantly, we can begin to see the patterns and relationships really contributing to shape issues. We can see new solutions. And we can follow strategies to positively *influence* Shape Intelligence. Our shape is eminently changeable. Shape Intelligence is flexible. It has had to be or our ancestors would not have survived. It is up to each of us to work with it, rather than fight against it, to improve our individual shape.

Key Point

Shape Intelligence takes in and stores vast amounts of information. Everything from (1) what your mother did during her pregnancy with you; (2) what, how, and when you were fed as an infant and child; (3) how much you eat, what you eat, and when you eat it; (4) whether you have restricted calories, fats, or carbohydrates in the past; (5) what you drink and when; (6) how much, what type, and how frequently you exercise; (7) how much sleep you have gotten; (8) the types of stress in your life, and trust us, much, much, more. When it comes to natural weight, much of what we would consider inconsequential, is viewed as anything but by this intelligent system. This system does more than simply store and remember discrete facts. It learns from its experiences, anticipates the future, and makes best guesses about what shape and weight might better prepare us for this anticipated future. Shape Intelligence also responds to emergent threats (like food restriction) and novel situations (like pregnancy) in creative ways, using the stored information as a guide. Shape Intelligence is always learning. As you engage in new behaviors or make changes in your environment, it will learn from them and then respond accordingly. With the correct changes in behaviors and environment the result will be a shift in your shape; a healthy shift you get to keep and enjoy.

Closing Dialogue

Health Scene Investigator: Now, how then do we explain a person's shape?

Apprentice: It would seem that we must start by assuming that Shape Intelligence has a very good reason for deciding upon a person's particular shape. We must then attempt to discover what things in a person's diet, lifestyle, or environment might lead it to make this decision.

Health Scene Investigator: Exactly so. Do you know what these things might be?

Apprentice: I am sorry to say that at this point I do not. I have evidently been paying too much attention to how much people eat.

Health Scene Investigator: Not to worry. I will teach you to better use your scientific imagination and to see possibilities that you have previously missed. Before we get to these possibilities, it is important that we learn to focus our powers of observation on vital clues.

Chapter 8

Shape Assessment

It is of the highest importance in the art of detection to be able to recognize out of a number of facts which are incidental and which vital.

Sherlock Holmes

Opening Dialogue

Health Scene Investigator: Let's return to *Survivor*. Do you remember Big Tom?

Apprentice: Yes I do. He was on two different seasons of *Survivor*.

Health Scene Investigator: You are correct. In *Survivor Africa* he made it till day 37 and lost 62 pounds. In *Survivor All Stars* he made it till day 36 and lost another 42 pounds. With all of this weight loss how did Big Tom look and what was his health like?

Apprentice: As I recall, Big Tom's shape was changed to a degree; however, he did not become lean and muscular. And like the other participants he was struggling to function by the end.

Health Scene Investigator: That matches my recollection. This illustrates a very important lesson. As a culture we are highly focused on weight. Yet in this case, weight loss did not shift Big Tom's shape to look like Brad Pitt's. Can you think of facts that might be more vital than weight?

Apprentice: I can't but I would imagine we would want to look for evidence that tells us whether the weight loss corresponds to a person looking better, worse, or unchanged. I think we would also want to observe whether there is evidence that could tell us whether health is staying the same, worsening, or improving.

Health Scene Investigator: Exactly so. The evidence you described I would categorize as vital, while weight alone is simply an incidental fact. Let me explain.

The Vital or the Incidental?

To investigate a health scene, we must gather and analyze evidence. In order to do this properly we must be able to determine which evidence is vital and which is incidental. We must be able to concentrate on objective details, but we must know which details are the important ones. Otherwise, we waste energy on facts that get us nowhere. Or, even worse, we focus on facts that interfere with our ability to solve a case. Weight illustrates this point.

HSI CLUE

Shape is about appearance, contour, form; it is what something looks like. Losing weight won't turn a stone into a statue. It only creates a less heavy stone. How do we transform stone into a statue? We change its shape, sculpting it. We remove weight in, just the right places. How might this apply to your body?

The vast majority of shape-related research focuses primarily, and in many instances exclusively, on weight. Most individual efforts are also focused on weight, generally speaking, on losing it. We are taught to rejoice over pounds lost. Most weight loss initiatives lead us to believe that the numbers on our scale are the greatest predictor of our current success and future health. Weight alone, however, is a very poor predictor of shape success or failure, of worsening or improving health. In order to appreciate why this is the case, it is important to understand precisely what weight tells us. Weight reveals the relative heaviness—mass—of an object. Weight does not tell us anything about how the object occupies space nor does it tell us anything about what the object might be made of. Let's discuss the first of these points.

Imagine a block of stone next to Michelangelo's statue of David. If the two weighed the same, would we confuse them? Of course not; there is a big difference between a stone and a statue and the difference in this case would be missed if we focused on weight.

We need to instead place our powers of observation on a more vital clue, the manner in which the stone and statue occupy space, their shape.

Shape is what gives objects, including our body, form and contour. Shape provides the visual characteristics we either find appealing or unappealing. Weight has nothing to do with this appeal. If we doubled the weight of the statue of David but kept its shape identical, most of us would find it equally as appealing. And if we caused the statue to weigh less (to lose weight) by altering its shape, we would destroy much of its intrinsic appeal.

Now let's discuss the second point. Weight also fails to tell us anything about the quality of the substance we are observing. Most of us would prefer a pound of gold over a pound of sand despite the fact that they both weigh the same. Why? Although these substances weigh the same, they are not qualitatively the same. Gold is of superior *composition* and thus holds the greater value.
[Editor's Note: Body Composition is discussed in the next chapter.]

These same principles apply to our bodies. Whether we are determined to lose weight because of a desire to look better, feel better, enjoy greater health, fit into old clothes, or any other reason, shape and composition lay at the heart of our desired outcome. These are the vital facts needed to investigate a health scene. They are also the vital clues that you will need to pay attention to in order to track your true progress and real success. Weight is an incidental, and sometimes misleading clue at a health scene.

When we mistake weight for a vital clue, the opportunity to be deceived about the health of an individual is quite high. With the exception of extremes like emaciation or severe obesity, weight is a very poor indicator of health. Focusing on loss of weight is equally as deceptive. We might lose weight and enjoy greater health; or we might produce worse health by losing weight. We might create a more visually attractive body by losing weight, but we also might not. We have investigated many health scenes where weight loss worsened shape. The same is not true for shape. The newest scientific studies agree that shape predicts both health and attractiveness much more effectively than weight. It is a far more vital clue.

Cases of the Incidental and the Vital

Let's examine several pieces of evidence that highlight the incidental nature of weight. The first clue is from two large epidemiological studies, the *Case of the Framingham Heart Study* and the *Case of the Tecumseh Community Health Study*. These studies have been monumental scientific undertakings which have followed tens and tens of thousands of people for decades. After analyzing the data, one group of researchers reported that weight loss was associated with an increased death rate. For greater amounts of weight loss the risk of dying continued to increase. This is hardly a testament to the value of weight loss as a marker of improved health. Now this is going to seem strange, but the same researchers looking at the data from these two large studies also reported that fat loss reduced the probability of dying. The reason for this seeming paradox is that weight is presumed to be a reasonable surrogate marker for body fatness; it is not. Weight and body fatness are not the same thing. They are two very different clues. As these two large community studies suggest, assessing one can lead us to one inference while assessing the other might lead us to infer something completely different.

HSI CLUE

BMI is often used as a way to estimate an individual's body fatness. It is not effective for this purpose. It overestimates "fatness" in athletes and some ethnic groups; while underestimating "fatness" in aging persons, the chronically ill, and pregnancy as just some examples. Far better clues are available.

The next piece of evidence is from a *Study in Hormone Replacement Therapy*. Post-menopausal women were given hormone replacement therapy using a combination of estrogen and progesterone. At the end of an 18-month period of therapy researchers observed that the women on hormone replacement therapy experienced no significant changes in weight. Despite the lack of observed change in weight, the women on this combination of hormone replacement therapy did experience (1) an increase in body fat percentage, (2) a decrease in muscle tissue, and (3) a shift in body fat from their lower body to their waist areas. They had become fatter and their shape had become more apple-like. These changes did not occur because weight increased; they occurred despite the fact that it didn't. Once again weight would lead us to draw a faulty inference. If we mistakenly thought of weight as a vital clue we would have been deceived. We would have closed this case file and been confident that the combination of hormone replacement therapy used in these women does not worsen shape over an 18-month period. But this was not what occurred. Shape did worsen. When we gather and assess more vital shape clues the case looks completely different: We detect an undesirable shift in shape occurring despite weight remaining unchanged.

Now let's examine the *Case of Lipodystrophy*. Lipodystrophy is a medical term that means fat wasting; though it can also be used to mean a specific pattern of shape change. It is observed most commonly in HIV+ persons. In fact, this type of shape change occurs so commonly in HIV+ individuals treated with highly active antiretroviral therapy (HAART) type medications that it now has a medical name—*HIV-associated lipodystrophy syndrome*. This syndrome is characterized by declines in fat in the arms, legs, and parts of the face, which often occur simultaneously with increases in fat in the neck, upper back, chest, and abdomen. Body fat is being redistributed—shape is changing—often significantly. These changes can occur even when weight is staying the same. Why is this important? It is important because a lipodystrophy type of shape change is a poor sign when it comes to health. This is true whether a person is HIV+ or not. Yet shape changes like these can be completely missed if the only clue gathered at a health scene is weight.

The last case we want to share with you is the *Case of Normal Weight Big Belly Syndrome*. Researchers whose results were published in the June 2008 issue of the American Journal of Epidemiology came to the conclusion that even when our weight is in a "normal" range we can be at a higher risk of dying if we have a big belly. The researchers based this inference on data they collected after following almost one quarter of a million people older than 51 years of age for nine years. No matter what a person's height and weight—even if they would result in the person being considered to be in the "normal" range—the odds of dying during

HSI CLUE

Imagine we have two men of identical heights and weights. One eats well, is physically fit, gets plenty of sleep and has a low amount of stress. The other doesn't. The result is that the first man has a trim waist and an athletic build. The second man has a bulging belly and poor muscle tone. Scientific studies using BMI consider both of these men as being of equal fatness. They have mistaken the incidental for the vital, and, as a result, lump both men together into the same health risk category.

the nine years increased if a person had a bigger waistline for their size. This was observed in both men and women, in smokers and non-smokers, in "healthy" people and those with chronic illness, and in all ethnic groups studied. It has been an obvious fact for a century that weight is what matters when it comes to our health. If we accept this obvious fact, then being "normal" weight should mean that we have a "normal" risk for dying. Yet what this study showed is that being "normal" is not always "normal" when it comes to risk of dying. People with a bigger belly were at a higher risk of dying than those with trimmer waistlines even when they had a theoretically "normal" weight. Weight would have deceived us; it could have left us feeling over confident in our health. In this case, waistline or belly size—a clue that gives us a clearer picture of how weight is distributed—proved to be a more vital clue.

HSI CLUE

In a 2009 study, the heaviest individuals for their heights were far less likely to have either dementia or cognitive decline. Being overweight or obese, at least according to BMI, appeared to have a protective relationship. When shape was assessed a different picture emerged. People with the biggest bellies were most likely to have dementia or cognitive decline. Weight told one story. Shape told the opposite one.

Many shape cases mirror these examples. Weight is a fact. It will be at a health scene and it is one of the easiest clues to gather. But just because it is easy to detect doesn't mean it is the most important clue. As the cases above illustrate, it's often a deceptive clue, leading to inferences that are incorrect. When we place our powers of observation on weight rather than shape, we are likely to be misled in many instances. We will have underemphasized something vital and overemphasized something which is far more incidental.

Weight is presumed to be a reasonable surrogate marker for health and body fatness when in fact it is not an accurate indicator of either. Weight can be going down because of wasting away, a finding that often accompanies diseases like cancer or AIDS. It can go down because of malnourishment, such as in *Survivor*. Conversely, it can go up because of a gain in muscle mass or re-hydration. In the first two instances it would give a superficial impression of winning when in fact the person is losing. In the last two instances it gives an impression of losing when again the opposite is true.

We tend to naively think of losing weight as being good or healthy. Science and medicine know better. When potentially toxic chemicals have been historically studied for side effects, it has been weight loss, not weight gain that they focus on, because science has long recognized that losing weight is a toxic side effect that can have disastrous health consequences. The context, why and how weight is lost or gained, matters.

As Holmes taught Watson, being able to recognize which clues at a health scene are vital and which are incidental is "of the highest importance in the art of detection…" Your success as a Health Scene Investigator will be predicated on your ability to make this determination. Will you get bogged down with, and led astray by incidental facts? Or will you be able to see through these to the more vital? Will you confuse weight as being vital? Or will you be able to recognize it for what it really is, an incidental clue? Like Holmes, the quality of your inferences will be a reflection of your ability to recognize which clues in a case are incidental and which are vital.

The Case for Shape Appeal

While a large degree of what we find appealing or attractive is a personal preference, defined in part by our individual tastes and the culture in which we were raised, there are certain considerations that seem universal when determining physical attractiveness. These include:

- General body shape and appearance
- Symmetry between the left and right sides of the body and face
- Erect body posture
- Appearance of health (skin, hair and nail qualities, no visible disease or deformity, etc.)
- Height (for males)

You will notice that several items on this list are not under our influence, such as height, while others are, at least to a degree. You will also notice that weight failed to make this list. The current obsession in the United States and Canada is a slimmer body frame, which usually gets mixed up with a body that weighs less, a mix-up that contributes to behaviors and goals that do not necessarily produce the shape that would actually be considered appealing and attractive.

A thin body frame has not always been the ideal. There have been times when a heavier body frame has been considered both more desirable and healthy within our society, and there are still cultures which consider a larger than average body frame as the most attractive. That said it is critical to understand that, whether the ideal is a slimmer or heavier body frame, in both instances, shape is a significant influence determining what is viewed as more or less attractive. The vast majority of persons within a culture that prizes a slimmer body frame will not view an emaciated body as attractive, nor would extremes of fatness be considered ideal in most cultures that value a heavier body frame. In both instances shape—how weight is distributed—would be a deciding factor. Because of this a person who might be categorized as obese based solely upon their height and weight might be considered very attractive by many people, even in our culture, if the person possessed an appealing shape, a high degree of body and facial symmetry, a pleasing posture, and a healthy appearance.

HSI CLUE

Irrespective of our weight and frame size, we all have it within our power to create a better proportioned shape, improve our posture, and enhance our health. This means it is within our power to significantly improve our attractiveness. To produce this shift in appearance we need to concentrate our efforts on the vital areas we can *influence* rather than being so focused upon our weight.

What shape is considered attractive? There appear to be some relatively universal shape proportions that significantly influence what is viewed as attractive; with these guidelines being understandably different for males and females. As a general rule males with a chest that is proportionately slightly larger than the average for men of their height and frame will be rated as more attractive than males with a smaller chest size. The waist-to-hip ratio is also a marker of male attractiveness with a ratio of about 0.9, the measurement around the waist being 9/10ths the measurement around the hips, considered visually attractive; while significant departures from this ratio are typically viewed as progressively less appealing. An athletic or muscular physique is also usually rated as more attractive; however, extremes of muscularity, such as is found in body builders, are not as appealing to a majority of the population.

While there is no universally agreed on weight that is considered as attractive for females even within the United States and Canada, there is a tremendous amount of agreement on the shape that is viewed as attractive. This agreement is also consistent across cultures and time. Similar to what has been found with males, but to an even stronger degree, waist-to-hip ratio is a significant indicator of the female shape viewed as appealing. For females, a ratio of 0.7, the measurement around the waist being 7/10ths the measurement around the hips, appears to define a desirable female shape across different cultures and eras. Sexual icons of vastly different body frames and weights including Sophia Loren, Marilyn Monroe, and Salma Hayek, as well as the Venus de Milo, all have waist-to-hip ratios estimated as being very close to this 0.7 proportion. While dieting will not guarantee this type of shape, and the rebound after coming off a diet can actually move a female further away from these proportions, the right type of strategies can create shifts towards this shape.

Next Steps

Tracking weight is easy; all we need is a scale. Unfortunately a scale won't tell anyone what type of weight is being lost or gained, whether shape is being shifted to more or less attractive areas, or whether someone is getting healthier or less healthy by the change in weight. To assess shape we need to look very specifically at where our weight is located. We can objectively assess this clue by using a tape to measure the areas listed in the table below.

MEASUREMENTS	Day 1	Day 30	Day 60	Day 90
Neck Circumference				
Bust/Chest Circumference				
Waist Circumference				
Hip Circumference				
Thigh Circumference (mid thigh)				
Bicep Circumference (mid upper arm)				
PROPORTIONS (Ratios) Waist-to-Chest Ratio Waist-to-Hip Ratio Waist-to-Thigh Ratio				

Measuring the circumferences of these areas requires a paper or cloth tape measure similar to what a tailor or seamstress would use. A spouse or friend can measure these areas for you. In a pinch, you can measure most of these sites yourself. Gather these more vital clues from your health scene and use changes in them, not weight, to track your progress.

While the above measurements and proportions are vital objective measurements, they don't in and of themselves tell the whole shape story. A man's chest circumference might stay the same, but because of weight training, the shape (and composition) of this area of his body might have changed profoundly for the positive. The same holds true for other areas. It is always important to place circumference changes in any one region in the context of (1) changes in the contour and definition (muscle tone) of the region, (2) overall changes in our whole body's shape proportions, and (3) diet, lifestyle, and environment changes we have been making. Ultimately, shape is something that can really only be aesthetically appreciated at the level of the whole, how each region relates to other regions, and to our overall proportions and symmetry. A mirror can be used to gauge this overall picture. Even better, an actual picture can be taken and then compared to future pictures you take every month. Taking pictures and creating a shape timeline with them can be a useful and powerful way to visually capture where we started and where we have traveled. We strongly recommend this exercise. When added to other assessments, it can be an extremely valuable clue. A bathing suit is a good attire choice for the picture. Whatever attire you do choose please make sure that (1) you wear the same attire each picture session and (2) the attire actually reveals, rather than hides, your shape.

Irrespective of other attractiveness traits such as weight and body frame, we can do things to shift our shape that will invariably lead to others viewing us as more attractive. Focusing on weight loss will not ensure a more attractive body nor does weight gain mean we will necessarily have a less attractive body. The only way to generate shape appeal—a more attractive body—is to sculpt a better shape. To look the way we want is not simply a matter of losing weight; it is a matter of removing weight from the right places, and quite often, shifting some weight to other areas.

Closing Dialogue

Health Scene Investigator: Now that we have discussed the above clues, can you list facts that are more vital than weight?

Apprentice: Yes, we need to assess the location where weight is stored and how it is proportionately related to the rest of our body. This requires gathering and analyzing evidence about circumferences and proportions. We also need to be able to observe the whole shape and how this shifts over time.

Health Scene Investigator: Excellent. Now let us move on to an equally vital fact, the quality of a person's weight, its composition.

Chapter 9

Body Composition Analysis

Here is my lens. You know my methods.

Sherlock Holmes

Opening Dialogue

Health Scene Investigator: When we left off our last discussion I mentioned that we would next discuss the composition of weight. Do you recall my mentioning this detail?

Apprentice: Yes, I do, although I am not certain I understand what you mean by this.

Health Scene Investigator: Let me provide you with an example. If two persons wanted to reshape their bodies and one lost 10 pounds while the other lost no weight, who would you rate as the more successful?

Apprentice: I would assume the first was more successful.

Health Scene Investigator: How is it you have arrived at this conclusion?

Apprentice: The first person was able to lose weight while the other person was not.

Health Scene Investigator: The weight loss is evidence of something, but we do not know what it is evidence of. Did they lose body fat? Or was the weight loss because of a loss of muscle tissue or dehydration? And what of the other person; if they lost 10 pounds of body fat but gained 10 pounds of muscle wouldn't that mean they were quite successful?

Apprentice: Now that you ask those questions I see that it is not possible to determine success with the limited information we have.

Health Scene Investigator: Exactly so. Determining success must be judged only after examining all vital clues. Although many people draw inferences similar to the one you originally suggested by looking only at weight, judging success is a matter of perspective and weight only affords a very limited point of view. We need some method to determine the quality of weight change before we can determine success. Let me explain.

The Need for a Body Composition Lens

When we search our memory for images of Holmes, a man with a magnifying lens looking for clues comes readily to mind. The lens was a tool he used to focus his already substantial powers of observation. With the point of view this lens provided, he could, quite literally, see things he would otherwise miss, and as a result, draw better inferences. When it comes to investigating shape scenes, most people rely quite heavily upon weight. Unfortunately, using a scale and observing weight is akin to Holmes looking at a crime scene with only his naked eye. He might be able to detect some superficial clues, but he is likely to miss hidden ones. To avoid this we, like Holmes, need a lens that allows us to better focus our powers of observation on the more vital clue of body composition To illustrate this point, let's look at a hypothetical example of two men who are equal in height and weight; both six feet tall with weights of two hundred pounds.

- Man One: Weight is 200 pounds. Percent Body Fat is 12% (total amount of body fat in pounds is 24 pounds). Fat Free Mass (Muscle, Bone, Fluid, and Organ Weight) is 176 pounds.
- Man Two: Weight 200 pounds. Percent Body Fat is 25% (total body fat = 50 pounds). Fat Free Mass (Muscle, Bone, Fluid, and Organ Weight) is 150 pounds.

While these two men *weigh* the same, the *composition* of their weight is very different. Now imagine a case in which the first man improves the quality of his diet and increases his commitment to weight training for six months. At the end of that time period we observe that he still weighs 200 pounds; however, when we use our lens to detect changes in body composition we also observe that his total body fat has dropped to ten percent (a decline of four pounds of fat) and his fat free mass has increased to 180 pounds. If the only clue we gathered were his weight, it would lead us to infer his diet and lifestyle changes were not effective. We would be wrong. We would have missed the fact that he replaced four pounds of body fat with four pounds of muscle, a very significant and positive change.

Now let's look at the health scene of the second man over a similar time period. We discover that he began taking a new medication. Six months later we observe correctly that his weight has not changed. Yet when we look through our body composition lens we observe an increase in body fat from 25 percent to 27 percent. He gained four pounds of body fat. We also detect a corresponding four pound decline in muscle mass. With the unaided eye his weight appears to tell us that the medicine is not worsening his shape. Aided by a lens that allows us to track changes in body composition, we come to a different conclusion.

In both of these hypothetical examples, weight is a superficial but deceptive clue. It misleads us and as a result we draw inferences that are incorrect. To prevent this type of mistake a health scene investigator needs a better lens; something that will help them to detect more difficult to spot, but ultimately more meaningful clues.

HSI CLUE

Researchers followed 4107 elderly men for six years. During this time there were 713 deaths. As has been the case in many studies underweight men were exceptionally likely to have died. Who else was likely to have died? With the exception of this underweight group, weight was not a valuable clue; shape and body composition were. The men with the poorest shapes (larger waist size in this study) and least amount of muscle were most likely to have died. Men with smaller waist sizes and an above-average amount of muscle were at the lowest risk for death.

Cases of Composition

To further illustrate the need for a body composition lens, let's discuss the *Case of Tamoxifen*. The primary clinical use of tamoxifen is breast cancer prevention. It is the world's best selling drug for this purpose. The reason it is used for breast cancer prevention is because of how tamoxifen interacts with estrogen. Some cancerous cells in breast tissue are sensitive to estrogen; if there is more estrogen, they grow faster, and if there is less estrogen, growth is slowed. Tamoxifen works by hindering estrogens from binding to the fat cells in breast tissue. This lowers estrogen activity, and hence, slows the growth of estrogen-sensitive breast cancer cells. Does shape or composition pay a price for this anti-cancer benefit?

HSI CLUE

In one study, roughly 19 percent of men and 25 percent of women were classified as obese based on BMI. When the composition of weight was evaluated the results were quite different. Using percent body fat as the criteria, approximately 44 percent of these men and 52 percent of the women were now revealed to be obese: Same group, different lens, and very different conclusions.

Estrogens have a feminizing effect on shape. This hormone helps produce the curves associated with the female shape. Its effects are evident when a young girl enters puberty. The rising level of estrogens are in large part responsible for shifting shape away from an androgynous child's shape to the more curvy female adult figure. The effect of estrogen on shape is also evident during menopause. Declining estrogen levels during menopause often result in a redistribution of weight from the hips and thighs to the abdominal area. With the drops in estrogen production some feminine curves are lost. These changes in shape can be accompanied with changes in weight. They can also occur with little to no weight change.

Tamoxifen is designed to hinder the body's ability to use estrogen. This effect is, in theory, most powerfully in breast tissue, but it occurs in other fatty tissues as well. We know that estrogen plays a very dramatic role in a woman's shape but has a far less influential role in weight. With that as the case, where should we focus our powers of observation? Should we only assess weight? Or would we be better served using a lens that allows us to look more directly at the type of tissue tamoxifen most strongly influences, fat tissue? When it comes to a drug that has its greatest effect on fatty tissue, investigating weight alone would seem to be an inadequate clue. Under the best of circumstances, weight is a non-specific clue. Shape is more vital. The same is true for composition. No studies to-date have been designed to investigate tamoxifen's effects on shape parameters such as waist circumference or waist-to-hip ratio, but several have investigated body composition. In these studies, which would, based upon their design, be more akin to circumstantial evidence than proof of cause, women taking tamoxifen were reported to have more overall fat. They also have greater amounts of belly fat and liver fat.

Could tamoxifen be a case where the failure to use an appropriate lens is causing medicine to miss something important; tamoxifen might be worsening shape or composition even under circumstances where weight is not noticeably changing. Assessing weight would not allow this clue to be detected. Assessing body composition might.

The importance of assessing composition is more evident in the *Case of Insulin*. Insulin is used to manage blood sugar levels in both Type 1 and Type 2 diabetics. Both types of diabetes have elevations in blood sugar in common; however, the nature of the cause of this higher blood sugar and the underlying physiology are quite different. Type 1 diabetics lack insulin, so in persons with this condition, insulin is used as a replacement therapy for something that is missing. Type 2 diabetes is a bit different. Persons with type 2 diabetes usually still make insulin, but their bodies don't respond appropriately. Insulin usually isn't missing in type 2 diabetes; it just doesn't work correctly. Although both Type 1 and 2 share the name diabetes, they are, in fact, very different diseases. What happens when we use insulin as a treatment for these very different conditions?

In both types of diabetes, giving insulin commonly causes a person to gain weight. Weight gain occurs so frequently with insulin therapy that it is a medically recognized side effect. Now let's ask an important question. Since the nature of the cause and underlying physiology differ in Type 1 and Type 2 diabetics, might the nature—the composition—of the weight gained also differ? When this question has been investigated using a body composition lens, the answer is yes. The weight gain in Type 1 diabetics given insulin is mostly muscle. In Type 2 diabetics given insulin it's mostly fat. When we look at weight, the results look very similar; insulin results in weight gain. When we use a lens that allows us to investigate the composition of the weight we observe something very different. The weight gain caused by insulin in Type 1 diabetics is disproportionately a gain in desirable weight, muscle.

HSI CLUE

Is your medication causing a worsening of your shape? This is a critically important question, since many North Americans take one or more medications. We will discuss this issue in more detail in chapter 16 but suffice it to say that many medications contribute to unwanted shape and composition changes. These unwanted shape changes could be occurring while weight remains unchanged, so assessing shape and body composition is a must when taking medications.

This is usually not the case in the Type 2 diabetics, where the weight gain caused by insulin is in large part body fat.

The *Case of Tamoxifen* and the *Case of Insulin* are not unusual. They are simply evidence of an essential fact; body weight and body fatness are not the same things. Changes in one cannot be used to accurately predict changes in the other. Unfortunately, a weight-centric view dominates the majority of scientific research on health-related topics including the side effects of medications. Science has focused on the incidental and easily observed. It is impossible to know what is occurring with the composition of weight if the only clue gathered is weight. A body composition lens is needed to assess this hidden clue. This lens allows us to alter our point of view and observe evidence we cannot see without it. Without this lens the inferences we can draw from any research, or health scene, is limited. With it, we can make far more accurate inferences about what works and what doesn't. We can, just like Holmes, be in the business of knowing things other people don't.

Cases of "Normal" Weight Obesity

The most widely used way to estimate body fatness is body mass index (BMI). BMI is determined by dividing our weight by our height squared (weight/height^2). It is a weight-centric perspective for judging body fatness. With what you currently know, would you guess it is a vital or an incidental clue at a shape and weight health scene? At extremes of very low and high weight, BMI can be a reasonable marker of body fatness and the risks associated with it. It will correctly categorize most, but not all people at these extremes. BMI will not correctly categorize body fatness at other weights. In fact, as the evidence below—the *Case of Normal Weight Obesity*—intimates, being "normal" weight but over-fat might actually be the norm in North America.

In 2007, a team from the prestigious Mayo Clinic announced that something they called *normal weight obesity* was extremely prevalent. What did they mean by this? What exactly is normal weight obesity? These researchers were saying that lots of people, who would be considered as having a normal amount of body fat when the only clue gathered and used to determine fatness was BMI, would actually be over-fat when a better lens was used. To arrive at this conclusion, the Mayo Clinic team found more than two thousand one hundred normal weight individuals, as determined by their BMI. Then they looked at them through a body composition lens. When they did this the result was, frankly, startling. More than 62 percent of these normal weight individuals were over-fat. A majority of the normal weight men had body fat percentages greater than 20 percent and a majority of the normal weight women had more than 30 percent body fat. In this case, BMI, calculated using weight and height, was a misleading clue. It mistakenly categorized these people as being normal when it comes to body fatness. A majority of them were anything but. Composition revealed this fact.

We find similar discrepancies, in many cases, where weight clues can lead us in one direction but composition clues lead us to an entirely different conclusion. To illustrate this point let's look at the *Case of the High Risk Breast Cancer Patients*. A study conducted on a group of pre-menopausal women determined that some of them were likely to be at an increased risk for breast cancer. Weight and heights were gathered for each of them and BMI was calculated. With this information all 30 of the women were categorized as being normal. Yet when the researchers used a better lens, one that allowed them to view the composition of the weight, a very different pattern emerged. Almost all of these women, 28 out of 30, had fat mass that was higher than, and muscle mass lower than anticipated. In other words, almost every one of these high breast cancer risk women was under-muscled and over-fat for their sizes. This clue was completely missed when only height and weight were measured. It was readily apparent when the health scene was investigated with a body composition lens.

We find a similar story in the *Case of the Under-muscled HIV patients*. HIV/AIDS researchers have noted that a significant relationship exists between amounts of muscle and progression of this viral disease. The trend over time is for a slow but progressive depletion of muscle mass. Muscle mass in one study was found to be only 54 percent of normal at the time of death—the persons who died of AIDS had lost 46 percent of their muscle tissue. This is extreme muscle loss. Even lesser degrees of muscle loss are strongly associated with poor outcomes in HIV+ persons; it is a clue that things are going downhill for the infected individual. With weight as our only clue, we can't observe what is happening with the amount of muscle. Things might look "normal." With a body composition lens, loss of muscle tissue is an easily spotted clue.

Assessing Body Composition

There is no readily available method for direct assessment of body composition. Instead, in both research and clinical settings, body composition is almost always estimated indirectly. Several different methods exist for estimating body composition; each having its own advantages and disadvantages. The most significant trade-off between most of these methods is cost/convenience verses reliability. Typically the least expensive and most convenient methods sacrifice a bit of reliability. Some common body composition assessment methods include use of (1) calipers to assess skin-fold thickness, (2) underwater tanks, (3) isotopes, (4) x-ray radiation, and (5) electrical current. Each of these methods uses specific prediction equations to estimate body composition at a whole body level from the data they collect. In terms of maximizing convenience and minimizing cost, while maintaining a high level of reliability, in our experience, the best lens for investigating the contribution different types of tissue make to overall weight is bioelectrical impedance analysis (BIA). This technology is perfectly suited for use in a doctor's office or gym setting, and it is the one we rely upon for investigating and tracking trends in shape cases.

BIA sends a harmless and imperceptible electrical signal through the body and then measures how the body modifies this electrical current. The theory behind BIA is that since different tissue, such as muscle and fat, are comprised of very different substances, there will be a measurable difference in how well or poorly they allow this electrical signal to move through the body. From the measurements obtained, an accurate estimation of the contribution muscle, fat and fluids make to our overall weight can be safely and quickly determined.

HSI CLUE

Aging in humans is associated with a progressive loss of muscle size and strength. This is called *sarcopenia*. It is associated with poor health outcomes, with higher degrees of sarcopenia being associated with frailty, falls, poor quality of life, and premature death. Sarcopenia can't be detected by paying attention to weight since many individuals with it are also progressively gaining body fat. It is easy to spot when the composition of weight is tracked.

Using BIA as a lens allows for an accurate estimate of the contribution several different tissue types make to our overall weight. When this testing method is applied correctly, it gives extremely reliable evidence of how the composition of weight changes, either for better or worse, over time. This determination can be invaluable in detecting shifts in the quality of our weight well in advance of actually detecting changes in our weight. This is important because the earlier desirable or undesirable shifts in body composition are detected, the more likely we will be able to spot the little things in our diets, lifestyles and environments that are contributing to these shifts, allowing us to make corrections and adjustments in advance of significant changes in shape.

Next Steps

Depending upon the resources in your local community, one or more body composition assessment methods might be available to you. There might be a place that offers BIA, a place that uses calipers to estimate body composition, or a place that does underwater weighing, as just some examples. Gyms are a great place to begin your search for what is available to you locally. Many gyms offer some form of body composition assessment. Other local options to investigate include hospitals, medical clinics, and health professionals who work with weight management. [Note: HSI Team members can assess body composition. See the Appendix section for locations of team member clinics.]

Our current body composition is important; the direction we're going is usually even more important. No matter which body composition assessment method is used, the most important thing to remember is that the real value in analyzing body composition is in monitoring how body fat and muscle amounts change over time. This is of far greater importance than the initial data obtained, and it's true no matter which method is used to get your results. To obtain evidence of how muscle and fat amounts are changing over time requires reexamining body composition periodically. In order to obtain the most accurate and reliable tracking data there are two important considerations.

HSI CLUE

In the *Case of the Army Rangers* and the *Case of the Minnesota Experiment* (chapter 4) lost weight was regained after the period of underfeeding ended. Weight regain was a clue. But the vitally important clue was that dieting caused a rebound increase in body fat to an amount far greater, about 40% higher, than had existed before these situations. This fact would have been missed if the only clue gathered had been weight.

Because each body composition assessment technique actually measures something different to estimate body fatness and muscle amounts, trying to accurately compare data and gain insight on how you are tracking over time is far less precise when different assessment techniques are being used and compared. Think of it as being a bit like comparing apples and oranges. While both are fruit they are not the same fruit. The same principle applies with different body composition assessment methods. We don't want to be comparing apples and oranges. If skin calipers, bioimpedence analysis, underwater weighing or some other method is going to be used the first time, make sure body composition is assessed using the same technique the next time.

Like many body functions, there are predictable changes that occur over a 24-hour period with body composition. These occur because of our circadian rhythms—rhythms we will discuss in more detail later in chapters 12 and 13. Because of these rhythms body composition would not be expected to be precisely the same at 7 a.m. as it would be at 7 p.m., as an example. While these circadian changes are small for body composition, they will introduce some degree of error into data. It is best to eliminate this potentially confusing variable by having body composition assessed at approximately the same time each time it is assessed. If body composition is going to be assessed the first time at 4 p.m. it should be reassessed at or around 4 p.m., give or take an hour or so, at subsequent visits; the same applies to other times of the day.
[Note: For menstruating women the same consistency of timing principle applies on a monthly level. Predictable variations in body composition occur at different points of one's menstrual cycle. It's, therefore, best to measuring body composition on the same day of the menstrual cycle each time it is assessed.]

Once you have two or more assessments, the information can now be used as a clue to how you are responding, for the better or worse, on a qualitative level to your unique diet/lifestyle/environment situation.

BODY COMPOSITION	Day 1	Day 30	Day 60	Day 90
My Weight (in lbs or kg)				
My Fat-Free (lean) Mass (in lbs or kg)				
My Fat Mass (in lbs or kg)				

Final Point

When you weigh yourself on a scale the number reflects everything that is on, or in, your body at that time. The scale can't distinguish the boots on your feet from the amount of fat in your body, or the fat around your waist from the muscles in your chest. Although this failing is obvious, our society unfortunately remains obsessed with the number on a scale. This weight-centric mindset is ingrained into our way of thinking. Sadly, it is not uncommon to encounter individuals who evaluate the "healthiness" of a food or activity based on how they believe it will affect their weight, with no thought to what it might be doing to their shape, body composition or health. As an example, some Type 1 diabetics don't take their medication—insulin—because of concerns over weight gain. This is called *diabulimia*. It is a rapidly growing medical problem. Failing to take insulin can result in a medical emergency. As mentioned in the *Case of Insulin*, while insulin can cause weight gain, in a person with Type 1 diabetes most of the weight gained will be healthy weight, it will be muscle and will result in a more attractive shape. The person will look better, feel better, and be healthier with this added weight. A weight-centric view contributes to the decision to practice diabulimia. What would occur if, as a society, we were instead focused on the shapes of our bodies, the composition of our weight, and our overall health trend? By becoming more invested in the view we get when we look through the lens of body composition we can move past the limitations found in a weight-centric view. We can begin to appreciate that weight is an incidental fact; the quality of that weight, its actual composition, now that's vital.

> **HSI CLUE**
>
> Significantly improving shape often requires adding more muscle tissue. Once sufficient muscle tissue is gained a tipping point, of sorts, is reached and shape will often shift dramatically.

Closing Dialogue

Health Scene Investigator: Has your perspective on success shifted?

Apprentice: Absolutely. We can only truly understand success by looking in detail at both shape and the composition of our weight and how these things change over time.

Health Scene Investigator: Very good. Now let me ask you another question. We have discussed body fat as being one of the aspects of composition; is all fat the same?

Apprentice: My general impression is yes; all body fat is, in essence, the same.

Health Scene Investigator: Never trust to general impressions. Concentrate yourself upon details. Detection is, or ought to be, an exact science. Treating body fat with exactness may, of course, seem a trifle, but there is nothing as important as trifles when one is investigating a health scene. With that understanding let us turn our powers of observation to the details of body fat.

Chapter 10

The Details of Body Fat

I am glad of all details, whether they seem to you to be relevant or not.

Sherlock Holmes

Opening Dialogue

Health Scene Investigator: They say that genius is an infinite capacity for focusing our attention and abilities on details. It's a very bad definition of course, but it does apply to investigative work. With that in mind, allow me to ask you a question: When it comes to body fat, what is your primary concern?

Apprentice: The amount—quantity—has been my primary concern.

Health Scene Investigator: Amount is certainly a vital clue, but is focusing our attention on amount sufficient, or, should we be looking at other details as well?

Apprentice: I am confused. You mean to say that there are other details?

Health Scene Investigator: Yes, that is precisely what I mean to say.

The Importance of Details

In *The Adventure of the Copper Beeches* Holmes informs us that he is glad of all details, whether they seem relevant or not. In *The Adventure of Black Peter* he admonishes an inspector Hopkins; telling him, "Tut, tut, my dear sir, you must really pay attention to these details." And in *A Case of Identity*, Holmes states, "Never trust to general impressions, my boy, but concentrate yourself upon details." Details were exceedingly important to Holmes.

HSI CLUE

Assume for a moment that we have two people with identical amounts of body fat. Person one has higher amounts of fat under the skin and lower amounts of fat inside the abdominal cavity. Person two has the opposite pattern. Are these two people at equal risk of disease? Are they both equally likely to be alive a decade from now? In other words, is it how much fat they have that matters or does location trump amount?

The enduring emphasis on weight—losing it or gaining it—in medical research, the media, and with the public, is an example of trusting to something that is more of a *general impression* than a *detail*. Shape and body composition are a far more detailed, and insightful way to look at a health scene. When muscle and fat are monitored as part of a body composition assessment, clues emerge that would otherwise be missed. Quantifying the amount of muscle and fat is an important detail. This detail is far too infrequently gathered when the effects of medications, foods, and other potential shape tipping points are scientifically studied. The result is incomplete information. Drawing conclusions from incomplete information would hardly be the way to approach a criminal investigation. The same is true when it comes to health scenes. Like Holmes, we want to know *all* of the details before we come to a conclusion. Knowing how much fat a person has is one of these details; knowing its distribution or location is another.

During the past few decades, science has uncovered many new details about fat. Fat makes and releases a variety of communication molecules. It appears to be a highly intelligent superorganism, albeit one scattered diffusely throughout the body. All fat isn't the same. White fat stores energy, brown fat burns it. Fat in different locations of the body can function quite differently. It can respond in highly localized manners. It can have its own fingerprint—fatty acid profile—as was discussed in chapter 7. Fat location can also tell very different stories about health risk. Two people with identical *amounts* of fat could have very different risks for heart attacks or diabetes, as examples, based on the *location* of the fat. One might be at a low risk, the other at a high risk. In this instance, location would be trumping amount—the 'where of the what' would be an important detail.

The idea that location might be important shouldn't come as a surprise. Many individuals directly experience location issues. Some of us, rather than gaining fat uniformly in all areas, will accumulate fat disproportionately in some areas and not others. The same applies when it comes to reducing it; we might find losing fat in some areas is far more difficult than in others. The area might be the belly, hips, thighs, knees, or upper arms, as examples. It might be several of these areas. Body fat appears where it wants to, can be gained or lost unevenly, and can cling tightly to places we most want it to disappear. It, in other words, behaves as if it has a mind of its own, not only when it comes to amount but also in terms of how the amount is distributed. This detail will be highly important to most people. It will impact how they look and the satisfaction, or lack thereof, they will have with their shape no matter what their weight. Location details also provide valuable health risk predictive information. They can also be a clue to what is contributing to shape changes. When it comes to fat, we don't want to trust to general impressions; we want to concentrate on the details. Medicine has been slow in coming to this recognition. As a result clues have been missed and mistakes have been made.

Location as a Shape Clue

Where we store fat is an important clue. Focusing our powers of observation on this detail, rather than simply the amount, can shift our perspective on what is, or has, occurred. This point is highlighted when we return to the *Case of Overfeeding Identical Twins* (investigated in chapter 5). Participating twins were overfed by 84,000 calories over a period of 100 days: Weight was gained. Some gained as little as 9, and others as much as 30 pounds. Much of this weight gain was body fat, and some was muscle. Four months after the overfeeding period ended, most of the weight and excess fat gained through massive overfeeding had been spontaneously lost. Eating close to 1000 excess calories a day for months on end didn't make these twins permanently fatter. This was an important finding. Another important clue emerged when the details of fat location were observed. The rebound effect from overfeeding slightly reduced upper body fat—fat inside and around the waist and trunk—below the levels it was before the overfeeding experiment. Not only were there no persistent effects when these twins were fed a massive amount of extra calories, the rebound effect actually produced a slight improvement in upper body shape; an improvement that would have been missed if location had not been considered.

HSI CLUE

An apple shape is considered high risk; a pear shape is a low risk shape. If two persons weighed the same amount but one had an apple shape and the other had a pear shape their health risk would be different. This same principle applies to amounts of fat. If two people have identical amounts of fat, but one stores it as belly fat and the other in the arms, hips, and legs, the latter would be at a lower risk for disease.

As newer technologies have allowed scientists to measure and categorize fat tissue by location there has been a growing appreciation that, while how much we have is important, the location is equally, and in some instances more important. This is illustrated in the *Case of Lipodystrophy* (mentioned in chapter 8). Lipodystrophy is a degenerative condition affecting fat tissue. It generally entails loss of fat from some areas and abnormal increases in others. The result is localized shortages and excesses. This redistribution of fat is seen with HIV-associated lipodystrophy (a common side effect of highly active anti-retroviral medications). This lipodystrophy is characterized by peripheral *subcutaneous*—below the skin—fat wasting. Fat is lost in the arms, legs, and parts of the face. The fat wasting in these areas is often, but not always, accompanied by increases in fat in the neck, upper back, chest, and abdomen. The net result can be a person with normal *amounts* but a very abnormal *distribution* of subcutaneous fat. In a worse case scenario, the fat redistribution might result in thin arms and legs, gaunt face, sunken cheeks, a rounder trunk, bigger belly and a buffalo hump. Even if they are losing weight, a person with HIV-associated lipodystrophy is usually dissatisfied with the way their shape is changing. This should not be a surprise; thinner arms and legs, with a thicker trunk, bigger belly, buffalo hump, and a gaunt face aren't cosmetically very appealing. It also might not be particularly healthy. A lipodystrophy type of shape change is associated with increased risk for heart disease and diabetes. It is a clue that, health-wise, things might be moving in an undesirable direction. Location, in this instance, is a highly relevant detail.

Lipodystrophy is not the only reason to be concerned with location details. Many of us will experience fat gain or loss patterns that are far from uniform. This point is highlighted in the *Case of the Disproportionate Loss of Peripheral Fat*. In this case, scientists measured subcutaneous fat at four different sites in 61 obese women before and after six months of eating only 1200 calories a day. Caloric restriction, as a sole strategy, reduced subcutaneous fat proportionally more in peripheral than in central regions. Weight was lost. The same was true for fat. But neither of these was reduced uniformly. The body seemed to be clinging more tightly to fat in some areas—belly and trunk—than in others.

Shape changes over a lifetime. Some of this is due to the cumulative effects of gravity. Some is due to age-related declines in muscle tissue. And some is due to changes in fat location. As we age we store more fat in our belly region, and, typically, less in our arms and legs. This change can be occurring even in the absence of noticeable weight changes. This was seen in the *Case of Menopause*. In this case, eight healthy women were assessed prior to menopause and eight years later—in the postmenopausal period. No change in weight was detected, but the location of the weight shifted significantly, with belly fat increasing by 28 percent. This study is not alone in showing that belly fat tends to increase with aging. Other studies have reported similar findings. Belly fat also tends to be more difficult to lose as we age.

The above cases illustrate the importance of paying attention to the location of fat. Amount of fat is an important fact but the "where" of the "what"—the pattern of fat distribution—can provide information that will be missed entirely if this detail is overlooked. Focusing solely on the amount of body fat can also lead to seeing but not observing, as Holmes might say. We would be accurately seeing a clue—amount—but failing to observe a potentially even more important one—its distribution.

HSI CLUE

Although LDL ("bad") cholesterol levels have, on average, slightly declined in the American population over the past three decades, during the same three decades population-wide triglyceride levels (blood fats) have increased significantly. What is causing this dramatic increase in blood fats? Might discovering what is causing it also provide clues to what is causing an increase in our waistlines?

Cases of Subcutaneous and Visceral Adipose Tissue

Most fat is located in adipose tissue; a specialized type of connective tissue made up of fat cells. Adipose tissue can be broadly divided into two categories—*subcutaneous* and *visceral*—based on its location. Lumping all adipose tissue together will give us a general impression about overall body fatness, but this impression can be misleading.

Two people can have identical amounts of adipose tissue, and yet, have widely different shapes and health risks depending on the relative quantities of the fat stored subcutaneously and viscerally. Different circumstances might cause equal gains in adipose tissue amount, but can have disparate effects on which type of adipose tissue is gained. The same can occur when fat is reduced. These are details, highly relevant details.

Subcutaneous adipose tissue was mentioned in chapter seven. It is the layer of fat just below the skin. It stores energy and provides insulation. To picture this type of fat it might help to imagine a steak. The outside layer of fat on a piece of steak is subcutaneous fat. It is the fat that would have been located between the cow's outer skin and the muscle (meat) that was beneath. Love handles, female breasts, and the fat we can pinch on arms, legs, hips and waists is subcutaneous fat. When calipers are used to estimate body fatness, they are, very specifically, measuring subcutaneous fat.

Unlike subcutaneous fat, which is stored, relatively speaking, on the outside of the body, visceral fat is stored *inside* of us. It is located in the internal cavities of our body, inside the chest, abdominal, and pelvic regions. It surrounds organs like the heart in the chest cavity or the intestines in the abdominal cavity. It is invisible to the naked eye, can't be measured when we use calipers, can't be felt when we do a pinch test, and can go undetected unless imaging technologies are used to look inside the body. The job of visceral fat is a bit less clear than that of subcutaneous, but part of its job is energy storage. It also has strong links to stress and sleep deprivation. Presumably at least one of its jobs is to provide a nearby (and readily accessed) source of stored energy for our internal organs during periods where higher stress is expected (or ongoing). Its links to sleep deprivation suggest it is a source of stored energy for times when we might sleep more, hibernate so to speak.

The general theme in research is that observing greater amounts of subcutaneous fat at a health scene is not, on its own, generally a reason for concern. Noticing changes in its distribution might be. The important clue is where we have subcutaneous fat. Having more on our upper arms, thighs, buttocks, or hips, far from being a poor prognostic sign, is associated with better health outcomes. It is too little, not too much, in these areas that carry added risk. With visceral fat the rule of thumb is more straightforward; increases are a poor prognostic sign. Visceral fat plays a big role in producing the apple shape that carries a higher health risk. It is visceral fat that directly contributes to a paunch or potbelly, an unhealthy shape no matter what our weight may be.

Amounts of visceral fat can, and sometimes do, paint a very different picture than weight or even total amounts of fat might paint. One instance where this is commonly the case is aging. Visceral fat tends to increase as we age. One year from now an average person will have greater amounts of visceral fat than they have today. A decade from now it will have increased even more. This is especially likely to be the case if the person is sedentary. This increase can occur with or without changes in weight or total amounts of body fat. Visceral fat is a detail that can't be gleaned from the general impression we might get from weighing ourselves. But its increase, combined with the age-related tendency to lose muscle, and shift subcutaneous fat from the arms and legs to the belly and trunk, can result in a big shape change.

The things that cause increases and decreases in visceral fat are not always identical to what cause increases or decreases in subcutaneous fat. In Chapter 7 it was mentioned that swimming in cold water might cause Shape Intelligence to make insulative adaptations. Subcutaneous fat serves an insulation role, so it makes sense that swimming in cold water might produce a different subcutaneous fat response than would walking or biking. The same theme holds for other situations and circumstances. If Shape Intelligence is given a different type of challenge, it might adapt differently: Chronic stress serves as an example. Stress, with the exception of cold stress, does not produce an increased requirement for insulation. So in terms of fat gains, we wouldn't expect an intelligent system to respond to it in the same way it would to cold-water swimming. Not surprisingly, it doesn't. Chronic stress tends to result in a disproportionate increase of belly fat, especially visceral belly fat. This internal location is apparently a more important place

HSI CLUE

Rats were fed diets containing lard, corn oil, or fish oil for six months. At no time during these six months did the weights of the rats fed different dietary fats differ; yet their body fat amounts and types did. The rats fed fish oil ended up with less body fat and less visceral fat than did rats fed lard or corn oil. If we truly wish to understand the effects of different dietary substances, paying attention to general impressions like weight, can cause us to miss clues that only become apparent when finer details are gathered.

to build up fat stores during circumstances characterized by high stress. What we do and what we experience will dictate to a large extent where we gain or lose fat. Because of this, paying attention to the details of where fat is gained, lost, or shifted is highly relevant. Only by understanding *what* Shape Intelligence is actually doing can we hope to decipher *why* it is doing it.

HSI CLUE

Studies indicate that people who try to control or maintain their weight through dieting rather than with exercise are likely to have major deposits of internal fat. This is true even if, from the outside, they appear to be thin or normal weight. Dieting can lead to a generalized impression of success; adipose tissue details might lead to a very different conclusion.

Noticing that we are getting fatter while disregarding where we got fatter can make it much more difficult to figure out why we got fatter. It can lead to poor inferences about the causes of the fat gain and lead us to choose solutions for changing our shape that don't address the underlying cause. Furthermore, getting fatter while disregarding where we got fatter, and why we got fatter, can lead to poor inferences about the possible health consequences. An increase in subcutaneous fat typically has a marginal impact on our health. Depending upon where the increase occurs, it might even lower our risk for disease. This is not the case for visceral fat. An increase in fat in the abdominal cavity has a very strong correlation with higher risk for heart disease, stroke, diabetes, sleep apnea, and the other health challenges that are commonly linked with increased weight. We must look past the superficial to detect this clue and make the correct inference.

Medicine uses body mass index (BMI)—a calculation using height and weight—as a way to guess about body fatness. It uses this guess to categorize people as thin, normal, overweight, or obese. While BMI tells us something about group risk, it is unreliable for predicting individual risk. It is also a highly unreliable means to accurately predict amounts of visceral fat. This was demonstrated in the *Case of Thin Outside, Fat Inside.* Dr. Jimmy Bell, a professor at Imperial College in London, England, and his team of scientists used magnetic resonance imaging (MRI) to detect internal fat in nearly 800 men and women. Forty-five percent of the women and 60 percent of the men, who would have been considered as "thin" or "normal" based upon their BMI, had excess amounts of visceral fat. They were, in the words of these scientists, "thin outside and fat inside." The superficial clue, the general impression that weight gave, was misleading. Cases like this suggest that the whole concept of how we decide who is and is not fat needs to be completely overhauled. When the superficial—weight—is used as a warning sign of poor health, it can miss the mark. It can falsely identify people as being of low risk, who are in fact at a much higher risk of heart disease and diabetes than are people who weigh far more. The same principle applies if body fat amounts are measured but the locations and types of fat are not. Detecting amounts and changes in the overall distribution of fat, as well as shifts in visceral and subcutaneous fat allows for better inferences.

Paying attention to the location details allows us to detect causes of shape changes that might otherwise be missed. A medication, as an example, might not cause gains in weight. It might not even cause gains in fat. But there are instances where it can still be causing shifts in the distribution of fat. One of these instances was mentioned in the *Case of Lipodystrophy* with highly active anti-retroviral medications. Adipose tissue details also allow for the tailoring of better solutions for producing improved shape. To reduce fat in one area might require one, or more, modifications in diet, lifestyle, or environment. To reduce it in another area might require slightly, or entirely, different strategies. From the perspective of Shape Intelligence, all fat is not created equal. Shape Intelligence makes best guesses about how much fat we need. It also makes predictions about where best to add it based on the nature of the challenge it is doing its best to solve. By paying attention to the details of subcutaneous and visceral fat, we are in a far better position to notice and better understand what it is doing.

HSI CLUE

Studies show that North Americans have had our muscles become more like marbled steak while our livers have become more foie gras-like. To produce these types of changes in a cow or a duck the food industry must make very specific changes to the diet, lifestyle, and environment of the animal. What can we learn from this?

Cases of Marbled Steak and Foie Gras

While most of the fat stored in the body will be stored in adipose tissue, fat can also be deposited in other places. We can have fat deposits in our arteries, liver, and muscles. We can also have it floating in the blood (triglycerides). In these locations fat would be correctly thought of as fat, but it would not be adipose tissue. Increases of fat in these locations are, in general, warning signs.

Most people are aware that fat deposits in the arteries—atherosclerosis—are a health concern. It is associated with increased risk for heart attacks and strokes. Fewer people are aware of the health risks of becoming more like a marbled steak or foie gras.

Intermuscular fat is fat stored on the inside of our muscles. Once again imagine a steak. The marbling we see is intermuscular fat. Marbling adds a fatty taste to the meat that, for the past few decades, consumers have preferred. In fact, grading of steaks into premium, choice, and select is based almost entirely on the degree of marbling; with extra marbling fetching a steak a higher grade, and hence a steeper price. Unlike feedlot cattle, wild game has minimal marbling. The same is true for beef from pastured cows; it has relatively little marbling. Highly marbled meat is not the natural order of things. But since greater marbling fetch higher prices, the cattle industry has adapted; altering its livestock rearing practices to produce more of the highly marbled steak we have been demanding.

The recipe for producing beef with more marbling includes (1) selectively breeding cattle to produce higher amounts (a genetic solution), (2) feeding them more corn and allowing them less pasture (a diet solution), and (3) keeping them as sedentary as possible by putting them on feed lots (a lifestyle solution). It's not hard to imagine that we get a less healthy cow when we breed it to be more fatty, feed it a fattening diet, and limit its opportunities to move. The same goes for us when it comes to our intermuscular fat amounts. As is the case with animals, high amounts of intermuscular fat in humans is a sign of poor health. Marbling of our muscles is associated with insulin resistance and diabetes. The previously mentioned HIV-associated lipodystrophy syndrome is associated with increased marbling. Like visceral fat, marbling is not an easy clue to observe directly; detection requires imaging technology. But educated guesses about the likelihood of marbling can be made. Just like with cattle, a sedentary lifestyle and a processed food diet appear to produce more marbling, and, the solution to preventing it is equivalent to what we see in nature; putting ourselves out to pasture so to speak; using our muscles more and eating less processed, better quality food.

Our muscles can marble. Fat can also be deposited in the liver. Extremes of this are known medically as *fatty liver*. An increase in liver fat is a significant health risk, and like increases in visceral fat and intermuscular fat, it is a poor prognostic sign. Foie gras is the food version of liver fat. It's made from the liver of a duck or a goose that has been specially fattened. Fattening is accomplished by feeding a grain-based diet, and then during the last several weeks prior to slaughter, force-feeding the bird corn mash. A wild duck may double its weight in the autumn, storing fat throughout much of its body and especially in the liver, in preparation for winter migration. Force-feeding corn mash produces a liver six to ten times ordinary size. Foie gras is considered a delicacy. It also highlights an instructive lesson between what is eaten and where fat gets stored.

Assessment

The gold standard for detecting and quantifying fat according to location is use of some type of imaging technology—CT scans, MRI, or ultrasound—that allows science to look deeper than the surface of the body. These technologies are being used more and more in research settings. As a result, fat location knowledge is increasing by leaps and bounds. These technologies have yet to find their way into mainstream medicine and are unlikely to do so in the near future. The vast majority of us will not have them at our disposal when it comes to assessing our individual cases. We will need to gather other clues.

Subcutaneous fat can be estimated by using calipers at multiple sites in the body. We can also do our own pinch tests in these areas. While imaging is the only precise way to detect visceral fat, at health scenes there are other clues that can be used to make a Holmesian inference—an *argument to the best explanation*—about visceral fat. One of the most important clues is waist shape. Even if the size of the waist isn't large, its overall shape can be an important clue. The so-called potbelly is an example of a stomach that, no matter the actual size, is almost certain to contain significant amounts of visceral fat. To assess stomach shape, it is important to pay relatively less attention to the total waist size and to focus your powers of observation on its front-to-back size. A thick trunk with a thin oval shaped midsection will measure out as a large waist size. Despite the large waist size, the shape is healthy; being caused by the side-to-size width of the trunk, which is mostly a result of muscle and

HSI CLUE

Shape Intelligence makes location specific decisions based on past and present experiences. Experiences that cause large increases or decreases in subcutaneous fat might have far different effects on visceral fat, intermuscular fat, liver fat, or blood fats. There are mysteries hidden in the details.

subcutaneous fat. Conversely, a similar or even smaller overall waist size, which has a rounder shape (a lower side-to-side and a greater back-to-front width), would be a clue to excess visceral fat, because to produce this shape—rounding effect of the stomach—usually requires an accumulation of internal fat. The key detail is the distance from the back to the widest point of the front of the abdomen. This can be assessed standing or lying as long as we are consistent. A growing distance between these two points suggests an increase in visceral fat; a decreasing distance indicates that visceral fat is shrinking in the stomach region.

The next clues to look for require lab work to identify the presence of signs of *metabolic obesity*. Metabolic obesity means any or all of a clustering of metabolic warning signs including high "bad" cholesterol (LDL), low "good" cholesterol (HDL), high triglycerides (blood fats), high blood sugar, insulin resistance, elevated blood pressure, and increased liver enzymes (a marker of fatty liver). Presence of one of these warning signs is suggestive of increases in visceral body fatness, intermuscular fat, liver fat, or all three. A clustering of more and more of these warning signs progressively increases the odds of higher amounts of fat accumulation in these areas. A person who weighs a lot but has no signs of metabolic obesity would statistically be at little to no increased risk for heart disease, diabetes, or early death. They would be expected to, despite the high weight, have relatively low amounts of visceral fat, intermuscular fat, and liver fat. They will give a general impression of being fat, but on the inside, where it counts, details will they are likely to be lean. Conversely, a person who is superficially thin, but with a clustering of these metabolic warning signs, would almost always have excessive amounts of hidden fat. They would be thin outside, yet, inside, where it counts, they would be over fat.

Final Points

Shape Intelligence is constantly deciding whether it should increase or decrease fat stores. As it makes these decisions it takes into account the different locations available for storage, their respective jobs, and the quality of fats it has available to place in these different locations. In a simplified sense, it might decide to send the fat in cold water fish (fish oil) one place (like our immune system where it can help us fight off infections), while if we were to eat the same amount of fat as trans fats (partially hydrogenated vegetable oils), it might send it to a very different site (like depositing it as visceral fat or liver fat). If we were to consume large amounts of corn-derived sweeteners (high fructose corn syrup and crystalline fructose) Shape Intelligence might make our livers more foie gras-like or it might increase blood fats. If we ate the same amount of sweetener as honey, neither of these two decisions might be made. If we stop using our leg muscles, Shape Intelligence might make the muscles in our legs more marbled, yet make no changes to our other muscles. These are just some examples; examples that allow us to observe a theme: As we look at the details of fat we see an intelligent system making very specific decisions when it comes to where to put what. By applying the same degree of detail when we think about body fat, extremely valuable clues emerge at health scenes; clues that would be missed if we treat all fat as being the same.

While there are unique individual differences in terms of how Shape Intelligence might choose to locate fat in any one person, there are consistent patterns. Because of this, shape can provide clues to the reasons why more fat is being defended and why it is being located in specific places, that neither weight nor an amount of fat alone could provide. In other words, when we observe diet, lifestyle, or environmental factors that consistently result in an increase in visceral, intermuscular, liver or blood fats (high risk locations), this teaches us something very different about shape and health than if we were to observe Shape Intelligence respond by increasing subcutaneous fat. In the following chapters, some of the cases will focus on body fat location details. These details allow clues to emerge that would otherwise be hidden. The expression *the Devil is in the details* refers to the notion that a mysterious element can lie hidden in the details. This is absolutely the case when it comes to fat and where it is stored.

Closing Dialogue

Apprentice: I had no idea that there were so many details about body fat. It makes me really question my past efforts at, well, trying to lose it. It makes me wonder whether I might have inadvertently been doing more harm than good when it comes to my shape and health.

Health Scene Investigator: That is an excellent insight. Now that we have discussed shape, body composition, and details of fat location, it is time to begin our investigation into health scenes in earnest. Let's begin by investigating sleep.

Apprentice: Sleep? What does sleep have to do with shape?

Health Scene Investigator: Improbable as it might seem to you, know the answer is a great deal…a very great deal.

Chapter 11

Sleep and Shape

I can see that you have not slept for a night or two. That tries a man's nerves more than work, and more even than pleasure.

Sherlock Holmes

Opening Dialogue

Health Scene Investigator: Let's discuss your case. Have there been any times in your life where over a period of a few months you observed a significant worsening of your shape?

Apprentice: Actually, yes. There was one such period. Why do you ask?

Health Scene Investigator: I ask because that time period might contain important clues to the types of events and circumstances that contributed to your current shape, your tipping points, so to speak. Now, what was your sleep like during that period?

Apprentice: My sleep…I hadn't been expecting you to ask about sleep. I was expecting you to question me about, well, my diet, for one thing. What does sleep have to do with this?

Health Scene Investigator: It is really quite elementary. Here, let me explain.

Can Lack of Sleep
Try More Than a Man's Nerves?

In 1910, not too long after the time of Holmes, North Americans slept about nine hours a night. By the mid-1970s average sleep time had dropped to seven and one half hours. By the late 1990s this number had dropped to below seven hours per night. As a society we are sleeping fewer hours today than humans did one hundred years ago. While some of us are getting enough sleep, many of us aren't. In 2008, the U.S. Centers for Disease Control and Prevention (CDC) reported more specific results based on a survey of 19,589 adults in four states. Ten percent of the adults responded that they didn't get enough sleep every single day of the prior month. Another 38 percent said they didn't get enough sleep at least seven or more days in the prior month. The CDC has also released nationwide data indicating that the percentage of persons who claim to sleep six or fewer hours each night increased from 1985 to 2006. This growth in the number of people who are sleeping fewer hours is occurring in persons of all ages.

The findings of the CDC are consistent with those of the National Sleep Foundation (NSF). In the 2007 Survey of Women, the NSF reported that in their efforts to "do it all," women in the United States were sacrificing sleep. When asked about their sleep, 60 percent answered that they only get a good night's sleep a few nights per week or less. Two out of three women responded that they experience sleep problems at least a few nights each week; 46 percent experienced sleep problems every night.

HSI CLUE

Volunteers were allowed free access to meals and snacks during two stays in a sleep laboratory. One of the stays they were allowed 8 ½ hours in bed; the other they were allowed only 5 ½ hours. When sleep time was reduced, intake of food at meals stayed the same, but snacking went way up, especially during night and normal sleep hours. What was it about sleeping a few hours less than normal that resulted in a "craving" for snacks? Why did snacking at night go way up?

Adults are not alone. Children sleep fewer hours, on average, today than they did 40 to 50 years ago. In one study, the percentage of children sleeping eight to nine hours per night decreased from 41 percent in 1960 to 23.5 percent in 2001-02. During this forty-year time period the incidence of childhood obesity has nearly doubled. It has also been rising in step with the reductions in sleep in the adult population. Is this just a coincidence or is there a relationship between how much sleep we get and our shape?

Circumstantial evidence, most of it from long-term observational studies, indicates that there is a consistent relationship between sleeping fewer hours and increased weight. This relationship exists for adults and children. It can't be explained by simply factoring in genetics, demographics, or social and lifestyle influences. And it appears to be linear, with progressively shorter sleep durations being associated with higher risk for obesity. Short sleep duration also predicts future weight gain. In a large group of people the individuals who are sleeping the fewest hours at the start of the observation period are the ones who are most likely to gain weight by the end of it. Observational studies provide circumstantial evidence. They are not designed to answer whether one thing causes another. But they can help us to determine whether something is or isn't a coincidence. The observed relationship between shorter sleep duration and a poorer shape appears to be more than a coincidence. Sleep deprivation impacts tens of millions of North Americans. Could it be a shape tipping point? Could getting too little sleep be causing Shape Intelligence to adapt, resulting in a defense of a higher natural weight? Could lack of sleep be doing more than just trying our nerves?

Sleep Self-Regulation and Sleep Debt

Conventional wisdom once held that the need for sleep did not accumulate. If a person were deprived of sleep for a few nights, all they needed was one good night of sleep, and they would be all caught up. This belief was an obvious fact. Actual facts disprove it. One good night of sleep is not enough to completely offset the equivalent of many nights of inadequate sleep. The need for sleep accumulates. It is self-regulated. Our body seems to care about how much sleep it gets. Evidence indicates that it keeps track of whether or not it is receiving the needed amounts. If it isn't, it changes its behaviors to get more. One of the changes it initiates is *sleepiness*; another is *microsleep*.

A propensity to sleep—sleepiness—builds the longer we have been awake. Sleepiness is to sleep as thirst is to water and hunger is to food. It is an intelligent bio-behavioral response aimed at pressuring us to get something the body feels it needs—sleep. For most of us, if we have been awake for 16 hours, sufficient sleepiness will build up to cause us to fall asleep for about eight hours. If we have been awake for 40 hours straight, a greater degree of sleepiness will have built up, which allows us to sleep for a greater amount of time than usual.

HSI CLUE

Feeling sleepy while studying, working, driving, watching TV, etc. is a common complaint. When asked, a person will usually admit that they aren't getting enough sleep. They are aware that they are sleepy, and, they seemingly recognize its cause, yet they often fail to do the one thing that will correct the problem— sleep more. Do you take steps to get more sleep when you notice you are sleepy during the day or while engaged in activities?

Many adults and children routinely experience daytime sleepiness. This is a direct clue that they need to get more sleep, just as chronically being thirsty is a signal that more water is needed. Sufficient sleep satiates sleepiness, as sufficient water satiates thirst. While a thirsty person will, typically, happily drink more water, the same is not always the case with sleepy people and sleep. Rather than experiencing sleepiness and realizing that this is a biological signal indicating that sleep is needed, sleepiness is often viewed as a sign of weakness or an indication that more caffeine is needed. The "thirst" for sleep is not quenched; it is resisted. Fortunately, a hallmark of self-regulated processes is redundancy: There are usually several ways to achieve a goal. We see this redundancy with sleep.

Biological pressure, including sleepiness, hunger, and thirst, are ways for complex adaptive intelligence to put pressure on us to acquire something it needs. These are corrective mechanisms, but they aren't the only corrective mechanisms. If we resist sleepiness, which many of us do, life tries to find other ways to get what it needs. In chapter 6 sleep eating was mentioned; food is eaten in a state akin to sleepwalking. Complex adaptive intelligence waits until the conscious mind, which is resisting eating, is asleep, and then takes control of eating behaviors for its objectives. Sleep eating is as an example of what can occur when we resist the pressure, hunger in this instance, being applied to get us to eat more. When we resist our sleep needs, complex adaptive intelligence can also take direct control. People who chronically resist sleeping a sufficient amount experience microsleep— brief periods of sleep lasting from fractions of a second to no more than a minute. The sensation of nodding off in a meeting or while driving, is an example of microsleep. During this brief period the brain is literally, and involuntarily, put to sleep. A person might be, but often isn't, aware that they just went to sleep. Microsleep is an example of the body taking over control of something that is normally volitional. It is a *life finds a way* solution to the challenge encountered when a person is "successful" in resisting sleepiness.

Sleep is self-regulated. Self-regulation implies that complex adaptive intelligence will be trying to find a way to acquire what it feels is important with or without our help. It also implies that the thing in question is decided and controlled for us. We don't get to vote on how much sleep we need; the amount will be determined for us. Each of us will have a specific target range for sleep, which will be adjusted based on circumstances, at least to a degree. This target range isn't the same for everyone and it isn't the same under all circumstances. It is adjustable. We see this with the aging process and average sleep needs.

Table 1: Average Sleep Requirements

Age Group	Sleep Requirements
Infants (ages 3 to 12 months)	14-15 hours
Toddlers (ages 1 to 3 years)	12-14 hours
Preschoolers (ages 3 to 5 years)	11-13 hours
Children (ages 6 to 10 years)	10-11 hours
Early teens (ages 11-17 years)	10-11 hours
Late teens through adulthood	8-9 hours

Averages tell us something about a group, but they don't necessarily tell us about all the individuals in the group. Just like with height, with some humans being tall and others short, there is a natural variance in sleep needs. Some of us will constitutionally be short sleepers; requiring far less sleep than an average person. Others will be long sleepers, needing more than an average amount of sleep. Most of us will be in the middle between these two extremes, closer to the average for our age. While it might be normal for a constitutionally short sleeper to sleep six hours a night, for an average sleeper this amount would be far too little. It would leave them feeling sleepy. Just like with height, where most of us will be close to the average, and very few of us will be seven feet tall, there are very few actual short sleepers—far fewer in fact than the millions of people who claim to sleep fewer than six hours a night. We each have our own set point for sleep, an amount that is normal for us, when it comes to sleep. While this set point is adjustable, we don't get to directly adjust it. Just like with dieting and weight, where we can temporarily get to a scale weight that is lower than our natural weight, most of us can sleep less than the amount we need. But just because we can sleep less doesn't mean it is good for us to sleep less, or that there is not a penalty or cost to us for doing so.

Evidence suggests that a part of our brain keeps track of how much sleep we need, and how much we get. If we need eight hours of sleep and only sleep for seven hours, we wake still owing one hour of sleep. Sleep researchers refer to this hour as *sleep debt;* the sleep the body is still owed. We could, in theory, repay this hour by sleeping an extra hour—nine hours—tonight. If, night after night, we consistently sleep a bit less than our actual sleep needs, sleep debt will accumulate, it will add up. Imagine that we need eight hours of sleep each night to repay sleep debt in full, but only sleep six hours a night Sunday through Thursday nights. In this instance, we would enter the weekend with ten hours of sleep debt. If we don't sleep enough extra hours on the weekend to pay off this debt in full, we start our next workweek still in debt. This debt will be added to any new sleep debt we accrue in the upcoming week. Over the course of a few weeks, if we are neglectful of our sleep needs, we might build up sleep debt equivalent to having missed several nights' worth of sleep.

Unlike our personal finances, where we can save surplus money, the theory of sleep debt predicts that there is no such thing as a surplus of sleep. The sleep account can never run in the black; it can only be in the red or balanced at zero. This means that we can't sleep extra today and save it for a rainy day. We can only fall asleep if we have a sleep debt and we can't stay asleep after the debt reaches zero. This model of sleep debt is an over simplification, with sleep self-regulation like most body functions being far more complex, but it illustrates a key point: Sleep debt appears to be carried over and to build up. Complex adaptive intelligence appears to keep track. It remembers, and it takes steps to make sure the debt is paid off. If all else fails, it will do its best to adapt intelligently.

The Case of Hibernation

Our body is constantly learning and adapting. What might a growing amount of sleep debt be teaching it? What type of adaptations might it cause? To answer these questions we want you to consider a situation in nature that occurs every year—the *Case of Hibernation.* Leading up to the period of winter sleep, weight is gained, almost exclusively as a result of increases in body fat. During the period of hibernation animals enter a state of prolonged sleep and gradually use up these body fat reserves. These two observations—fat accumulation prior to winter sleep and fat depletion during it—are readily observed.

Hibernation is an intelligent adaptation to a real world challenge. It allows animals to survive periods of relative food scarcity and harsher weather. The annual cycle of fattening is, in part, triggered by changes in the *photoperiod* (length of days). Shape Intelligence of a hibernator makes a best guess about how much fat is needed and it acts on this best guess *in advance* of when the extra fat reserves will be needed. Shorter days are the environmental cue that reminds it to set the wheels in motion for fat accumulation. A hibernator's shape change isn't only an issue of eating more food. It involves Shape Intelligence making an intelligent prediction about how much body fat is going to be needed and when it will be needed. It then acts on this prediction whether or not extra food is available. If, during the period leading up to hibernation, sufficient food is available, more food is consumed. The increased food intake makes accumulating massive amounts of extra body fat easier, but it isn't a necessary precondition for getting fatter. A hibernator can gain more body fat leading up to winter sleep even when food intake isn't increased. In fact, it can get fatter during this time period even if it is placed on a diet. If a hibernator is food restricted during the time period when it is preparing for winter sleep, its weight might not increase but its body fat still can. This fat increase occurs at the expense of other aspects of body composition like muscle; with Shape Intelligence robbing Peter to pay Paul, so to speak, by sacrificing muscle weight to build fat stores. This is an intelligent response to what is, frankly, an undesirable situation—a food shortage during the period when extra energy, as body fat, needs to be stored. A hibernator can survive

> **H S I   C L U E**
>
> In hibernators Shape Intelligence uses changes in day length as an integral part of its predictions about how much fat to store, where to store it, and *when* to store it. Winter sleepers defend less body fat as days lengthen and more as days grow shorter. Since the animal's survival relies on this shift in shape, we might infer that this is a highly intelligent thing to do. We might also infer that sleep appears to be intimately related to shape self-regulation.

winter sleep with less muscle but if sufficient fat stores aren't accumulated it has little chance of survival.

A hibernator has a seasonally adjusted set point for fat stores. It is the increase in the set point that is responsible for the fattening leading up to hibernation. The increase in food intake, assuming extra food is available, is an effect of the set point increasing. A bear, as an example, does not get fatter because it is eating too much; it eats more because its Shape Intelligence is directing it to get fatter. This is an important distinction. The amount of body fat being defended is adjusted upward leading into winter sleep; and downward by the end of winter sleep. Because the set point for body fat is lower by the end of hibernation, unlike participants on *Survivor* or dieters who respond as if they are starving when body fat stores are depleted, hibernators awake each spring feeling comfortable at their leaner shape. A hibernator has clear delineations during the year when it regulates its shape quite differently; defending more body fat in preparation for winter sleep, less after it, and easily switching between these two defended levels. In the *Case of Hibernators*, increased food intake leading up to winter sleep is an effect of a sliding natural weight setting; it is not a cause. Shape Intelligence makes changes to its predictions about how much fat it needs and adjusts metabolism, appetite, and other aspects of biology and behavior to ensure it acquires the target amount. The animal does not get fat because it is eating too much and exercising too little. It gets fatter because its Shape Intelligence has temporarily changed the rules of the shape game because getting fatter is essential for survival. After the need for the extra body fat reserves has passed, a leaner shape is defended in the spring and summer.

Hibernation physiology offers an instructive insight into how the defense of a specific natural weight can change seasonally. Shape is not set or unchangeable. It is adjustable and it will be adjusted based upon the circumstances. Shape self-regulation in preparation for hibernation is evidence of an intelligent system adjusting it for a particular purpose—survival. It is also evidence for something else: In a hibernator the self-regulation of sleep and of shape is not two independent and unrelated biological phenomena; they are intricately linked. With that in mind, do you think it is possible that some part of our brain might think that when our sleep debt has grown to a certain point we might pay all of it back by, well, hibernating? And if this were the case, how might it prepare us for this period when we would be expected to be sleeping more? Might it fatten us up?

Scientists have discovered genes for hibernation in humans. This suggests we might have at least a limited ability to hibernate. Humans have also preserved a mechanism for perceiving seasonal changes in day length and for extending sleep duration during periods of long nights. This was seen in a study where volunteers spent fourteen hours in darkness—from 6 pm to 8 am—and 10 hours in light everyday for at least a month. On the first night the volunteers slept for eleven hours. They continued to sleep for extended periods of time for the first several weeks. By about three weeks they settled into a stable routine of two hours of quiet rest, followed by a bit more than four hours of sleep, then another two hour bout of quiet rest, followed by another bout of four plus hours of sleep, and a third bout of quiet rest prior to waking. The net result was eight and a half hours of sleep and a bit less than six hours of quiet rest. Assessments of brainwaves and physiology indicated that the period of quiet rest was a previously uncharacterized physiological state—neither sleep nor waking. This type of split sleep punctuated by quiet rest has been observed in mammals living in the wild during long winter nights. In this study, humans reverted to this quiet rest, sleep, quiet rest, sleep, quiet rest, wake schedule almost as soon as they were placed in an environment with more hours of darkness than light. The volunteers also remarked how refreshed they felt after sleeping in this manner, in effect stating that they had never before felt so awake during the day; findings that were verified by testing. Many languages, including medieval English, have words, which roughly translate as first and second sleep, for this split sleep pattern. Some languages even have words for the quiet rest that punctuates either side of a split sleep period— a rest period often described as something between sleep and waking. The ubiquitous number of languages with words for first and second sleeps suggests that, rather than being unusual, in a pre-industrialized world, a repeating quiet rest-sleep pattern might have been the norm during some parts of the year.

Humans have genes linked to hibernation. We have a mechanism that allows us to extend sleep duration during the same types of environmental cues that trigger hibernation. Using this mechanism appears to leave people feeling more rested. Scientific studies, some of which will be discussed below, indicate that sleep deprivation produces biological and behavioral changes that favor fat accumulation. The *Case of Hibernation* provides the theoretical basis for the interrelated nature of sleep and shape self-regulation. It suggests the observed bio-behavioral changes seen in sleep-deprived persons just might be intelligent and purposeful adaptations.

The Case of Post-Pregnancy Weight Retention

Some woman will have persisting worsening of shape that roughly coincides with having a baby. Many years later, if questioned, they will correctly identify the general time period when shape worsened. When asked why, in almost every instance, pregnancy will be blamed. Pregnancy is a big thing. It is obvious. As such, it's not surprising, given what we discussed in chapter two, that it gets the blame. But is pregnancy really the tipping point in the *Case of Post-pregnancy Weight Retention*? Or is there some other clue that we are missing, something less obvious?

HSI CLUE

Estimates suggest that an average woman accrues four hundred to seven hundred hours of sleep debt during the first year after having a baby. Shape changes that occur in the time period around pregnancy are usually blamed on pregnancy. Could this growing sleep debt be contributing?

There is little doubt that becoming pregnant changes a woman's shape and produces weight gain. In fact, pregnancy offers a vivid example of Shape Intelligence in action, temporarily shifting a woman's shape for a defined and intelligent purpose—reproduction. Pregnancy-induced shape changes begin to reverse themselves immediately following delivery. This makes sense: There is little reason for Shape Intelligence to keep the shape changes that were only required to support having a baby after a woman has had the baby. What Shape Intelligence gives, the pregnancy shape, it subsequently takes away when there is no longer an intelligent reason for it. As a result, many women will have a shape and weight very similar to the one they had prior to becoming pregnant one year after giving birth. But some women will weigh 20, 30, or 40 pounds more one year after having a baby than they did prior to becoming pregnant. Medicine views this as having *retained* the weight they gained during pregnancy. Why didn't Shape Intelligence take away the weight gained during pregnancy once it was no longer needed for reproduction? Or did it take it away?

Many of the women who experience so called weight retention no longer look pregnant. They might retain weight; they don't retain a pregnancy shape. This is an important clue. While they might weigh more, and in some cases much more than they did before becoming pregnant, they often won't be confused with being a pregnant woman. How can this be explained? What if pregnancy weight were being shed at roughly the same time that some new factor was causing natural weight to increase? If this occurred, it would be tempting to view the weight as being retained, because the changes would be canceling themselves out, yet in reality, the new factor, not pregnancy, would be the real cause. Do women, in general, and women who weigh much more after pregnancy than prior to it, face any novel challenges during this post-pregnancy time period that might require shape adaptations?

Let's return to the NSF 2007 Survey of Women mentioned earlier in this chapter. Only about one out of four women of childbearing age in this survey claimed to experience more than a few nights a month of poor sleep. While that is by no means a trivial amount, it paled when compared to pregnancy. Forty percent of women claimed to have many nights of poor sleep during pregnancy. The picture was bleaker during the postpartum period; 55 percent of women claimed to experience many nights a month of poor sleep after having a child. These results are not surprising. New parents, especially new mothers, rarely get enough sleep. Some new mothers get one to two hours less sleep than needed most nights during the first five months after delivery. They often continue to get fewer hours of sleep than they require, getting 30 to 60 minutes less sleep than needed, until the baby is two years old. The result can be a sleep debt that rapidly grows into the hundreds and hundreds of hours. During the tail end of pregnancy, and even more so after pregnancy, Shape Intelligence encounters a new challenge—chronic sleep deprivation.

> **HSI CLUE**
>
> A study called Project Viva investigated women's sleep one year after giving birth to their children. The women who were sleeping the fewest hours six months after having a baby were significantly more likely to weigh much more one year after delivery than they weighed prior to becoming pregnant.

Could post-pregnancy weight retention be, at least in part, caused by lack of sleep? One recent study identified a relationship between the amounts of sleep women get during this postpartum time period and how much they weigh a year after delivering their baby. The women who slept the fewest hours were the ones most likely to have failed to return to their pre-pregnancy weight. They were the weight retainers. The relationship observed in this study suggests the possibility of a vastly different explanation for post-pregnancy weight retention. The real culprit might not be pregnancy; it might be lack of sleep. If sleep is to blame, a sensible solution is to sleep more. While this area requires more research, we have observed cases where new mothers, who were struggling with regaining their pre-pregnancy shape, experienced a tipping point of sorts, in a positive direction, once they began to get as much sleep as they needed.

The Case of Sleep Apnea

Tens of millions of North Americans suffer from sleep disorders, one of the most common of which is sleep disordered breathing (SDB). SDB is a continuum of sleep disorders characterized by breathing difficulties during sleep. Snoring is a mild form of SDB. Sleep apnea, a condition characterized by pauses in breathing during sleep, is a more severe form. A person with sleep apnea stops breathing many times during the night, with each interruption fragmenting sleep and interfering with the ability to get a good nights' sleep. Estimates suggest that 10 to 20 percent of adults have sleep apnea. The vast majority of affected individuals, perhaps as many as nine out of ten, go undiagnosed and untreated. One of the most consistent historical observations in persons with sleep apnea has been that many of them are overweight or obese. Extra weight is often blamed as being the cause of sleep apnea. Is it?

While many overweight or obese individuals will have sleep apnea, others will not. And while most normal weight individuals will not have sleep apnea, a fair number will. So weight tells us something about group risk for sleep apnea, but its precision leaves a lot to be desired for individuals. Shape appears to do a better job predicting who will and won't have sleep apnea, but still suffers from lack of precision. This is not the case with visceral fat. In one study the amount of abdominal visceral fat was able to predict who was a simple snorer and who had sleep apnea with one hundred percent accuracy. In another study, individuals above a certain amount of visceral fat all had sleep apnea. More than simply being related to weight or shape, sleep apnea appears to quite specifically be related to visceral body fat. Is the increased visceral body fat causing sleep apnea? Is the sleep apnea causing an increase in visceral fat? Or do we have more of a chicken and an egg situation?

It's certainly plausible that weight and visceral fat are contributing to sleep apnea. It is also possible that sleep apnea is causing gains in visceral fat, and hence weight. And it just might be that both circumstances are occurring simultaneously and that additional factors are involved. What is known is that as individuals progress along the continuum of sleep disordered breathing, from snoring to mild sleep apnea to severe sleep apnea, on average, massive amounts of weight are gained. Sleep apnea also predicts future weight gain. A person with untreated sleep apnea, compared to a person of equal weight, is far more likely to gain weight over the next year. In this case, sleep apnea appears to precede weight gain, which suggests that it might be causing the increase in natural weight. Presumably this is because the struggle to sleep is causing severely fragmented sleep, and as a result the affected person does not get enough sleep during the night to meet their needs no matter how long they are in bed.

> **HSI CLUE**
>
> In the year leading up to a diagnosis of sleep apnea men and women in one study gained a massive amount of weight (on average 14-19 pounds each). Most of the weight was fat. People of a similar weight without sleep apnea had stable weights over the year. This evidence suggests that sleep apnea came *before* weight gain. It might have been causing it.

If sleep debt were causing shape changes in a person with sleep apnea, we would expect to see treatments that allowed a person to sleep better to improve aspects of shape. Do we? The medical treatment for sleep apnea is an apparatus that supplies continuous positive airway pressure (CPAP) during sleep. CPAP does not cure a person of sleep apnea; it allows them to breathe more normally and as a result to sleep better, and hence, pay off sleep debt more efficiently. Does therapy with CPAP affect shape? In scientific studies regular CPAP use tends to melt away visceral body fat. It gets rid of the very thing that has the strongest relationship with severe sleep disordered breathing, hmmm. This suggests that sleep apnea, and perhaps other sleep disorders might be hidden causes of worsening shape or increased body fatness. It also suggests the possibility that part of the solution to improving shape, if sleep quality is an issue, just might be getting the appropriate therapies that will allow us to sleep better.

Cases of Intentional Sleep Deprivation

The most direct evidence that lack of sleep can cause unwanted shape changes is from the clues left when scientists have intentionally sleep-deprived volunteers—*Cases of Intentional Sleep Deprivation.* Total sleep deprivation for one to a few days causes measurable changes in information molecules related to shape self-regulation (leptin, ghrelin, and insulin). These changes are in a fattening direction. Appetite also increases substantially with just a single night of sleep deprivation. Recovery from this acute sleep loss reverses these metabolic and appetite changes. These changes, and their subsequent reversal, are exactly what we would expect if Shape Intelligence had decided to defend more body fat with the sleep loss, and then changed its mind after the sleep debt was repaid. Longer-term partial sleep deprivation studies have observed similar clues.

HSI CLUE

When people are deliberately deprived of sleep during research experiments, they initially notice the effects on their alertness, mood, physical performance, and sleepiness. After a few days they get used to feeling sleepy—they adapt—and being tired feels normal. Because of this tendency to get used to not getting enough sleep, most of us are very poor judges of how tired we really are.

In partial sleep deprivation studies volunteers spend a few days to a few weeks in sleep laboratories during which time sleep is permitted but limited. Participants might be allowed as few as four hours and as much as six hours of sleep each night. In the studies conducted to date, changes in biology and behavior suggestive of a decision to increase natural weight have been reported. Information molecules related to shape—insulin, leptin, and ghrelin—change in a direction associated with fat accumulation, appetite and hunger generally increase, and people increase their intake of calorie-dense foods and snacks, especially at night. These changes would be expected to promote weight and fat gains if they were maintained over time. They are reversed when volunteers are allowed to extend sleep sufficiently to repay the sleep debt accrued during the nights of partial sleep deprivation. This means that the changes in biology and behavior that result from six nights of sleeping only four hours a night, are corrected when the volunteers are subsequently allowed to sleep twelve hours a night for six nights. This is compelling evidence.

Two studies presented at SLEEP 2009—the annual meeting of the Associated Professional Sleep Societies—provided even more compelling evidence for the fattening effects of partial sleep deprivation. In the first of these studies researchers had 92 adults spend two nights of unrestricted sleep (10 hours in bed), followed by five nights of restricted sleep (4 hours in bed), and then four nights of 10 hours in bed. During the 11 days of this study, weight increased on average by about three pounds. A group of well-rested control subjects did not experience any weight gain over the same 11 days. In the second study nine overweight volunteers spent five and one half hours in bed for one two-week period (partial sleep deprivation) and eight and one half hours in bed for another two-week period (full night of sleep). At least three months separated each of these two experimental periods. During both study periods participants were fed a moderately calorie restricted diet. The short-term calorie restriction resulted in weight loss, with similar amounts of average weight loss during both the partial sleep deprivation and full night of sleep conditions. Body fat was also monitored and revealed an important finding that would not have been detected if weight alone had been measured. When allowed to be in bed for 8 plus hours a night during two weeks of moderate calorie restriction, 57 percent of the lost weight was body fat. During the two weeks of partial sleep deprivation, although these participants lost a similar amount of weight, only 26 percent of it was body fat. Equivalent calorie restriction caused similar losses of weight no matter how much (or little) time was allowed for sleep in this experiment, but during the two weeks of partial sleep deprivation far more of the weight loss was muscle and much less of it was fat. Sleep deprivation seemed to cause the body to cling more tightly to fat.

Cases of Intentional Sleep Deprivation provide direct evidence that getting insufficient sleep affects aspects of the bio-behavioral system involved in shape self-regulation. All of these changes are in directions that would make us highly susceptible to fat accumulation. The evidence also informs us that a significant reduction in sleep time results, on average, in some degree of weight gain and that this weight gain can show up quickly. Lastly, observations indicate that weight might not be the best clue for what is truly going on under circumstances of sustained sleep inadequacy. Body fat appears to be far more impacted than weight by partial sleep deprivation. The totality of evidence suggests that lack of sleep might cause Shape Intelligence to alter its decision about what shape to defend. It learns and adapts, updating its body fat predictions, and as a result we might just end up fatter than we were before we experienced a period of less sleep. While this is bad news, clues from *Cases of Intentional Sleep Deprivation* also offer hope.

In the studies that have allowed the participants to extend sleep sufficiently, to fully repay the accumulated sleep debt, the obesogenic bio-behavioral changes caused by partial sleep deprivation are reversed. Information molecules, appetite, and food behaviors return to what they were prior to the period of partial sleep deprivation. The studies, which have extended sleep duration to allow for complete recovery from partial sleep deprivation, are encouraging. They suggest that the changes in our biology and behavior caused by sleep deprivation are correctable if sleep hours are extended sufficiently to repay the outstanding sleep debt in full. Could extending sleep duration also reverse any shape changes caused by lack of sleep? Scientific studies have not been conducted to answer this question. Some experts have called for these type of controlled studies; studies designed to measure the effect of sleep-promoting interventions on appetite and shape.

While formal studies have not been completed yet, our client case files suggest they would observe transformative shifts in shape and appetite occurring after a person starts to sleep as much as their body allows. An informal "test" conducted by *Glamour* magazine in 2009 also provides support for the power sleeping more might have to positively affect our shapes. Sleep experts helped seven women make over their sleep habits. The goal was to find out whether getting more sleep could make a difference in the shapes of these women. The women were asked to make one simple change—get at least seven and a half hours of sleep every night. They did not restrict calories, follow any elaborate diet, or dramatically increase the amount they exercised. In fact, they were asked to keep their diets and exercise habits the same. Did getting more sleep change the shape of these women? In the words of Jenny Stamos Kovacs (the author of the *Glamour* magazine article) "Did it ever! Week by week, we were amazed by the results the women reported. At the end of 10 weeks, the six of the seven participants had dropped between six and fifteen pounds. These were not the only changes. One of the women had "shaved almost five inches off her waist, hips, bust and thighs—even though, at 5'4" and 133 pounds, she wasn't overweight to begin with." Another woman (Natasha Crawford), even though she was only able to meet the goal of sleeping at least seven and a half hours a night a few nights a week, "…still lost a total of two and a half inches off her waist, bust and hips." These are dramatic changes: Sleeping more seemed to be a tipping point for shape improvement. Would faster or greater results have been observed if they had extended sleep duration even more? What might have occurred if they had actually hibernated? We don't have the answers to these questions, but we do encourage you to run your own experiment—extend your sleep hours—and find the answers for yourself and your shape.

Solutions

William Dement, MD, is the founder and director of the Stanford University Sleep Research Center. He is also the author of a book titled *The Promise of Sleep*. Dement is a leading authority on sleep. He has reported that four out of five undergraduate, nursing, and medical students sampled at Stanford University are severely sleep deprived. His findings appear to be a microcosm of a larger epidemic sweeping North America: The vast majority of us are not getting enough sleep. In his work, Dement mentions that in most instances the accumulation of a massive sleep debt happens so gradually that the persons it is affecting completely misses the boat on the cause of their sleepiness and fatigue. They mistakenly blame their tiredness on all manners of other things—a virus, depression, overwork, stress, and getting older, as examples. They seem to look everywhere in search of an explanation, but miss the mark on the real issue; the issue being that they have been chronically sleeping a bit less than their body really needs. This matches our experience. The changes in energy levels, daytime performance, health and shape that result from too little sleep are easily blamed on the wrong things. If we were to focus specifically on shape and weight, the changes that sleep deprivation cause don't always jump right out at us after a few days or even weeks of getting insufficient sleep. They can be incremental and easily missed changes. They tend to affect body fat more than weight. And even those who notice a change in shape occurring tend to focus on obvious facts—increases in appetite and how much food is eaten, both of which, as mentioned, can be effects of sleep debt.

We notice that we are getting fatter and realize we are craving starchy snacks and fattening foods. We see that we are consuming more calories. And we blame the change in our shape on what we are eating and on our lack of willpower to resist fattening food. But in this case of insufficient sleep, the root problem is not eating more. Eating more is an effect; an effect caused by a sleep quantity or quality problem. We are not getting fatter because we are eating more; we are eating more because our body is trying to get fatter. And, while this is a subtle difference, it is a vitally important difference. Correcting this issue isn't a matter of eating less; it is a matter of sleeping more.

HSI CLUE

Several quotes from the participants in the *Glamour* magazine article give clues to the power of sleep. One participant stated, "My stomach is getting flatter and my love handles smaller." Another said, "The changes in my body fascinate me, because I really haven't changed anything except my sleep habits. I eat the way I always have and exercise the same amount, maybe even less because my schedule is tighter now that I have to go to bed earlier!"

Most of us woefully underestimate how much sleep we need: We need more than we think we need. Daytime sleepiness is a clue that we need more sleep; its absence is not a reliable clue that we don't. Just because we don't feel sleepy, doesn't mean we don't need more sleep. In health scenes we have investigated, we routinely discover that people are relatively disconnected from how sleepy they really are. One reason for this is that we adapt to chronic sleep deprivation quickly. After a few days of being slightly sleep deprived, feeling a bit sleepy starts to feel normal. If slight sleep deprivation continues, our body might feel the need to rise to the occasion, so to speak, and adapt in ways that allows us to sleep fewer hours. While our body's ability to adapt will allow us to function with fewer hours of sleep, part of this adaptation might be an increase in body fat. We won't be feeling as sleepy as we probably should, but the cost for not feeling our true sleepiness is paid by our shape. Sleepiness, in our experience, can figuratively be put in a closet—hidden away—so that we can make it through our days and won't be pulled out until we start to sleep more.

Another reason that people can be disconnected from their sleepiness is that many things can mask it, hiding it from us. We can live a life propped up by caffeine, stimulants, or nervous energy, and, as a result, won't fully experience the depth of our sleepiness until caffeine is unavailable, the stimulant is stopped, or the weekend or a vacation comes. We all know people who can't function without coffee, or who sleep much more on a weekend than during the workweek, or while on a vacation from work or break from school. These are strong clues that we have some sleep debt to repay even if we might not normally feel sleepy. While these clues, as well as others, can provide valuable insights into whether lack of sleep is an issue, the most reliable clue is whether sleep can be extended. The general rule of thumb is that if a person can sleep more, they need more sleep.

Sleep researchers have consistently found that almost everyone, whether they consider themselves sleep deprived or not, has no problem sleeping more than their habitual amount if they allow themselves to. This is strong evidence that our accustomed amount of sleep isn't enough. Many of us will have an ability to sleep for extended periods of time, and when we do, we will feel much more sleepy than normal. We blame the extra sleepiness we feel on getting more sleep. We think that getting more sleep is *making* us sleepy. This is a misinterpretation. It would be like thinking that drinking more water when we are thirsty makes us thirstier. A better interpretation is that the extra sleep is unmasking a problem the body has been working hard to cover up. The prevailing theory is that it is physiologically impossible to sleep too much. If you can sleep, you need sleep. Sleep can never run in the black; it can only run in the red. So sleeping more can't make a person sleepy; it can only repay existing sleep debt.

Our body is a complex adaptive system. In our experience it can adapt to chronic sleep deprivation by hiding our sleepiness from us until it feels like it is a *good time* to catch up. This good time is days when we get more sleep. Feeling much sleepier after sleeping more than our habitual amount is a signal that there is still more sleep debt to repay; quite often a large amount more. If we accrued a large sleep debt from months or years of sleeping less than we need, it will not go away with a few good nights' sleep, any more than hunger went away in the volunteers in the Minnesota Experiment with a few big meals. Just as hunger did not normalize until weight had been regained and body fat was approximately 40 percent higher than pre-calorie restriction, sleepiness persists, and often increases, once we begin to repay sleep debt in earnest.

Let's return to Dement, the renowned sleep expert. What solution does he offer to his sleep deprived students? In a nutshell, Dement instructs them to get as much extra sleep as possible. If they are in the habit of sleeping for seven hours a night and think they probably need eight, he might ask them to sleep for ten. He asks them to do this for as many nights as it takes till they cannot sleep for ten hours any more. At this point, they might only be able to sleep for nine hours a night, so now the homework becomes sleep nine hours a night. At some point, students who follow these simple instructions reach a point where daytime sleepiness and feelings of fatigue vanish; and are replaced by a feeling of being wide awake and alert all day long. The crux of Dement's advice is straightforward. To pay off sleep debt a person should get as much extra sleep as possible.

In a sense, paying off sleep debt is no different than paying off a large credit card bill. We can't pay off past credit card debt by only keeping pace with the amounts we are spending now. We have to pay off more than we are spending to make headway.

Our advice is identical to Dement's: Sleep for more hours than you habitually do. Ideally sleep for as many hours as your body will allow. If your schedule permits, and your body allows, sleep for 14 hours a night. Continue to do this until your body won't allow you to sleep for extended durations. In our experience a person with low sleep debt totals might catch up in a few weeks. They won't be able to still sleep for 10 hours a night much less 14. A person with a mountain of sleep debt might not be all caught up even after a few months.

To extend sleep durations we want to allow our body to fall into a sleep cycle when sleepiness first occurs. Falling asleep earlier than normal is often a matter of catching the natural windows of opportunity when the body is primed for sleep. We refer to this as *catching the sleep bus*. The opportunity for sleep seems to come like a bus, arriving at certain times and leaving at certain times. If we get on, we'll fall asleep. If we miss this bus, we might need to wait for the next one to arrive. The sleep bus does not always pull into the station, so to speak, and park there. It can come and it can leave without us. If we miss the sleep bus, we might have to wait for the

HSI CLUE

The "Sleep Diet" used in *Glamour* Magazine included:
1. Get a *minimum* of 7½ hours of sleep every night
2. If your schedule allows, sleep even more.
3. Go to bed and wake up at the same time each day.
4. Begin preparing for sleep at least 45 minutes before you plan on closing your eyes by doing some type of relaxing pre-sleep activity. TVs, computers, cell phones, etc. should be turned off and lights dimmed.
5. No caffeine after 2:30 pm and no alcohol for at least three hours before bedtime.

next bus to arrive, which in our experience might be one to two hours later. Allowing ourselves to go to sleep when the sleep bus makes its first stop for the night can entail preparing for and going to sleep earlier than we might ideally desire. If we are serious about repaying sleep debt, it is critical that we catch an earlier sleep bus. If we experience sleepiness at 9:30 p.m., the time to go to bed, to get on the bus, is 9:30 p.m. If we miss this first opportunity for sleep, the next sleep bus might not arrive until after 11 pm. Getting on this later bus might not allow us to sleep the extended hours we need to before our morning commitments call us.

We mentioned that there have not been any scientific studies on what happens to shape if a person follows this type of protocol—when they, in a sense, hibernate. Some experts have called for these types of controlled studies; but none have been conducted yet. Can a large sleep debt cause an increase in body fatness? Can repaying this debt reverse this change? These questions have not been scientifically answered. Theories in this area are unproven. But just because it is unproven, does not mean you have to wait. You can run your own experiment now. Many of our clients have run experiments similar to what Dement suggests. They have put aside notions that the need for sleep is some form of weakness. They have slept more; more than they thought they could or should sleep. In many instances this one change has been a tipping point to a better shape (and resulted in improvement in many other areas including work, school, exercise performance, and health).

HSI CLUE

One study observed that people who habitually slept the fewest hours were 5 times more likely to have signs and symptoms of eating disorders than were people who habitually slept for longer amounts of time each night. This evidence suggests that signs and symptoms of eating disorders might be a clue that a person is not getting sufficient sleep.

While extending sleep duration is appropriate for inadequate sleep occurring because of neglect, medical support is often required if a person has a sleep quality disorder (such as sleep apnea). If you have any suspicions that you might have a sleep quality issue, discuss this topic with your physician. Trying to improve shape while having untreated sleep apnea, as an example, is a recipe for disappointment. With appropriate treatment, and better sleep, improving shape isn't such an uphill struggle.

To summarize, evidence suggests that it is possible that something about not getting enough sleep might cause our body to defend more fat—increase its natural weight. Appetite and metabolism change to make getting fatter easier. Body fat accumulation seems to become easier in a similar manner to what occurs in a hibernator in the fat accumulation phase of hibernation. Visceral fat tissue might be particularly susceptible to increasing when sleep is inadequate. We have observed cases of sleep-deprived individuals getting fatter despite their best efforts at eating well and exercising appropriately. And we have seen a reversal in this struggle once they began to get more, or better quality, sleep. If Shape Intelligence is defending more body fat because we are sleep deprived, the path to shape improvement is addressing the real issue: The solution, in this case, is to extend the amount of time spent sleeping, it is to, in a word, hibernate.

Closing Dialogue

Apprentice: I always knew that sleep was important; I just had no idea how important.

Health Scene Investigator: You are not alone. Most of what science knows about sleep has been learned in the past 25 years. Most of what has been learned about the interrelationship between sleep and shape has been discovered within the past decade. And there is still much to learn. Let's return to my earlier question. You had a period in your past when, over a few months, you observed a significant worsening of your shape. What was your sleep like then?

Apprentice: Looking back at my health scene now, it is apparent that I was not getting sufficient sleep. In fact, this period was the one time in my life when I slept the fewest hours. Do you think extending my sleep now might help?

Health Scene Investigator: It just might. It is certainly an experiment worth running. Now let's move onto another vital area…our body clock and its interactions with shape.

Chapter 12

Lighting and Shape

Everything comes in circles—even Professor Moriarty... It's all been done before, and will be again.

Sherlock Holmes

Opening Dialogue

Health Scene Investigator: What would happen if you went food shopping on your way to work for the day?

Apprentice: Much of the food I purchased would likely spoil.

Health Scene Investigator: And what would occur if you consistently dropped your daughter off at school at noon instead of at 8 a.m.?

Apprentice: She and I would both get in trouble with the school.

Health Scene Investigator: Exactly as I suspected...very important clues.

Apprentice: I must be missing something. I don't understand why those questions are important for investigating a health scene.

Health Scene Investigator: What you just related to me was that when you do the correct things—buying food and dropping your daughter at school—at the wrong time, it creates a mess; spoiled food and school troubles, specifically. Timing is important in our daily lives; it is no less important for our body. Because of this we want to know what occurs. We also want to know when it occurs. Let me explain.

Everything Comes in Circles

In *the Valley of Fear* Holmes tells us that everything comes in circles. We see evidence of this in nature. Cycles of day and night, waxing and waning of the moon, and seasonal changes are examples of things that come full circle at different time scales. Human physiology is intimately connected to these naturalistic cycles. It has a day and a night, a waxing and waning, and different seasons. It is in perpetual motion, constantly changing, but changing in a way that repeats at predictable time intervals. It's all been done before and will be done again. This principle, rhythmic change, can be seen with weight.

HSI CLUE

Sleep-wake cycles are one example of a rhythm that repeats every 24 hours. Blood pressure, cholesterol, pulse rate, temperature, pH, metabolism, immune function, bone remodeling, and detoxification are different in the day than the night. Women have robust monthly rhythms and all of us have annual biological rhythms. Shape self-regulation also has a rhythm; it repeats daily, monthly (in menstruating women) and over the course of a year.

Our weight does not stay constant; it constantly fluctuates. The daily fluctuations in weight were used for humorous purposes in Helen Fielding's book *Bridget Jones's Diary*. Bridget's March 7th diary entry was as follows: "130, 128, or 131 lbs.?? Aargh. How can I have put on 3 lbs. since the middle of the night? I was 130 when I went to bed, 128 at 4 a.m. and 131 when I got up." While Bridget's weight fluctuations on this night might not be typical, fluctuations of weight within a few pounds over the course of 24 hours are normal. They also follow a repetitive pattern. We generally weigh more at night than during the day. The same rhythm holds for body composition; there are small but detectable and consistent day-night rhythms in muscle tissue, body fat, and water weight. In all of these areas, amounts increase as we move towards and into night and decrease during the day. In women, if we continued to observe weight over the course of several months, we would detect another rhythm—a menstrual cycle rhythm. Weight increases detectably during the premenstrual phase, reaches a peak during the first half of menstruation, and declines post menstruation. If we were to stretch our observations out even longer we would detect an annual rhythm. Weight tends to increase as days shorten and decrease as days lengthen. The high point of this annual weight rhythm coincides with the holiday season in the Northern hemisphere. Bridget experienced this seasonal rhythm.

On January 1st she weighed 129 lbs; noting in her diary this was "post-Christmas." Over the course of the year she loses and gains lots of weight, but when the holidays arrive once again, we find her back at her peak weight—a weight of 131 lbs. It's all been done before, and will be again.

There are subtle, yet perceptible, differences that can be detected over the course of a day, a month (in menstruating women), and a year in shape and metabolism. We have a day and a night shape, and a winter and summer shape. These shape differences cycle. They repeat like clockwork, or in the case of yearly changes, like calendar work. Human function is intimately and inextricably entwined with rhythms, layered one on top of another. Figuratively speaking, we are clocks and calendars.

Human Clocks and Calendars

To fully understand human function it is not sufficient to look at the *what*. We must also understand the *when*, the timing or rhythm of things. Almost every important function in our body has at least one rhythm; many have multiple rhythms. The most studied biological rhythms are *circadian rhythms*—rhythms with a period of about 24 hours. These are not our only rhythms; we also have rhythms that repeat on both shorter and longer time scales. Annual rhythms represent one of these longer biological rhythms.

The hypothalamus—the same part of our brain involved in self-regulation of thirst, appetite, sleep, activity, temperature regulation, sex drives, and shape—is the location of a group of neurons that act as a 24-hour biological clock. Many experts believe that this group of neurons acts somewhat like a *master body clock* for circadian rhythms. Daily changes in lighting conditions orient this body clock in time. If our eyes are exposed to correctly timed light and darkness, the master body clock synchronizes our body, and all of its functions, to the sun's schedule. If we are exposed to bright light late at night and darkness in the morning this body clock orients itself differently in time. Changes in lighting are also the critical external signal used by calendar mechanisms, which are at least in part located in our pineal gland. As was discussed in the *Case of Hibernation* (chapter 11), changes in length of days—photoperiod—are used by hibernators to anticipate what changes might be needed in physiology and behavior, and to initiate these changes in advance of when they are required. External lighting conditions are used as ways to orient both human body clock and body calendar functions in time, and to shift aspects of our physiology in ways that best match the particular time of the day and year.

HSI CLUE

Some people are morning people; others are night people. Many of us fall somewhere in the middle. In one study of persons with bipolar disorder, night people were significantly fatter than day people. What could our preferences for when we are awake and asleep have to do with how fat we are? Night people are also at a higher risk for some diseases, and shifting to a day schedule tends to improve the health of night people. Why?

Lighting conditions have profound effects on physiology. This can be seen in the *Case of Polycystic Ovarian Syndrome*. Polycystic Ovarian Syndrome (PCOS) is the most common hormonal disorder among women of reproductive age, estimated to affect five to ten percent of women. This syndrome was unknown prior to 1935. It appears to be a 20th century health issue. PCOS has very strong associations with shape. Women with this syndrome, no matter what their weight, usually have proportionately high amounts of belly fat. Like most complex health problems PCOS is almost certainly a multi-factorial problem, with aspects of diet, lifestyle, and the environment interacting in unique ways with individual genetics to determine whether and how women will experience this syndrome. It is, like many chronic degenerative conditions we face today, complicated. Lighting conditions are one of the complicating factors. Scientific studies in animals provide direct evidence of the role light and lighting might play in PCOS. Constant lighting will produce polycystic ovaries, as well as signs and symptoms consistent with this syndrome, in several different types of animals. In animals that are very susceptible because of their genetics, as little as 14 hours of continuous lighting a day will trigger this condition. Evidence has also indicated that removing aspects of the calendar tracking ability (pineal gland) makes animals susceptible to polycystic ovaries. Lighting conditions are an environmental tipping point for PCOS in some animals: Whether the same might be true for humans has yet to be investigated.

PCOS is not alone, lighting conditions can influence cancer in animals. In the *Cases of the Implanted Cancer* scientists took breast cancer cells and grafted them onto laboratory rats. They divided these rats into two groups. One group was placed in an environment with 12 hours each of light and darkness every day. The other group was placed under continuous light for 24 hours a day. They lacked one thing—darkness. The lack of darkness produced by constant light exposure caused the breast cancer cells to grow much faster. In another similar experiment two groups of rats were exposed to normal lighting conditions during the day; however, one group was exposed to darkness at night and the other group lived in dim light conditions during normal darkness hours. Compared to the constant light in the previous experiment, dim light seems like a relative trifle: It was anything but. Failure to get darkness, even if lights were dimmed at night, resulted in cancer growing at a faster rate and far fewer of the rats surviving cancer.

In these animal studies, and others like them, lighting conditions were a tipping point which made a big difference in whether PCOS occurred, cancer grew, and even whether the animals survived or died from cancer. The effects of lighting are not limited to animals. Circumstantial and direct evidence suggests that it influences human health. The *Case of Digestion* is an example. Two scientific studies on our ability to digest food under different lighting conditions were conducted. In one, volunteers were exposed to either bright or dim light conditions, while the researchers measured the volunteers' ability to digest a meal. The bright lighting conditions had a beneficial effect on digestion. In the other study, volunteers were again exposed to bright or dim light conditions. This time digestion was better with dim light exposure. Why did the same *what*—bright and dim light—produce opposite results? The answer is because the *when* of it changed. In the first study the volunteers were exposed to either bright or dim light from 7 in the morning till 3 in the afternoon. They either were (with bright light) or weren't (with dim light) exposed to naturalistic lighting conditions. In the second study the *when* was changed. The volunteers were exposed to bright or dim light conditions from 5 at night until bedtime. This time dim light produced the more naturalistic lighting conditions. Bright light was not always helpful for digestion, nor was dim light always harmful. The important variable was whether or not the lighting conditions

HSI CLUE

Many of us live lives characterized by light pollution. We rarely experience sunrise and sunset, and are inside under artificial lighting during most of our days. Much of the light exposure we do get is poorly timed: We might not get enough bright light in the morning, but get too much at night. Sleep environments might never get completely dark. When it comes to lighting conditions, we have changed our environment, and as a result, it is changing us.

were evolutionarily appropriate for that time of day. In the *Case of Digestion* it wasn't just what was done that mattered; it was when it was done.

Lighting conditions have been linked to cancer, heart disease, and other chronic health problems. There is abundant direct evidence that lighting affects (1) sleep, (2) mood, (3) circadian rhythms, (4) appetite, and (5) metabolic function. What can we infer from the evidence? The clues tell us one thing unambiguously: The *what* and the *when* of lighting conditions are powerful environmental influences on human function and health. Light and darkness might seem trivial: They aren't. We are clocks and calendars. The health and shape outcomes we produce are clock and calendar dependent. It is important that the correct biological events occur; it is equally as important that they occur at the correct time and in the proper sequence. Timing matters and lighting conditions play a disproportionately large role in timing.

The Principle of Synchronization

Scientific studies suggest that the group of neurons in the hypothalamus—*light-sensitive* circadian pacemaker—is not our only 24-hour clock. Many tissues in the body keep time, including the liver, heart, stomach, and fat cells. They also shift the tasks they do in a time-dependent manner. The liver, as an example, prioritizes certain biological activities in the early morning and others late at night. The same is true of bone remodeling. Processes that remove old bone dominate during dark hours; processes that add new bone dominate during daylight hours. Time dependency occurs with many hormones—cortisol and melatonin serving as examples. Adrenal glands release high amounts of cortisol between 7 and 9 a.m., and very low amounts during darkness hours. Cortisol's peak punctuates the start of daytime physiology, readying us to face the day. Melatonin is on a roughly opposite schedule, with high amounts released by the pineal gland between 10 p.m. and midnight and little released during daylight hours. It is a darkness hormone, signaling the onset of nighttime physiology. The schedule of both of these hormones is influenced by lighting conditions. These are not isolated examples: They are the tip of the iceberg when it comes to circadian changes in human physiology.

Tissues and systems in the body schedule some tasks at certain times and others at other times. Since our body is a whole system, not separate and independent parts, what one tissue or system does, and when it does it, affects other aspects of the whole. Because of this, it isn't sufficient for the liver to schedule and perform all of its tasks independent of what is occurring elsewhere in the body. Some of what it does might need to be coordinated with bone remodeling. If it isn't, its jobs and bone remodeling both suffer. The same principle applies to timing with respect to cortisol, melatonin, or any other timed function in the body. Healthy function isn't simply a matter of doing the right thing; it is a matter of doing it at the correct time with respect to every other biologically relevant event. This requires coordination; it requires being in sync. And being in sync is a matter of setting all of our different body clocks to the same biological time.

The importance of timing is apparent in the *Case of the Timed Hormones*. Two groups of female hamsters with a genetic tendency to obesity were placed in constant lighting conditions for ten days and then lived the next ten weeks under short day length conditions—10 hours of light and 14 hours of darkness—while allowed free access to food. This lighting and darkness schedule is sufficient to cause these hamsters to become obese; indicating the power lighting conditions can have over shape. But the scientists took an additional step in this study. During the first ten days both groups received daily injections of two hormones—cortisol and prolactin. One group was injected with prolactin immediately after getting a shot of cortisol; the other group got their prolactin injection 12 hours after the cortisol shots. In this case, the same hormones were given; the only difference was when one was given with respect to the other. What happened? The group that received the injections of these two hormones timed together remained lean. The other group became, from a hamster perspective, physically and metabolically obese. Under the lighting conditions used in this experiment, altering the timing of one hormone with respect to another produced completely different shape results and the results persisted long after the experiment had ceased.

HSI CLUE

Synchronization of biology and behavior with the environment allows a living organism to anticipate periodic events, such as the appearance of darkness or winter, and to engage in appropriate changes *before* the external conditions have shifted. Perhaps nowhere is this as visible as with body fat regulation within migratory animals or animals that engage in hibernation; animals whose survival absolutely requires shifts in their shape in anticipation of periodic environmental changes.

HSI CLUE

The timing of appetite can be a vital clue to rhythm synchronization. When our 24-hour rhythms are in sync, appetite is synchronized to naturalistic light-dark cycles. We wake early in the sun's day and experience significant appetite within 30 to 60 minutes after waking. A robust morning appetite is a clue that our body clock is in sync. Having little to no appetite in the morning, but being hungry late at night, is a clue that rhythms are out of sync.

Timing of biological events matters in animals; it also matters in humans. But just because timing is important doesn't mean things always stay in sync. The science of biological rhythms refers to a situation where physiological events are mistimed as *internal desynchronization*. Disruption of tissue timing can occur when food intake, sleep cycles, or timing of light exposure are suddenly altered. Rotating shift work can cause internal desynchronization. Flying across multiple time zones disrupts timing of biological events. Jet lag experienced after these trips is due to the abrupt change away from our normal reference point for time, and the resultant confusion in timing this produces. Shift work and frequent travel are associated with elevated risk for many diseases, presumably, in part, because they disrupt timing— they are a severe form of *body clock stress*. Shift work also has strong associations with weight gain. The *Case of Intentionally Disrupting Timing* suggests that these links are more than coincidental.

One of the most powerful methods for disrupting the coordination of biological timing is to drastically alter when we eat, sleep, or are exposed to light/darkness. In this case, instead of eating and sleeping at their normal times, the volunteers carried out these activities of daily living twelve hours out of phase. This would be the rough equivalent of traveling across twelve time zones. They maintained this schedule for eight days. At the end of the study period leptin levels had moved in a fattening direction, blood sugar had increased, tissues had become less sensitive to insulin (insulin resistance), and blood pressure had worsened. Signs and symptoms of metabolic obesity developed quickly when body clock orientation in time was abruptly and significantly shifted.

Abruptly altering the timing of our daily activities to a significant degree throws the body into a state, at least temporarily, characterized by internal desynchronization. Shift work, flying across many time zones, or large changes in when we carry on activities of daily living—sleeping, waking, eating, and exposure to light/darkness—will cause mistiming of biological events.

In the case of shift work, mistiming might last as long as we continue to work these hours. In the case of flying across time zones, aspects of biological timing can still be disrupted weeks after the experience of jet lag has faded. Shift work and long-distance travel are big things; desynchronization can also occur because of many circumstances that occur routinely in the modern world, including bright light exposure at night, or day-to-day inconsistency in sleep-wake times, meal patterns, or lighting conditions. An example is the common occurrence of going to sleep and waking much later on a weekend than on weekdays. This creates a minor form of jet lag.

When we are experiencing any significant degree of internal desynchronization, changes occur in both biology and behavior, which, if sustained, would be fattening. Internal desynchronization has links to many chronic diseases including cancer, diabetes, heart disease, and ulcers. It is also associated with increased risk for obesity. Desynchronization is one side of the rhythm coin; the other side is being in sync. Lighting conditions are the critical time-giving cue that set and synchronize light-sensitive body clocks. Lighting (photoperiod) is also the vital time-giving cue for keeping our body calendar in sync with the seasons. When we eat, which will be discussed in the next chapter, is the time-giving cue for *food-sensitive* body clocks.

Lighting conditions influence body clocks and calendars. This makes evolutionary sense. Humans evolved in a world where the sun was the dominant time-giving cue for daily and seasonal light-sensitive rhythms. Our physiology is still predisposed to orient itself to the sun's schedule as long as our exposure to light and darkness roughly coincide with a solar day. Like the solar day, our body has a night and day. As darkness becomes dawn, physiology shifts from night to day routines. As day turns to dusk, and dusk to darkness, it is a signal for the reemergence of nighttime physiology. Our body also has seasons. Changes in the length of day (and night) act as a timing cue for our calendar functions. As day length decreases, it is a cue to flip the pages of the calendar from summer to fall to winter, and as days lengthen the calendar flips to spring and back to summer.

Body clocks and calendars are involved in the regulation of appetite, metabolism and shape. Integrating Shape Intelligence with activity, feeding, and sleep-wake cycles makes evolutionary sense. It would have allowed ancient humans to coordinate their daily activities with those of the body in a way that matched the one reliable source of light they had—the sun. It also would allow them to match their physiology with seasonal fluctuations in food availability that occurs, in large part, because of the sun's annual cycle. In the modern world, where light and food are available around the clock and around the year, this coordination is no longer necessary for survival, but it remains as part of the legacy we inherit from our earlier ancestors. Perhaps because of this, the best health and shape results seem to occur when all of the different biological events in our body are coordinated with each other and with the sun's schedule. This requires synchronization. And synchronization is, to a significant extent, determined by lighting conditions. The general rule of thumb is that lighting conditions that more closely mimic the light and darkness schedules encountered by pre-industrialized humans— naturalistic lighting—allows for better body clock and calendar function. As lighting conditions diverge further and further from being naturalistic, as they have done in the modern world, shape and health suffer.

Body Clocks and Shape

Body clock orientation in time has a pronounced effect on shape and metabolism. This is evident in the *Case of Clock Mutant Mice*. The Clock gene encodes an essential component needed for the function of the master body clock. Mice that lack this gene have more difficulty orienting to a 24-hour day. They eat large quantities of food and become obese. And they develop signs and symptoms of metabolic obesity—high cholesterol levels, excessive fat in the liver, and insulin resistance. There is a direct relationship with disrupted body clock function and poor shape in these animals. The identification of this link between body clock orientation and shape in animals has resulted in some scientists questioning whether there might be a similar relationship in humans.

In the *Case of Intentionally Disrupting Timing*, scientists were able to move aspects of biology in a fattening direction by doing the equivalent of shifting all activities of daily living normally done during daylight hours to nighttime, and shifting sleep to daytime. The volunteers in this study became extreme night people, and apparently this shift, in when we do things, was fattening. Shift work is a real world example of this type of reorientation in time. Unlike in the study, which only lasted eight days, people who do shift work usually do so for extended periods of time. Studies of shift workers have revealed that they are more likely to be overweight or obese. Rotating shift work is also a risk factor for future weight gain. Shift work is associated with disappointing weight loss results following weight loss surgeries. Shift work appears to be fattening. This type of evidence has led some researchers to suggest that living a nocturnal life, a lifestyle pattern that disconnects us from naturalistic lighting cues, might be a factor involved in body fat accumulation. The *Case of Freshman Weight Gain* provides circumstantial evidence for this hypothesis.

An urban myth, of sorts, informs us that during the first year of college, students gain 15 pounds. The newest evidence indicates that college freshman, as a group, do gain weight, just not this much (though many individuals do gain in excess of 15 pounds). Changes in diet, alcohol use, and academic stress are often discussed as possible causes. Perhaps they are. There is another change that accompanies college life that is rarely discussed. Many college students become night people. They go to bed later. They wake later. They get more bright light late at night and less early in the sun's day. More calories tend to be eaten in the evening hours and fewer are eaten early in the day. These might seem like small things, but for body clocks this is a big shift in orientation. Becoming a night person causes us to become desynchronized from the sun's schedule. It reorients body clock rhythms in time, and based upon what science has discovered about biological rhythms, this would be expected to have far from trivial effects of biology and behavior.

We have witnessed many cases of undesired shifts in shape with a move to a nocturnal schedule. We have seen this in college freshman, in shift workers, and in other individuals who become night people. And we have witnessed desired transformations in shape when a person moves from being a night person to becoming a day person. Our investigations into health scenes have resulted in a broader hypothesis than simply a connection between nocturnal living

HSI CLUE

A common complaint of flight attendants, especially during their first six months on the job, is weight gain. Business frequent flyers also commonly complain about weight gain. Conventional wisdom is that they need to do a better job eating and exercising to prevent this worsening of shape. The fault is theirs for failing in some way. But what if body clock stress were the real culprit? How might this change the way we thought about these complaints and what we did to help?

patterns and shape. We believe that chronic rhythm disruption is hidden in the background of the lives of many night people. This rhythm disruption might be the key factor when it comes to weight gain and fat accumulation in shift workers and college freshman. While living a nocturnal life might be one way to inflict rhythm disruption, there are other ways. The *Case of Dr. Mark* illustrates this point.

About a decade ago, because of job demands, Dr. Mark (Percival) spent six weeks flying across the United States and Canada evaluating 35 different medical clinics. He was constantly changing from one time zone to another. Before he began his travels Dr. Greg cautioned him, based upon his understandings of body clock function, that his shape, weight and health might suffer some consequences from the constant rhythm disruption—the body clock stress—this travel schedule would produce. Dr. Mark was unconvinced. He would eat well and exercise. Would this be enough to counter this amount of added body clock stress? We would soon find out. Six weeks later Dr. Mark returned: He was 15 pounds heavier and atypically lethargic, despite having attempted to do all the right things while traveling. Six weeks of this degree of body clock stress proved to be too big of a tipping point for him. His shape, which had been relatively stable for 25 years, shifted.

Dr. Mark's case is not an isolated instance. Body clock stress can be a tipping point for a significant worsening of shape. Whether it is because of frequent traveling across time zones, shift work, moving to a more nocturnal living pattern, or some other lifestyle or environmental factors that throw our body clocks out of sync; rhythm disruption can be an exceedingly powerful shape tipping point. Fortunately, shape changes caused by chronic rhythm disruption can be largely reversed when we get into sync. Dr. Mark was able to shed much of the fat accumulation within several months after getting back in rhythm, so to speak (or as close as he gets with his ongoing travels). One of the ways we get in rhythm is by improving our lighting conditions. The impact this timing cue has on eating patterns and shape is illustrated in the next three cases.

Let's begin with the *Case of Night Eating*. Night eating is a syndrome characterized by low to no appetite in the morning, eating a large amount of total daily food intake after the evening meal, and waking to eat or snack. Night eating is hypothesized to be a causative factor for worsening shape. The evidence for this hypothesis will be discussed in more detail in the next chapter. For now we would like to share a case with you. This case was reported in the medical literature. The person was identified as Ms. B. She was a 51-year-old, overweight, depressed woman. She was also a night eater. Her night eating and depression were worsening despite continued treatment with an antidepressant medication. She was treated with bright light therapy in the morning for 30 minutes a day over a two-week period. Her night eating and her mood improved. One month after ceasing morning bright light therapy her night eating had reappeared, while her mood remained improved. She was given 12 more sessions of morning bright light therapy and this time her night eating completely vanished. Lighting conditions improved her mood and shifted her eating habits.

The second case is the *Case of Phototherapy and Weight*. This is also a case from the medical literature. In this case four overweight women were treated with bright light (phototherapy) between 7 a.m. and 9 a.m. for ten days. After this initial treatment, they continued to have phototherapy twice weekly for another four and one half weeks. Three of the four women spontaneously experienced weight reductions ranging from 3.3 to 5.3 pounds.

The last case is the *Case of Light Therapy and Exercise*. Exercise can improve shape. The evidence for this is overwhelming. Can tinkering with lighting influence the shape results produced by exercising? In an attempt to answer this question scientists assigned 25 overweight or obese individuals to six weeks of moderate exercise. Some of the subjects just exercised. Others exercised and were exposed to bright light every morning. Weight decreased significantly with exercise whether the subjects received bright light treatment or not, but the amount of fat only decreased significantly in the exercising subjects who were exposed to bright light in the morning.

These are isolated cases and small studies. Yet, when they are added to other clues, what argument to the best explanation can we make? We know that biological rhythms are vital for health. We know that lighting conditions, and other lifestyle and environmental factors can interfere with or improve these rhythms. In some animals, changing lighting conditions affects shape. We know that shift work and other occupations that reorient our body clock in time increase the risk of being obese. The Clock gene directly affects shape in animals. Rhythm disruption can result in changes in biology and behavior that promote fattening. Desynchronized rhythms are a consistent finding in persons with eating disorders and among obese individuals. We have witnessed shifts in shape for the worse when people chronically disrupt their rhythms, as well as shifts for the better when they get back in sync. The best explanation for these observations is that body clock functions are a vital determinant of our shapes. If this hypothesis is true, lighting conditions, since they are such a vital timing cue for keeping body clocks in sync, should be a tipping point for the better or worse when it comes to shape. In our experience, for some people, they are.

The Case of Body Calendars and Shape

Calendar functions shift the shape of many animals. Hibernating animals and migratory birds are examples. Prior to hibernation or migration, many animals will adjust their natural weight in a way that allows them to be prepared for the upcoming circumstances. By defending more body fat a hibernator will have enough stored energy to survive winter sleep and a migratory bird will have enough energy saved away to make a long flight. In both instances body fat must be accumulated before it is actually needed. To accomplish this task Shape intelligence must have some way of knowing *when* to begin advance preparations. Shortening days provide this signal; alerting it to initiate the needed changes in metabolism and fat storage.

Emerging from body calendar research of hibernating and migratory animals has been an appreciation that the natural weight of these animals is continuously readjusted as the photoperiod shifts. A striking example of this seasonality of shape is the golden-mantled ground squirrel. In the wild these animals show a substantial seasonal variation in body fat stores. In labs a similar annual rhythm of fat gain and loss is maintained, occurring even when food is kept constant all year. Evidence like this is inconsistent with a theory that blames shape and weight entirely on caloric intake. Instead it is consistent with a theory that suggests these animals have some form of Shape Intelligence that is constantly adjusting natural weight across the seasons in an effort to produce very specific shape outcomes. Equally telling is what occurs when food is restricted in these animals. When they are placed on a diet they lose weight. When they are allowed free access to food they regain the weight.

We would expect this temporary weight loss outcome and rebound weight gain based on past cases we have discussed. But when they regain the weight they do not return to the weight they were before the diet, they return to a weight that is appropriate for the present point in their annual cycle. If they are dieted after the holidays and break the diet in the spring, they don't regain all the fat they lost; they only regain as much fat as they would normally have and need in the spring. The opposite occurs if they are dieted in the late summer and break the diet in the late fall. They regain much more fat than they lost because it is appropriate for them to be fatter going into the winter. The same phenomenon is observed if body fat is removed surgically; the animals replace it, but they do so precisely to match what they would normally need for that season. Whether it is the ground squirrel, other animals that hibernate, or migratory birds, in the animal world natural weight is tightly linked to calendar functions. It should not be a surprise to observe such precision in shape self-regulation in these animals. After all, adjusting body fat stores to match the demands created by the environment is essential for survival.

HSI CLUE

An eight percent increase in meal size has been observed at the time of the full moon relative to the new moon in a study involving nearly seven hundred adults. In both men and women several hormones involved in shape regulation have lunar rhythms. In women with regular menstruation patterns a marked decrease of waist-to-hip ratio occurs around the time of ovulation. Shape regulation appears to be rhythmically linked to lunar cycles.

Even among animals that are not known as hibernators, shape and body composition shift as days lengthen and shorten. Rats are nocturnal animals. Cattle, like humans, are day creatures. Neither is a true hibernator. Yet rats exposed to prolonged periods of long days are heavier and shift fat storage to internal depots—they become fat on the inside. In Holstein cattle short days lead to fattening; long days produce more muscle. In our experience we appear to be more like cattle, with short days—winter in the northern hemisphere—being fattening. This can be detected in the *Case of Holiday Weight Gain.*

We know that humans gain weight seasonally. While reports vary as to the amount of seasonal weight gain, it is clear that most people find it easier to gain weight in the fall and winter. We typically blame this weight gain on the holidays—on what and how much we are eating. This matches our intuitions. It is obvious.

HSI CLUE

Consistent exposure to bright light during winter months improved mood and vitality of office workers. The benefits were not just observed in workers with seasonal mood disorders; even "healthy" workers benefited. Lighting conditions have pronounced effects on how we feel and function. We might not be consciously aware of these effects, but light will, nevertheless, be impacting us.

But let's ask a question. Food plays a big part in the gatherings over the 4th of July holiday period. Why isn't everyone complaining about weight gain during this summer holiday? Could it be we are falling for an obvious fact; blaming our winter shape results on the wrong thing? Is how much, or what, we are eating the only reason we gain weight over the winter holidays? Or could it be that part of the explanation is that calendar functions are making it easier to gain weight and get fatter when days are shorter?

[Note: We have consistently observed that is easier for people to improve their shapes more rapidly (and to a greater degree) in the spring as days are lengthening and much more difficult for them to do so in the fall and early winter as days are shortening.]

Scientific studies have found that hormones like leptin, testosterone, growth hormone, insulin, DHEA, cortisol, and melatonin, all of which are involved in shape self-regulation, change with the seasons. The same is true for enzymes involved in fat storage and utilization; they shift with the seasons. Many of our body functions, including body temperature, cholesterol, blood pressure, and blood sugar regulation also have seasonal rhythms. Our physiological functions indicate that we are seasonal creatures. The *Case of SAD* illustrates the degree to which many of us are affected by changing calendars.

People with seasonal affective disorder (SAD) almost always have body clocks that are out of sync, with many biological events occurring at the wrong times with respect to each other and to the timing of the outside world. SAD is also a calendar condition; occurring in tandem with shorter days. Scientists have observed that the calendar functions of people with SAD change with the seasons, in a manner parallel to that seen in mammals that hibernate. This has led to a hypothesis that the root of this health problem might well be a problem of evolutionary biology. The bodies of people with SAD might be predisposed to want to hibernate, but modern life prevents these people from following this predisposition. The most recognized characteristic of SAD is low mood; it is not the only seasonal change these individuals experience. Increases in appetite, shifts in when a person is hungry, carbohydrate cravings, sleepiness, decreased desire for activity, and worsening shape, also commonly occur in combination with winter blues. SAD is more than a mood challenge; it affects many aspects of biology and behavior. How is SAD treated? It can be treated using a specific type of light therapy intended to mimic a naturalistic dawn (dawn simulation). Bright light in the morning, usually delivered using a light box, is a very effective therapy. Vitamin D—the vitamin we make from sunlight hitting our skins—can improve symptoms. All of these interventions can improve how a person with SAD feels. All three interventions have one thing in common; they are related to lighting.

The *Case of Bulimia* provides another link to clocks and calendars. Body clock issues are commonly encountered in persons with bulimia. There is also a distinct seasonal change in both mood and purging behavior in many affected individuals; with both tending to worsen in the late fall and winter. It has been hypothesized that the reason for this might be a lack of daylight. To test this hypothesis 22 women, with both seasonal worsening of mood and binge/purge symptoms, were treated daily for four weeks with morning bright light for 30 to 60 minutes. Depressive symptoms decreased by more than fifty percent and the frequency of binges by almost fifty percent. Several of the participants ceased binge/purge behavior completely and remained abstinent of binge/purge episodes. Light, an intervention with a known effect on clocks and calendars, shifted biology and behavior.

In the animal world, changes in the length of days triggers changes in shape. In humans, physiology and shapes shift in subtle, yet predictable ways with the changing of day lengths. Lighting conditions influence seasonal mood and eating behaviors in some individuals. People tend to gain several pounds over the winter holidays; pounds they often find difficult to lose. The duration of the photoperiod appears to have a strong impact on shape.

The Solution: Naturalistic Lighting

With lighting conditions (as well as meal timing and sleep-wake schedules) the key things to keep in mind are (1) day-in, day-out consistency, and (2) following naturalistic schedules similar to what pre-industrialized humans experienced. Early humans evolved in a world where the only two significant sources of light—sun and moon—were naturally occurring and varied in predictable and gradual ways. The body evolved to use changes in naturalistic lighting to prepare itself for the different demands that are caused by days and nights, menstruation in women, and the changing seasons. Our bodies are still designed to respond to these time-giving cues. Based on the evidence we have been able to uncover, the following five things are needed to produce the best body clock and calendar results.

1. Bright light early in the morning,
2. Exposure to naturalistic lighting during the day and across the year,
3. Sufficient sunlight on our skin to make enough vitamin D to meet our individual requirements,
4. Dark nights,
5. Waxing and waning of the moon.

In an ideal world we would experience the lighting equivalent of sleeping under the stars and spending our days outside. We would begin the day with a gradual increase in lighting intensity over a period of one to two hours; waking just after dawn as light intensified enough to rouse us from sleep. Most of the day would be spent out of direct sunlight, but with our eyes able to detect the naturalistic changes in the sun's intensity as it travels across the sky. At some point during the day, depending upon our skin complexion, season, and latitude, we would get enough direct sunlight on our skin to make the vitamin D we need to be healthy and lean. We would experience sunset and the shift to nighttime physiology this transition initiates. Night would have a lighting intensity similar to what would be caused by stars. We would be exposed to the waxing and waning of the moon. Our schedules, and hence our exposure to light, would be characterized by day-to-day consistency. We would rise and sleep at about the same time each day over the course of a few weeks, but our sleep-wake schedule would adjust itself gradually as the length of the sun's day changed, causing us to sleep for a bit longer during the long nights of winter than we do during the short nights of summer. This is what our body was designed for: Most of us don't live this life.

Lighting conditions affect all of us, but some of us are more susceptible to its effects than others. Fluorescent lights—one type of artificial lighting—cause measurable stress responses in some people; yet not in others. Some of us will need several hours of naturalistic light during the day to sleep well at night or lift our moods. Others might only need 30 minutes. Some of us will be severely affected by seasonal changes; others of us will manage short days much more readily. No matter where we might be on the continuum of susceptibility to lighting conditions, improvement in this area can be a tipping point for better health. If you are like some people we have worked with, it might even improve your shape.

While there are many things one can do to improve lighting conditions, the two most important are getting (1) bright light early in the morning, and (2) more hours of complete darkness at night. Early morning naturalistic light positively influences all biological rhythms that are synchronized by light. It is a make or break time for body clocks. And it can be a huge tipping point for improving how we function, especially in the winter months. There are three options for improving morning light quality. The first, and preferred option, is to get outside for 30 to 60 minutes between 7 and 9 a.m. daily. If the above is not feasible, use of a *light box*—a device that emits high intensity light—between 7 and 9 a.m. is an option. The third option is to use what you already have available to make your morning environment as bright as possible: Open drapes; turn on all available lights; sit near windows, and put the TV on. Thirty minutes represents the minimum, in terms of how much time to be exposed to bright light in the morning. One hour is a better target amount, but if more time is available there is no need to limit morning bright light to only an hour.

> **HSI CLUE**
>
> Clues to light and darkness issues include:
> (1) Little or no appetite for breakfast,
> (2) Late night hunger,
> (3) Food binges,
> (4) Cravings for carbohydrates,
> (5) Sleep issues,
> (6) Mood problems,
> (7) Trouble getting going in the morning,
> (8) Chronic digestive issues.

Whichever option is chosen, the *when* of morning light exposure matters—the time of exposure is important, as is day-to-day consistency. We want to make sure that our first bright light exposure occurs shortly after waking, preferably before 8 in the morning. Strong pulses of light early in the sun's day will reset our biological rhythms and synchronize them to the sun's cycles. If we wait till later, and don't get our first exposure to bright light until after 9 a.m., it tends to push most people's body clocks towards a nocturnal schedule, making them night people. Later and later exposure tends to shift body clock to more and more of a late night orientation. Day-to-day consistency of timing is also important.

If one day, morning bright light occurs at 7 a.m., and the next day it occurs at 9 a.m., this is, from a body clock perspective, akin to flying across two time zones. Rather than synchronizing our body clock, inconsistency can jet lag it.

In addition to morning bright light, it is important to periodically punctuate our days with exposure to naturalistic light. This allows our eyes to send a signal to the light-sensitive parts of our brain that lighting conditions are continuously changing. It also tends to orient us more firmly to the sun's schedule. This can be accomplished, at least to a degree, by sitting close by a window and using it as our principle source of illumination during the day. It can also be accomplished by going outside for at least five minutes every one to two hours during the day.

Actual darkness—lack of light—is a requirement for optimal body clock performance. The human body is evolutionarily adapted for daytime light and nighttime darkness. We need both. Without periods of darkness, light ceases to be a meaningful time giving cue; losing its ability to synchronize the body clock. Bright light in the morning shifts the body into daytime physiology. Darkness produces the shift to nighttime physiology. Without it the body remains in a sort of limbo between night and day physiologies, unable to completely shift gears into nighttime mode until the environment is dark. Once we have shifted to night physiology, we remain in it as long as darkness remains uninterrupted by light. The earlier in the evening the shift to nighttime physiology occurs, and the more uninterrupted time we spend in darkness, the more likely the body is to complete all of its important nighttime duties. If we don't spend sufficient time in nighttime physiology, some things can't get done, and health suffers.

While bright light in the morning is an important time giving cue, the same *what*—bright light—can be very disrupted if the *when* occurs at night. Much of this disruptive effect can be eliminated if we are more careful with the wavelengths—colors—of light we expose ourselves to at night. Light is made up of many colors. We can see them in a rainbow or with a prism, both causing light to refract in ways that reveal its hidden colors. Most people are aware of the health risks associated with one of these colors—ultraviolet (UV) light. Too much UV light exposure will cause sunburns and is associated with skin cancer. Far fewer people are aware that other colors of light have biological effects. Of all of the colors of the rainbow, the blue light wavelength has the strongest impact on light-sensitive rhythms. It appears to be the most important wavelength to get exposure to in the morning; it is also the most disruptive wavelength if exposure occurs at night. In an ideal world we would get sufficient blue light exposure in the early mornings to set our body clocks, we would get much less as dusk approached, and we would get none for the several hours prior to bedtime. The first part of this is accomplished by morning exposure to bright light; the latter part only occurs if our evening, late night, and sleep environments are blue light friendly (as low in blue light as is possible).

The goal is to minimize blue light exposure at night, especially in the hours immediately prior to bedtime. Since incandescent sources of lights (including candles and fireplaces) emit proportionally lower amounts of blue light, they are the preferred sources to use for nighttime illumination. Using only enough of these light sources to create a dim environment is preferable to using more of them, or brighter versions of them, to create a brighter nighttime environment. Since televisions and computer monitors emit significant amounts of blue light, the ideal solution would be to avoid these at night. This is not a realistic solution for many people. An alternative, and highly effective strategy, is blue light blocking. Orange lenses or tinting block blue light. An orange tinted light bulb will emit less blue light than a regular light bulb. Sunglasses with orange lenses will screen out blue light wavelengths. Polaroid lenses will usually also block out a significant amount of blue light. Special antiglare screens for blocking blue light emissions from TVs and computer monitors are available. Wearing orange-tinted sunglasses, or so called blue blockers, is a low cost and easy step. We strongly recommend this solution for people who spend any significant amount of time watching TV or using a computer during night hours.

The other important area to focus attention on is the sleep environment. An ideal sleep environment is *cave-like*. Simple steps to

HSI CLUE

Constant light (or darkness) isn't good for body clock accuracy. The reason for this is complex but basically boils down to one principle: Constant lighting conditions are devoid of time-giving cues. They don't send a signal our eyes can detect and respond to. This is why naturalistic lighting, including its opposite, darkness, is so vital for body clock health. Contrast, rhythmic change in illumination, is required for time keeping.

make the sleep environment darker include (1) having drapes/curtains that are dark enough to block outside sources of light pollution, (2) removing electronic devices which produce illumination (3) getting rid of night lights, (4) moving the head of your bed to the darkest corner of the room, and (5) wearing a mask over the eyes during sleep if there is still ambient light. For people who wake at night to go to the bathroom, or for some other reason, switching on a light can counter many of the benefits of other positive steps taken to improve nighttime lighting. If you are likely to switch on any lights after lights out, please replace these with bulbs that don't emit any blue light. Red or orange-tinted light bulbs are typically blue light safe. There are many small steps we can take to improve our individual lighting conditions. We can make a decision to be outside close to sunrise or sunset. We might use breaks at work or school as opportunities to go outside, even if for only a few minutes, to orient light-sensitive body clock to the sun's constantly changing intensity. We might make our sleep environment more cave-like, or our home blue light friendly at night. A small step can be as simple as buying some blue light blocking glasses and committing to using these while watching TV or using a computer any time after 8 at night. There is no shortage of opportunities for improving the quality of light and darkness in our individual environments. The only limits are on our individual willingness and creativity.

Closing Dialogue

Health Scene Investigator: What have you learned?

Apprentice: I learned that a person could be doing the right things for their shape and health, but if they did them at the wrong times, they would have a shape and health mess on their hands.

Health Scene Investigator (laughing): Well said.

Apprentice: I also must admit that I have quite a few lighting issues to address myself. I can make improvements in many areas.

Health Scene Investigator: Most of us can. But it is not where we are that matters so much as which direction we are heading. With light and lighting even a few small changes in our environment and habits can get us moving in the right direction. But lighting conditions are not alone. One other factor is also critical for body clock function. Let us turn our attention to this other time-giver—when we eat.

Chapter 13

Meal Patterns and Shape

It is nearly nine, and the landlady babbled of green peas at seven-thirty.

Sherlock Holmes

Opening Dialogue

Health Scene Investigator: It is 10 in the morning and I notice that you are eating a muffin. Didn't you eat breakfast today?

Apprentice: Well, I was in somewhat of a rush…

Health Scene Investigator: I see. Is this typical?

Apprentice: I have to admit that it is. I know that breakfast is supposed to be an important meal but I don't usually make the time to have it.

Health Scene Investigator: Hmmm, tell me more about your meal patterns.

Apprentice: I am not sure what you mean.

Health Scene Investigator: I want to know when you eat, how long you go between eating, and how consistent you are in eating meals at the same time day-to-day. We have learned that both *what* and *when* of lighting and darkness are important. The same is true for food. What we eat matters; so does when we eat it. Let me explain.

The Case for Meal Timing

In the *Adventure of the Three Students*, Holmes, in essence, asks Watson why their evening meal is late. Holmes's primary consideration at this point is hunger. Hunger aside, does it really matter if we have an evening meal at 7:30 p.m. or eat it sometime after 9 p.m.? What we eat is important. Is when we eat it also important? Would it make a difference if Holmes and Watson ate the same thing earlier in the evening as opposed to later at night?

HSI CLUE

Many biological processes including hunger, how much and what is eaten, energy expenditure, metabolism, shape hormones, and even the creation, transportation and storage, of sugars, cholesterol, and fats, are under the influence of circadian rhythms. These rhythms, and hence shape self-regulation, are influenced by light exposure; they are also influenced by when we eat.

Most of us are conditioned to overemphasize *what* we do and under emphasize *when* we do it. As we discovered with lighting, because of its interactions with body clocks and calendars, when was important. Decisions about when to eat seem like an ordinary thing. Many of us give relatively little thought to the timing, frequency and regularity of our meal patterns. We squeeze food into our busy lives—some as meals and some as snacks. We do what is convenient for our schedule, but we don't take into account what might be convenient for our body and its schedule. Could this inattention to meal patterns be affecting our shapes? Could this seemingly ordinary event—not so much what we eat but when we eat it—have extraordinary effects? The answer to this question is yes.

In Chapter 12 (*Adventures of Light and Lighting*) the principle of synchronization was discussed. We discovered that it isn't sufficient that the right biological and behavioral things are done; they must also be timed correctly. Lighting conditions play a large role in timing. Exposure to the same thing—light—at different times could produce extremely different responses. Bright light early in the day could help synchronize body clocks, but bright light late at night could disrupt timing, causing internal desynchronization. What we do matters; when we do it also matters. This principle also applies to eating.

When we investigate shape cases, we want to know what times, especially of the morning and evening, a person experiences hunger. But we don't stop there. We want to know what time they eat, how long they go between meals, and whether day-to-day meal patterns are consistent. We want to know whether they snack, and if so, how often. We want to know all of these things because the same thing eaten at different times can have different effects.

The Case of Food Sensitive Body Clocks

Many tissues keep time. Some, like the hypothalamus, are incredibly sensitive to lighting conditions. Light is used to orient these body clocks in time. These body clocks are said to be light sensitive. Other body clocks orient themselves in time based on when food is eaten. These so-called food sensitive body clocks are kept in sync, or disrupted, by the timing of eating episodes. The importance of meal timing is apparent when we turn our powers of observation to *Cases of the Implanted Cancer*. In this case (from chapter 12) we discovered that lighting conditions could influence the growth of, and the survival rates from, cancer. Lighting that was more naturalistic slowed growth and improved survival. Lighting conditions that deprived the animals of nighttime darkness, and hence the time giving cues that a shift from light to darkness provides, accelerated cancer growth and increased death from cancer. These types of effects are not limited to light. Meal timing also influences cancer growth and survival in lab animals, and it does this even when lighting is causing severe body clock stress. In one experiment mice with implanted tumors had their exposure to light advanced by eight hours every two days. These experimental conditions are the equivalent, from a body clock perspective, of flying across eight time zones every other day. The result is a form of chronic jet lag. These mice were under severe body clock stress; a stress that shifted clock gene rhythms in the liver and abolished them in the tumors, a stress that also accelerated the growth of their cancer. By altering meal timing—not what the animals ate, but when they were allowed to eat it—the rhythms of clock genes in these tissues were returned to a more normalized pattern, and more importantly, cancer growth was slowed. This is not an isolated scientific observation. Limiting food access to a particular time of day (or night) has profound biological effects all the way down to the rhythms of tissues and the expression of body clock genes. We are clocks and one of the vital factors that affect timing-related function, including shape, is when we eat.

The prevailing notions of weight essentially inform us that weight is largely an issue of how much food is eaten. According to this theory it shouldn't matter when it is eaten. Does it? In the *Case of Modifying the Time of Feeding* it did. This case involved mice. Mice live a schedule that is the complete opposite of ours; they are night creatures and we are day creatures. When we would normally be sleeping (at night), they are active. When we are active (during daylight hours), they are sleeping. If food is available mice will eat most, if not all, of their calories during their active hours—during the dark hours after the sun sets but before it rises. Scientists decided to investigate what would occur if the time when mice ate were shifted. Two groups of mice were fed identical foods; one group had access to the food during the 12 hours mice are normally active; the other group had access to the food during the 12 hours mice are normally sleeping. For the next six weeks the two groups of mice consumed the same amount of calories. They also exercised a similar amount. If the only things that mattered, when it comes to weight and body fatness, were how many calories were eaten and how many were burned during exercise, the two groups of mice should have finished the experiment weighing the same amounts and with equal amounts of body fat. This was not what was observed. The mice that ate their calories during their normal sleep hours gained almost two and one half times more weight and ended the experiment with about eight percent more body fat than the other group. Modifying the timing of when calories were eaten, even when the amount of calories eaten did not differ, led to a dramatic difference in weight and body fatness. Timing of calories was a critical variable. In mice, eating the same amount of calories during the 12 hours between sunrise and sunset produced very different shape and weight results compared to eating an equal amount of calories between sunset and sunrise. Because mice and humans live opposite schedules, this experiment would be the human equivalent of eating all of our calories at night. Would shifting our calories to the nighttime also affect aspects of human biology? The answer is yes. This has been apparent in the many studies that make up the *Case of Ramadan.*

The fasting month of Ramadan is the ninth lunar month of the Islamic calendar. During Ramadan eating and drinking is permitted in any quantity desired as long as the foods and beverages are consumed after sunset and before dawn. Because food intake is not restricted in quantity or type but only in timing, Ramadan provides a perfect opportunity to investigate the effects of nocturnal eating. The common theme in Ramadan research is that the shift in the timing of food away from daytime and into darkness hours creates wide-ranging changes to human physiology and behavior.

Among some of the more notable observations are (1) worsening of daytime mood and increased daytime lassitude, sleepiness, and napping (2) a reduction in mental, physical and social activities during the day and an increase in these activities at night, (3) alterations in the timing, and in many instances the quantities, of information molecules and hormones including those involved in stress, sleep, digestion, appetite, body fat, and muscle self-regulation, (4) changes in the efficacy of some drugs, and (5) worsening of the symptoms of several clinical conditions. Ramadan shifts someone into a night person. Ramadan only lasts 30 days, after which Muslims return to daytime meal patterns. With this return most of the changes caused by Ramadan are spontaneously reversed. A person reverts to being a day person, and physiology and behaviors return to a daytime rhythm. This is direct evidence of how altering the timing of eating dramatically shifts biology and behavior. When food is eaten exclusively during darkness hours, the same types and amounts of food have different effects than they do if eaten during the day.

HSI CLUE

Adults who eat breakfast are mentally and physically more efficient for longer periods during the day. People who eat breakfast are more successful at losing weight and sticking to a diet. Athletes who eat breakfast train more effectively. People who eat breakfast are more likely to rate their health as better. Missing breakfast increases the chance of heavy machinery and factory accidents.

Some of our body clocks are more strongly influenced by light; others by meal timing. Both of these timing signals are important. It is also important that they are coupled together. As a general rule of thumb humans seem to get the best long-term shape and health results when the rhythms of all of body clocks are in sync with each other and with the sun's schedule. This means we tend to do better when we get daytime light and nighttime darkness *and* when we eat all or most of our food during daylight hours. When both of these timing cues are misaligned with the sun's schedule (when we live nocturnal schedules), or if they conflict with each other (being awake during normal daylight hours for work or school, but skipping breakfast and eating late at night as an example) the shape and health results we produce tend to suffer. Presumably a large part of the reason why is because these patterns create a form of body clock stress. When faced with chronic body clock stress, Shape Intelligence appears to alter its setting for how much weight and fat to defend, and adjusts bio-behavioral defenses (including hunger and activity) to obtain its revised shape goals. The timing cues provided by light and darkness can lessen body clock stress or create it; they will either be helping to keep our body clocks in sync or disrupting them. Light is a powerful time keeping cue, but it is not the *only* time keeping cue. Meal timing is also vitally important.

Adventures in Meal Timing

Let's begin our investigations of meal timing with the *Case of Breakfast*. Most of us would acknowledge that eating a good breakfast is an important lifestyle habit. Scientific evidence supports this piece of conventional wisdom. After reviewing 47 scientific studies on this topic several scientists concluded that:

- Breakfast eaters are less likely to be overweight.
- Breakfast consumption may improve memory, test grades, and school attendance.
- Breakfast as part of a healthful diet and lifestyle can positively impact a child's health and well-being.

These same researchers also concluded that breakfast skipping is highly prevalent in North America and Europe. The facts tell us that the percentage of children, adolescents, and adults consuming any breakfast has declined over the past four decades. The facts also tell us that, even among people who claim to eat breakfast every day, the quality of foods consumed has shifted for the worse. Instead of breakfast being a balanced meal it might be a bagel, muffin, or donut: Something is being eaten, but it has more in common with a snack food than a meal. There is widespread agreement that breakfast is an important meal. Yet fewer and fewer of us are making the time to eat it, and when we do, what we eat is often decidedly not meal-like. These trends have paralleled the expansion of our waistlines. Circumstantial evidence suggests this trend is more than a coincidence.

Observational and epidemiological studies indicate that regular breakfast eaters are more likely to be leaner, while breakfast skippers have a high probability of being fat. The heaviest people, even when they do eat breakfast, donate less time to eating breakfast, eat smaller amounts of food, have less varied breakfasts, and have breakfasts higher in simple carbohydrates and lower in fiber and nutrients. This much is certain: Scientific studies consistently detect a strong relationship between breakfast habits and shape. This relationship is evident in the National Weight Control Registry. This registry is a database of persons who have reduced their weights substantially and been able to maintain the lower weight. Approximately 78 percent of persons who report long-term success claim to regularly eat breakfast every day of the week and only 4 percent of the successes in this database report never eating breakfast. This is reasonably compelling evidence that eating breakfast every day is, at the very least, a characteristic in the majority of people who have succeeded in improving their shapes. It is not proof that eating breakfast is a cause of this success. It might be; it might not be. It is circumstantial evidence because it is collected after-the-fact. Asking people what they have done, or are doing, with respect to breakfast, can help us detect potential relationships. To really test for cause, breakfast must be used as an intervention, and the response to the intervention must be monitored. This type of study provides direct evidence. In one such study the direct evidence indicated that eating (or skipping) breakfast strongly influenced how much was eaten.

Scientists designed a study that used eating or skipping breakfast as the intervention. In random order, women either ate or skipped breakfast every day for several weeks at a time. When breakfast was eaten it consisted of a bowl of whole grain cereal with low-fat milk, which was eaten between 7 and 8 in the morning. Eating breakfast resulted in better cholesterol and insulin levels. This is an important observation. Improving these physiological processes is strongly associated with better health and a more shapely body. But this was not the only change the scientists detected. During the weeks they were eating breakfast daily, the women spontaneously, without any conscious efforts on their part, ate less food. This is a very important clue. Most people take it for granted that the solution to weight and shape challenges is to eat less. It's the sensible answer. Rarely, if ever, is this sensible answer examined in a thoughtful way. We are led to believe that, when it comes to how much we eat, we are in conscious control. When this premise is examined in a more thoughtful manner, it collapses like the proverbial house of cards. The amount of food we eat is in part dictated by the complex bio-behavioral defense system that self-regulates our shape. It is probably also in part influenced by our reward system. But the key point is, because of these systems, eating less is a lot easier said than done. A conscious decision to eat less than our appetite dictates is difficult to execute for a week, never mind for a lifetime. With each passing day that we intentionally eat less than our appetite dictates, hunger gnaws at us more intensely. Eventually, we become like the participants in *Survivor* or the volunteers in the Minnesota Experiment: We are hungry all the time and the hunger is not satisfied even when we eat a big meal. This increase in hunger is part of the complex bio-behavioral defense of shape. This is not what occurred in this breakfast intervention. The women spontaneously ate less and they did not get hungrier. They were not eating less than their appetites dictated; they were eating less *because* their appetite dictated that they eat less. This might seem like a subtle difference. It is not. Eating less because we are trying to fight our hunger and eating less because we don't feel hungry could not be more different. It's hard to fight our appetite; it's easy to live with less hunger.

HSI CLUE

In a person whose body clock is in sync with the sun's schedule, appetite kicks in shortly after waking in the morning. In night eaters, it doesn't. Hunger is delayed. Hunger rhythms and night eating behavior can be shifted by consistently getting morning light exposure between 7 and 9 in the morning.

Mice gain weight and get fatter when they eat all of their calories on a schedule that is the opposite of the one they have been evolutionarily adapted to follow. Skipping breakfast appears to increase how much we eat. In our experience, it also shifts hunger sensation rhythms to a more nocturnal schedule. Breakfast skippers usually don't experience hunger in the early morning, they experience it later in the day and at night. As a result they tend to follow eating schedules that shift a significant amount of their calorie consumption into evening hours. In Chapter 12 we mentioned a case where this tends to occur— the *Case of Freshman Weight Gain*. Many college students go to bed later. They wake later. They skip breakfast. They eat late at night. They become night people. Some experts have hypothesized that there might be something about living a nocturnal schedule that is fattening. Could there be a shape cost that is paid when we reorient our body clock later in the day, because of when we wake and sleep, or when we eat and don't eat? The *Case of Night Eating* suggests that there just might be.

An obesity researcher named Dr. Albert Stunkard first noticed the relationship between night eating and heavier weight in 1955. A number of obese patients he was working with had no appetite in the morning. They skipped breakfast, ate modest lunches and dinners, and then ate a great deal of food during the evening and night. None of the leaner individuals he used as comparisons had similar meal patterns. He labeled the pattern of meal behavior he observed in these obese patients *Night-Eating syndrome*. Stunkard's original observations, and many observations since, indicate that night eating is common in obese individuals and rare in leaner persons. It is also associated with a high susceptibility for future weight gain, and has been linked to poorer outcomes in attempts to improve shape. Is it the cause in these relationships? Research into this area indicates that many night eaters believe that night eating *preceded* their weight gain. Stunkard, the most famous researcher on this topic, is also of the same belief; after night eating for a few years a person *becomes* obese; it is involved with causing the weight gain.

A person with night-eating syndrome typically has little to no appetite for breakfast, so they don't each much if any food early in the sun's day. They also tend to eat large amounts of their total food intake from dinner through bedtime. Many people with this syndrome will even wake at night and eat or snack. As a result the person has uncoupled much of their food intake, and hence the timing cues meal patterns provide, from the sun's schedule. Their hunger sensation rhythm (the timing of when they feel hungry) is shifted to later in the day, runs into the late evening, and can even have shifted into sleep hours. Is there a shape cost for this uncoupling?

Humans are active during the day and sleep at night. Many rodents, including mice and rats, are nocturnal. They are on opposite schedules from us in terms of sleep-wake cycles, activity, and eating. Because of this difference a day eating mouse would be the equivalent of a night eating human. A specific genetic type of mouse—EP3R-deficient—is a day eater and is the experimental model for night eating in humans. In this genetic strain of mice the day eating shows up at an early age and so does extra weight. These mice become over fat and weigh more than an average mouse when allowed free access to a normal rat chow diet. Almost all of the extra weight is body fat (visceral, subcutaneous and liver fat). The experiments with these day eating mice suggest that shape suffers when meal timing is uncoupled from what would be the normal sleep-wake and activity schedule for a species.

Scientists have also tracked changes in weight in humans with and without night eating. In one study obese night-eating women gained, on average, a bit more than eleven pounds of weight over a six-year time period. Over a similar six-year time period, obese day-eating women experienced an average weight gain of only two pounds. Just as was the case in the animal model of night eating, night eating in humans appears to be fattening.

While the *Case of Ramadan*, the *Case of Breakfast*, and the *Case of Night Eating* provide a significant degree of circumstantial evidence, the most direct evidence that the timing of when we eat influences shape comes from the *Case of Breakfast vs. Supper Calories*. In this case participants were allowed to eat all of their daily food either at breakfast (within one hour of awakening) or supper (not before twelve hours after awakening) as one big single meal. The amount and rate of weight loss was significantly greater when all daily calories were consumed at breakfast. The breakfast group lost an average of about two pounds a week. Weight loss in the supper group was minimal; and in several cases individuals actually gained weight on the same amount of calories that, when consumed at breakfast, were producing weight loss. What we eat affects our shape. We will investigate the evidence for this inference in chapter 19. When it is being eaten also matters.

Adventures in Meal Frequency

The timing of when we eat might be a vital determinant of our shape. The same appears to be true for the frequency with which we eat. If we eat more frequent meals most of us will improve our shape. If we skip meals or go long periods of time between meals, we might worsen our shape, even if we are eating similar amounts of food. The idea that the frequency of meals might influence shape is called the *meal frequency hypothesis*. In this section we will explore evidence that has given rise to this hypothesis

The meal frequency hypothesis proposes that body fatness is in part a function of having fewer (but usually larger) meals, as opposed to more frequent smaller meals. It is theorized that the relatively longer duration between meals that results from having fewer meals a day signals the body in a similar, but weaker manner to what would occur during periods of food scarcity. The result is a biological defense mechanism against scarcity, which we know as body fat. This hypothesis is based on a combination of circumstantial and direct evidence. Circumstantial evidence on the role of meal frequency in shape has existed for several decades.

Observational studies have found that there is a relationship between how frequently a person eats and their weight. Eating two or fewer meals a day is statistically related to being overweight or obese; eating three or more meals a day with being leaner. Successfully reducing body fatness (and keeping the improved shape) is also, to an extent, explained by eating fewer low quality snacks and more of our food as high quality meals. The circumstantial evidence indicates that a reduction in meal frequency—eating fewer but larger meals—is fattening. Does any direct evidence support this inference?

By varying the frequency of meals participants eat daily, while keeping calories identical, studies have provided direct evidence that meal frequency can influence aspects of metabolism, hormones involved in body shape regulation, and cholesterol levels. Direct evidence indicates that eating more frequent meals makes a big difference in keeping appetite in check. But what about shape; is there any direct evidence that meal frequency might directly affect it?

> **H S I   C L U E**
>
> Jorge Cruise, author of the *3-Hour Diet* is a big proponent of meal frequency. His book recommends that we:
> 1. Eat breakfast in the first hour after rising,
> 2. Eat every 3 hours during the day,
> 3. Stop eating 3 hours before bedtime.
>
> Cruise believes that this 3-step meal timing approach positively influences shape. Anecdotal reports from his readers suggest that he is correct.

In animal experiments, direct evidence indicates that when food is divided into smaller, more frequent meals rather than fewer larger meals, for a given amount of weight gained, more of the weight will be muscle and less will be fat. In this instance meal frequency has a stronger and more immediate effect on body composition. The direct evidence in humans comes from several different research studies. In one, eight young men were fed an identical amount of calories every day for two weeks. One group ate all of their calories in two meals each day, the other in six meals a day. Both groups were placed on similar activity routines. The men eating all of their calories in two meals a day experienced a small, but *progressive* weight gain throughout the study. The men eating more meals a day did not. Several other studies have examined the effects of varying meal frequency, while holding calories constant, on body composition during dieting. In each instance, body composition was better when more meals were eaten. The *Case of Starved Boxers* illustrates this point. Twelve boxers were placed on a diet. Each boxer got to eat

1200 calories a day for two weeks. The calories were divided into two meals for some boxers, while others had the 1200 calories divided into six meals. Both groups lost an identical amount of weight. Both groups also lost some muscle mass. We expect these results to occur when calories are withheld. But the men who ate the 2 meals a day lost *significantly* more muscle than did the men who ate more frequently. The increased meal frequency preserved muscle when calories were restricted.

Another piece of direct evidence is the *Case of 7, 5 or 3*. Boys and girls aged six to sixteen years were placed on three different meal plans. Plan A reduced the number of meals to three a day. Plan B increased the number of meals to seven a day. Plan C stayed on the original meal frequency—five meals a day. This experiment in meal frequency lasted for one year. While no statistical differences were detected in how much food was eaten daily under the three different meal frequency conditions, shape differences were significant in the older boys, and even more so in the older girls. In the boys aged 11-16, and even more markedly in the girls aged 10-16, eating three meals a day resulted in significant increases in body fatness. Eating five or seven meals a day over the same year resulted in essentially no change in body fatness. In this study there was no obvious shape advantage gained by eating more than five meals a day, but there was an advantage when daily food intake was spread over five meals as opposed to three meals.

In cases we have investigated, improving meal frequency can often times be a tipping point for improved shape and body composition. In adults this seems to be especially likely to occur among persons who habitually eat only one to two meals a day. We encourage clients to increase the number of meals they eat a day to a minimum of four and we let them know that we feel like best results are likely to be obtained by eating five meals a day. In an ideal situation the time between each meal would be relatively evenly spaced throughout waking hours with the last meal occurring three to four hours prior to sleep. Meals would also be eaten at approximately the same time each day. When this type of small, but every few hours and consistent day-to-day meal frequency pattern is followed, hunger rhythms reorient to match. We, in other words, start to get hungry for small meals at the times when we have been regularly eating them. This does several important things.

First, it takes the guesswork out of when food is coming into our body. One of the often overlooked aspects of our meal patterns is whether day-to-day they are consistent or irregular. Do we eat two meals one day and four the next? Do we eat at approximately the same times every day or are our meal times inconsistent and all over the map? Research into this area has found that having more consistent day-to-day meal patterns improves cholesterol levels, insulin sensitivity, and aspects of our metabolism. Why would it do this? We believe that if we are irregular in our eating patterns, it leaves our body guessing when food might be eaten. This might not seem like a very big deal; it is. An important appreciation that has emerged out of research into body rhythms and health is that predictability allows our body to do its many complex jobs more efficiently. Digesting and assimilating food is complicated; it requires coordinating many different things—stomach acid secretion, mechanisms to protect us against this acid, digestive enzymes, and much, much more. Getting all of these processes lined up and ready is easier to do when our body can predict in advance when food is coming. It can't schedule these tasks when our meal patterns are inconsistent or erratic. Instead, it will be left guessing, responding to food rather than planning for it. No matter how many meals are eaten a day, or when they are eaten, we encourage you to make a commitment to eating at approximately the same times each day.

> **HSI CLUE**
>
> If constantly leaving our body guessing about when food is coming results in poorer health and an increased susceptibility to weight gain, we should see statistically poorer health and increased rates of obesity in one group—rotating shift workers. This is exactly what has been observed in studies.

While eating more frequent meals is a desired outcome, snacking more frequently is not. Many of us snack because we are bored, stressed, or in need of some type of reward. We might snack even if we aren't hungry. Some people will even feel out of control with their snacking habits. Eating more frequent smaller meals will go a long way towards curing a snacking habit. It will establish more robust hunger rhythms and dampen the tendency to snack between these surges of appetite.

Our investigation into meal frequency has left some fairly significant clues. We have circumstantial evidence that shape is related to meal frequency. Meal frequency directly influences hormones involved in shape regulation. Short-term studies suggest that our weight and body composition are affected by how frequently we eat meals. It appears that there is something about eating fewer meals that causes Shape Intelligence to respond by prioritizing accumulation of body fat at the expense of muscle. This is consistent with our observations. When a person subsists on two or fewer meals a day, goes long periods of time between meals, or eats erratically, they tend to defend a higher proportion of weight as fat. Why might this be the case? Let's return now to the meal frequency hypothesis.

H S I   C L U E

The goal isn't to simply eat more frequently or to graze; it is to eat *meals* more frequently. What is a meal? A meal consists of sufficient helpings of one or more nutritious foods to keep us satiated for about three hours. A large candy bar, potato chips, or a bagel is not a meal. It is a snack. A bowl of soup, a salad, a sandwich, or other substantial serving of real food eaten at a *planned time*, when we are typically hungry constitute a meal.

It has been proposed that this response might be a biological defense mechanism. From an evolutionary perspective the ability to get fat is a survival advantage. It protects against times when food is scarce. But how does Shape Intelligence know when to be prepared, when defending extra body fat might be intelligent? If it waits until a famine occurs, it might learn to be better prepared for the next famine, but future preparation wouldn't be much good in the present situation. It would make more sense to look for some early warning signs; clues that the food supplies might be a bit uncertain in the future. Do you think it is possible that infrequent or irregular food intake patterns might act as one of these early warning signs?

We believe that meal skipping, going long durations between eating, and irregular eating habits cause Shape Intelligence to feel that there is some uncertainty about when or where the next meal will come from. We know how nature handles uncertainty over the key resources needed for survival. A camel is an excellent example. It has evolved to solve the uncertainty of water posed by its environment by storing extra water internally. A hibernating animal is evidence of a solution to the uncertainty of food that occurs seasonally. The animal stores more energy—body fat—as a contingency against this uncertainty. Migratory birds are another example. Because large amounts of energy will be needed and food supplies will temporarily be uncertain, migratory birds deposit large amounts of fuel in advance of their journey. The weights of migratory birds can double leading up to migration and this expansion of weight occurs rapidly. Weight gain can be as much as an increase of 15 percent in a single day. Our conscious behaviors can demonstrate a similar "I'd better be prepared" response to an anticipated period of food or water scarcity. When we know a big snowstorm or hurricane is expected many of us go to the super market and stock up on food and water. This is the intelligent thing to do. The sensible solution to uncertainty is preparation. Do you think that storing some additional body fat might be a sensible response to infrequent or irregular eating? If it is, the solution is equally sensible. The solution in this case would be to convince Shape Intelligence that food availability is anything but uncertain. How do we do this?

Meal Timing and Frequency Action Plan
The three critical issues with meal timing and frequency are:
1. Shifting more calories earlier in the day (preferably consuming all of our calories during the hours between sunrise and sunset),
2. Eating four to five meals daily,
3. Striving for day-to-day consistency with meal timing.

There are different ways to accomplish the above. One way is to follow an approach similar to that suggested in the *3-Hour Diet* by author Jorge Cruise. Cruise recommends that:
1. Breakfast be eaten in the first hour after rising,
2. A meal be eaten three hours after breakfast and at three-hour intervals thereafter,
3. The last food of the day is eaten at least three hours before bedtime.

Our experience indicates that this approach to meal timing, or ones similar to it, can be a tipping point to better shape results, increased energy, and often improved health. But there are a few things to keep in mind when working on improving meal timing.

The first of these has to do with breakfast: It is a make or break meal for body clock orientation. Eating a good breakfast shortly after waking, preferably prior to 8 a.m., makes it easier to accomplish every other meal-timing step. Skipping breakfast puts us behind the eight ball right off the bat. It causes us to miss the single most important window in the day for positively influencing food sensitive body clocks. It directly results in more calories being consumed later in the sun's day, and indirectly contributes to nighttime eating. Skipping breakfast, or eating it later in the morning, also makes it harder to eat enough meals in the day to optimize meal frequency's effects on shape. But it is not simply a matter of eating something for breakfast; the goal is to eat *real food*.

HSI CLUE

Persons who struggle with shape are often not hungry in the morning and very hungry in the late evening. Having no appetite in the morning and high amounts of hunger after supper or late at night is a clue that meal patterns are desynchronized from natural cycles of light and darkness. Shifting our shape is often dependent on synchronizing appetite and light-dark rhythms. This is done by eating breakfast, getting exposure to bright morning light, and minimizing exposure to bright light in the evening.

Many breakfast foods are poor choices from a food quality perspective. They have too much sugar, too little fiber, and are highly processed. The goal with breakfast is to eat real food—foods similar in preparation and nutrition to what our grandparents, grandparents would have eaten for breakfast. Chapter 19 is dedicated to food quality. It discusses what to avoid and creates the framework for choosing higher quality food. Part of the reason people don't eat real food for breakfast is because they are confused about what is and isn't real food. Part of the reason is lack of planning, preparation and being too rushed. And part of the reason has to do with cultural conditioning—our notions about what is and isn't a breakfast food.

Most of us have been conditioned to believe that certain foods are breakfast foods, while other foods are lunch foods, and still others might be dinner foods. Ready-to-eat cereals, donuts, muffins, bagels, pastries, and their ilk are for breakfast. Real foods, a serving of fish, brown rice, vegetables, soup, as examples, are for lunch or dinner. These are 20th century notions. Prior to the last century, in Europe and North America, food was food. Any food could be eaten at any time of the day. This is still the case in much of the world. Choosing to eat so-called lunch or dinner foods for breakfast can be an important step in eating a better breakfast.

While Cruise recommends eating every three hours after breakfast, and this might be an ideal timing interval, even taking steps to add one or two meals to a schedule where meals are eaten infrequently can be a big step in a positive direction. There are a few things that make eating more frequently easier to accomplish. One of these is eating enough food to keep us feeling full for three to four hours, but not so much that we still feel full when it is time for the next eating episode. If we eat too much, we might not want to eat five hours from now never mind in three hours. Finding out what amount of food is sufficient to keep us full enough, but not too full, can take a bit of self-experimentation, but in general, an amount of food that would fit in the palm of our hand is a good starting point. The next thing to keep in mind is that eating more frequently almost always requires planning. It generally doesn't just happen on its own. Most of us don't have lives like the children at the boarding schools mentioned in the *Case of 7, 5 or 3*: No one is scheduling and providing meals for us five times a day. We might have to fend for ourselves for at least a few eating episodes a day.

It's a lot easier to eat frequent meals when they are already prepared and only require eating, than when they have to be prepared or we have to go out of our way to get them. Because of this, the odds of eating frequent meals go up when we plan and down when we don't. When it comes to planning what you will have available, keep in mind that a meal does not have to always consist of many different items. The critical issues are the quantity of what we eat (it must be sufficient) and its quality (discussed in chapter 19). From the perspective of Shape Intelligence, we don't need to eat the equivalent of a restaurant meal or family dinner to be considered a meal; we only need to eat sufficient real food to convince this intelligence that a meal-like amount of food was in fact eaten. Even eating a sufficient quantity of one or two items of real food—a handful of nuts, a large bowl of yogurt or soup, a baked potato, a serving of meat or fish—can serve this purpose. Meals don't have to be complicated to count; simple one or two item meals work as long as we eat a sufficient quantity of food.

While eating more frequent meals is a desired outcome, snacking more frequently is not. It's important to understand the difference between the two. A snack is defined by either its size or its lack of nutritional value. Small serving sizes, even if the food were very healthy, would be a snack if the amount of food eaten didn't keep us satisfied for at least three hours. Snack foods and desserts, including chips, crackers, ice cream, cookies, candy, etc. aren't meals no matter how much of them we eat.

HSI CLUE

Some people prefer being night people. They might claim it agrees with them and that they feel better on this schedule. This might be true for some of these people; it might even be true for most of them. We certainly would not want to dispute anyone's real world results without investigating their unique health scene. What we will say, however, is that scientific evidence and our personal investigations into many cases, indicates that some night people get better shape and health results when they shift their schedules to become day people.

The last thing to consider is when the last food of the day is eaten. Our biology, including metabolism, is much different during the day than at night. The same thing eaten at breakfast and at midnight would interface with two entirely different metabolisms. While this represents an oversimplification, day-night differences in body clock function predispose us to use calories consumed early in the day and store those consumed at night. Because of this, the notion of avoiding eating for at least several hours prior to bedtime is a sound one. We have had hundreds of cases where this single change has produced a positive influence on shape (and digestion). A good starting point can be having dinner as soon as possible after your workday ends. Even eating an hour earlier than your normal routine might make a big difference. After this last meal of the day the goal is to not eat anything else until breakfast. There are four things that make accomplishing this easier: The first is breakfast, the second is eating sufficient overall food during the day and early evening, the third is morning light exposure, and the fourth is earlier bedtimes.

Eating breakfast lifts a great deal of the pressure to eat at night. In a simplified sense, we tend to eat a relatively fixed amount of *calories in a 24-hour period. If we eat our fill during day hours, we* aren't hungry at night; if we don't, we are. By eating breakfast we directly shift some calories earlier in the day— calories that won't be eaten at night. And we orient food sensitive body clock rhythms to earlier schedule, which also shifts hunger rhythms to an earlier schedule. Food is not alone in this effect to shift hunger rhythms: Early morning light exposure tends to shift body clock in ways that decrease late night eating. Hunger occurring later in the evening can be a clue that a person needs more sleep or an earlier bedtime. We have consistently observed that persons, who complain of late night food cravings, have these vanish if they go to bed earlier.

What we do makes a difference; when we do it matters, and so too does day-to-day consistency. Our body needs us to be consistent so that it will know what to expect and when to expect it. If we are consistent it can plan accordingly and prepare itself for digestion and all other food-related activities. If we aren't, it can't. Shape Intelligence will be looking for patterns in our daily behaviors; if we are consistent with our meal patterns it will reorient hunger rhythms to match the times when food is being eaten. It is trying to learn, it is up to us to teach it.

Note: Please visit our website www.healthsceneinvestigation.com to get meal suggestions, to find additional tips on creating better meal patterns, and to let the HSI community know what solutions you have found to make eating smaller more frequent meals easier.

Closing Dialogue

Apprentice: As you explained this subject I saw myself in much of it. I have been a classic breakfast skipper and I routinely wait until I feel famished before I eat. I have been really hungry at night for years, but never made a connection that this might be because of things I was not getting earlier in the day, like a balanced breakfast and morning sunlight. This is fascinating and I am excited to try it!

Health Scene Investigator: I think you will find that, as is the case with most things, it is quite elementary once one knows what clues to look for at a health scene.

Apprentice: And by eating exactly what I do now while improving my meal patterns I can improve my shape?

Health Scene Investigator: Let me answer your question this way…in my experience it is well worth your while to run this self-experiment. We have investigated two things that influence body clocks—light and meal timing. It was mentioned, in passing, that abrupt changes in the *when* of these time giving cues produces body clock stress. It is now time to turn our attention to the topic of stress in more detail.

Chapter 14

Stress and Shape

I wonder how a battery feels when it pours electricity into a non-conductor.

Sherlock Holmes

Opening Dialogue

Health Scene Investigator: Do you see that broken table over in the corner?

Apprentice: Yes, I do, how did it break?

Health Scene Investigator: I placed all of the weight lying next to it on top.

Apprentice: Why would you have done that?

Health Scene Investigator: I am carrying out an experiment. The first part of the experiment proved conclusive. The table collapsed under the added weight. Now, please do me the kindness to place that same weight on this table next to me (points at a table).

Apprentice: If you insist. (Proceeds to place weight on the table and nothing happens.)

Health Scene Investigator: What do you observe?

Apprentice: I can't say I really observe anything.

Health Scene Investigator: One important thing has happened, and that is that nothing has happened. The table supports the weight.

This is one material fact. There are other clues. I already mentioned one, the other table collapsed under the same weight. Look at both tables and tell me what difference you observe.

Apprentice: Well, one thing I notice is that the broken table has much thinner legs and the one where nothing happened has very stout legs.

Health Scene Investigator: Precisely so. We can infer that being stouter allows a table to withstand the added pressure weight places on it. I think this might be a very important clue for understanding shape.

Apprentice: I must admit I am confused. What do these tables and the weight we placed on them have to do with shape?

Health Scene Investigator: Allow me to explain.

Pouring Our "Juice" into Non-Conductors

The modern world is replete with factors and situations that have the potential to place pressure on us; to, figuratively speaking, drain our batteries. The usual word given to this pressure is *stress*. Each of us has pressure placed on us. This pressure might be related to our jobs, families, relationships, finances, or any of dozens of other factors and situations. But stress is more than what is done to us; the concept of stress also includes our responses and adaptations to these pressures. What types of stress are placing pressure on you? How is your body adapting?

The physical shape life takes on Earth is assumed by scientists to be influenced by the pressure gravity places on us; with this source of stress causing adaptations in size, shape and body composition. These effects are seen experimentally in the *Case of Manned Space Stations*. Astronauts manning space stations endure long periods at microgravity (gravity less than the Earth's). What happens to their shape? Muscles atrophy (shrink), bone mass decreases, and weight is lost. In a nutshell, when gravity decreases so too does the pressure it places on our body. Shape Intelligence adapts to these circumstances quickly by, in a sense, making us less substantial. In theory, living in gravity greater than the Earth's would produce an opposite adaptation. Greater gravity would mean added pressure. As a result people living in a world with greater gravity would be expected to be more substantial than us, stouter, more muscular, with thicker bone structure. This is a logical adaptation. Do you think that it might also be logical to adapt in ways that make us more substantial when we experience high amounts of other forms of pressure?

We evolved to live in a world with the Earth's gravity. It is an old stress. Other types of stress that are as old as humankind includes social stress, hunger stress (dieting), and cold and heat stress. The modern world also has many newer forms of stress that didn't exist even five decades ago, never mind millennia ago. These include (1) being stuck in traffic (mental-emotional stress), (2) flying across time zones (body clock stress), (3) credit card debt (financial stress), (4) spending hours in front of a TV or computer screen (nervous system stress), (5) working all day under artificial lighting (lighting stress), (6) being bombarded by electromagnetic fields (EMF) from power lines, cell phones, wireless devices and other EMF sources (EMF stress), (7) living near an airport or busy road (noise stress), (8) consuming highly processed nutrient-depleted foods (nutritional stress), or (9) being exposed to toxic chemicals in air, water and foods (chemical stress). These are just some of the types of stress we face today. Modern life can be stressful in ways that are similar to the stressors faced by ancient humans and stressful in many brand new ways. All of this adds up, with each additional source of stress placing us under more pressure. Stress causes adaptations. This is seen with gravity. Is it possible that other factors and situations we face every day that collectively fall under a category of stress might be affecting our shape, possibly even before they leave us feeling a bit like a drained battery?

> **HSI CLUE**
>
> Some of us expose ourselves to very stressful activities or situations, acting as if they are penalty free: With a bit of rest we'll be good as new. But stress leaves a scar of sorts. It uses up something that can't be replaced. One lesson from stress research is that we can live either a short highly stressful life or a longer lower stress life.

A Study in Stress

Circumstantial and direct evidence indicates that stress and shape are interrelated. In the last two chapters, body clock stress was mentioned as an example of a stress that is linked to worsening shape. There are many other examples. People with greater job stress are predisposed to gaining more weight. Military veterans suffering from post-traumatic stress disorder are at an increased risk of being overweight or obese.

Individuals who are exposed to long-term stress, caused by sailing around the world, get fatter, with most of the added fat accumulating in the belly area. Stressful life-events often proceed periods of weight gain. Financial stress and relationship stress are both linked to weight gain, especially in persons who are already overweight. Psychological stress at the time of incarceration predicts future weight gain among female prisoners.

HSI CLUE

If a rat is placed in an extremely frigid environment, it will die. By placing it in a colder, but not frigid environment first, it acclimates to cold and survives temperatures that would have previously killed it. This acquired tolerance to cold eventually runs out. The rat dies if left in the frigid environment; it even dies if moved to a moderately cool one. It is tempting to believe that once we are adapted to a certain stress we would be able to perpetually tolerate it. But in many instances, we can't and don't.

In medical research one of the most commonly used models of stress is the *Case of Voluntary Caregivers*. Voluntary caregivers are unpaid individuals, usually spouses or relatives, who assist a sick or disabled person with their activities of daily living. A husband or wife giving care to a spouse who has Alzheimer's disease would be an example of a voluntary caregiver, as would parents taking care of a child with a severe disability, cancer, or other chronic or terminal illness. Anyone who has been a voluntary caregiver can attest that it is stressful mentally, emotionally, and physically. This type of stress is associated with worsening shape. In one study, women who were voluntary caregivers for husbands with Alzheimer's disease gained significantly more weight over the next 15 to 18 months than did similar women who weren't caregivers. In another study, parents of children with cancer were more likely to both gain weight and to experience far greater weight gains than parents with healthy children. In these cases, the amount of weight the caregivers gain is strongly correlated with the degree of mental and emotional stress they experience. While this is circumstantial evidence, it does suggest that there is a relationship between stress and worsening shape.

Another example that illustrates the influence stress might have on shape is the *Case of Sexual Abuse*. Sexual abuse combines elements of physical, mental, emotional, and social stress. Do you think Shape Intelligence might take it into account when making decisions about what shape should be defended moving forward? In one study, women with a history of sexual abuse lost significantly less weight on a low calorie diet and had a much more difficult time adhering to the program. Research also reveals that women with a past history of sexual abuse are much more likely to eventually become obese, and they have disproportionately high rates of eating disorders. We have had clients who have reported gains of 50 to 100 pounds within one year after being sexually abused. In these cases, sexual abuse seems to have been a tipping point for worsening shape.

The next case is the *Case of Social Stress*. Many animals choose to live in groups. Dogs and wolves form packs. Birds, ocean-going mammals (dolphins, whales, and seals), primates (monkeys and apes), grazing animals (cows, deer, elephants, and horses), and felines (like a pride of lions) also live in groups. Rodents (rats, mice, hamsters, and squirrels) will spontaneously opt for socialization and form colonies. The drive to socialize is as innate as the drive to eat or reproduce for these animals. But being part of a group doesn't always benefit all members equally; life at the top tends to be good, while life at the bottom can be stressful. This dynamic is seen in primate groups in the wild.

HSI CLUE

In a study of adolescent girls, those who ranked themselves at the bottom of the social totem pole were more likely to gain weight compared to peers with a more positive view of their social standing. Is it possible that, like primates, adaptation to social stress entails shape changes?

One of the biggest sources of stress in the lives of wild primates is self-inflicted social stress. Like us, they face social pressures, but they face unequal social pressures. Some are bullied. Others are the bullies. Some are under far more threat, which requires constant vigilance; others create this threat. The amount of social stress is largely caused by where on the social hierarchy an individual is located. In a stable group the most stressful place is at the bottom. Dominant males take out their frustrations on the weaker males at the bottom of the social hierarchy. They may also decide to make the lives of those on the bottom miserable for no reason. Subordinate females are more likely to be victimized than are dominant females. In primates, social stress is associated with a very specific pattern of shape change—an increase in visceral fat. Factors that increase social stress, including bullying, being victimized by aggression more frequently, and spending less time in affiliative social interactions (tending to offspring, interacting with friends, etc.) result in an increase in belly fat, as well as signs and symptoms of metabolic obesity (high blood sugar, heart disease, etc.).

HSI CLUE

A group of men gained weight after experiencing significant life events. Some tried to diet the weight away; others didn't. The men who didn't diet eventually reacquired their previous weight. Among the men who dieted, in the words of the researchers, "the gain in body mass following few or many life events seemed to be permanent." What might this teach us about stress and shape? What might it teach us about using dieting as a way to counter this weight gain?

Primates are not alone. A hamster that experiences social stress will gain weight and get fatter. Like primates, it adapts to social stress by increasing its natural weight and altering its shape. A hamster will also adapt to non-social forms of stress in the same way—by becoming fatter. For many animals, social stress is a powerful shape tipping point. Evidence suggests that it might be fattening in humans as well. Poverty is a surrogate for social stress; not surprisingly the poor are far more likely to be obese and to suffer from obesity-related illness than are those with higher socioeconomic status. Evidence also suggests a link between poverty and the same type of shape changes detected in primates subjected to social stress: Being poor has a strong correlation with having increased amounts of belly fat. Our perception of social stress also appears to be related to future weight gain. Among adolescent girls, those who ranked themselves at the bottom of the social totem pole were more likely to gain weight over time than their peers with a more positive view of their social standing. The *Case of Overfeeding Identical Twins* is further evidence for the link between stress and worsening shape.

For any pair of genetically identical twins, if all aspects of diet, lifestyle, and environment are the same, shape of one twin will closely resemble the other. If the shape of one identical twin ends up being very different from that of the other, there must be a logical reason why. In one study of identical twins with different shapes, the investigators concluded that the best explanation for the difference in visceral fat amounts between identical twins was the amount of *psychological* and *social stress*. The twin that experienced more stress had a worse body shape even if the weight of both was equal. Similar to primates, not only was social stress linked to a worse shape, it was linked to a very specific shape pattern—bigger bellies.

Because of the strong links between stress and belly fat, scientists have investigated the mechanisms that might explain this link. During times of higher stress, the body produces more of a hormone called cortisol. Current evidence indicates that belly fat is more sensitive to cortisol than are other types of fat tissue. Visceral fat can even actively self-regulate how much cortisol is available locally. In animals, increased cortisol directly increases belly fat. In humans the direct effects of cortisol are well established because it, and similar molecules, is used as medications. Known side effects include gains in belly and trunk fat (central fat accumulation) and losses in muscle. The gains in fat amounts usually outpace the losses in muscle weight, with the end result being an easily detected gain in weight over time. The effects of cortisol on shape are especially pronounced when far too much cortisol is in the blood, whether because of an excessive dose give as a medication or because of some internal issue, such as Cushing's syndrome, that causes the body to produce high amounts of this stress hormone. Individuals with Cushing's syndrome gain weight, usually rapidly, but even bigger shifts occur with shape. Belly and trunk fat increase, the face tends to become rounder (moon face), and fat accumulates on the upper back and neck (buffalo hump). While these areas are gaining fat, the arms, legs, and buttocks often lose fat and muscle. The overall shape change is unmistakable.

Scientific studies reveal links between many different types of stress and shape. The known effects of cortisol provide a plausible explanation for how stress affects shape, in general, and belly fat, specifically. The evidence suggests that stress can have a big effect on our shape, but sometimes this effect doesn't show up until after a stressful period is over. This point was illustrated in the *Case of the Army Rangers* (discussed in chapter 4). This case was a study on how healthy, lean young men adapt to multiple forms of stress. The soldiers were subjected to exercise stress, calorie-deprivation stress, sleep deprivation stress, and cold stress. During Ranger training, while calories were being restricted and exercise levels were high, the soldiers lost weight and body fat. But five weeks after the end of Ranger training, the average soldier had 140 percent of their starting body fat. Stress left a scar, so to speak. It caused Shape Intelligence to adapt. Because calories were being restricted and the soldiers were being forced to be very active, this adaptation was not visibly apparent with respect to shape until after the stressors were removed—until the recovery period when Shape Intelligence finally had access to food and rest. This case illustrates an important principle. The effects of stress on shape are not always immediately evident. It takes time to learn, adapt and recover. The reason we are noticing a change in our shape this month might be because of something stressful that happened last month. This dynamic can make it harder to spot the real culprit.

From the clues we have discussed, and many other clues from our stress case files, stress seems to worsen shape and directly contribute to body fat accumulation—in some instances dramatic accumulation. The specific type of shape change that tends to be experienced with stress is a central pattern of body fat accumulation, an increase in belly fat. Sometimes the change in shape occurs while stress is ongoing; other times it occurs *after* the stressful event is over. Because of the interrelationship of stress and shape, if we are serious about improving our shape, we also want to be serious about reducing our stress.

Detecting Sources of Stress

Stress isn't only something that arises because of social situations and it isn't solely a mental-emotional phenomenon. Many things can cause stress. If we experience something as stressful, it will be. But even things we don't view as stressful can still be. If an event or circumstance interferes with the ability for our body to function normally, it will cause stress, and it will do this even if we don't think of it as particularly stressful. We saw this in the *Case of Dr. Mark* (discussed in chapter 12). He didn't think it would be significantly stressful to spend almost two months flying back and forth across two to three time zones, multiple times a week. It still was. Chronic disruption of body clocks interferes with the ability of the body to function. As such, it is stressful. Findings in stress research indicate that while certain things might always produce stress, almost anything, if it is intense enough, persists long enough, or hits us when we aren't ready, can cause stress. With this in mind, let's work on improving our stress detective skills.

In general usage, the word stress, or the feeling of being stressed out, is a sort of catch all for a host of perceived difficulties or challenging situations. We might feel stressed out because of an irritating colleague, a demanding boss, or an upcoming exam. Financial issues might cause us to feel more stress. Someone we care about might be sick or

HSI CLUE

People who effectively manage stress are far more likely to experience and keep positive shape changes. This was observed in a study of more than 2000 people. Those who reduced their weight by 44 pounds or more had one thing in common. They improved their ability to cope with taxing circumstances.

injured, causing us to experience mental-emotional stress. We might feel stressed because we are late for something and are stuck in traffic. There are many circumstances and situations that most of us will correctly recognize as stressful. There are also many things that we might miss. Things we think of as stressful represent the starting point for detecting sources of stress in our lives, not the ending point. Stress experiments reveal that widely different things including exercise, temperature changes, bright light, noise, injury, drugs, and toxic substances can produce stress. Almost anything can produce a stress response. Even things we generally think of as beneficial—as good for us—can produce a stress response if exposure is prolonged, too intense, or comes when we're unprepared for it. Let's look at a few real world examples to highlight these points.

Health suffers with too little rest. It's stressful. Since this is the case, it seems obvious that we should consider rest to be a "good" thing. Certainly too little of it isn't good for us. But is there such a thing as *too much good*? Stress research tells us the answer to this question is yes. Prolonged rest, such as bed rest, just like too little rest, produces a stress response. When it comes to rest there is a just right amount. As we move further away from this amount in either direction the stress response gets activated in bigger ways. Many real world things are like rest; too little won't be enough, but more isn't always better. This is the Goldilocks principle. In the story *The Three Bears,* Goldilocks encountered three bowls of porridge, one was too cold, one was too hot, and one was just right. The goal is to find the *just right amount* for us in all the things we do and experience. The just right rule of thumb applies to duration, intensity, and frequency. Exercise is an example.

Exercise follows the Goldilocks principle. Being sedentary isn't good for us, but neither is exercising all day. The goal is to move for long enough amounts of time, but not for too long. Prolonged duration of doing, or being exposed to many things, including exercise, increases the likelihood that it will cause stress. The intensity of things also influences the stress

HSI CLUE

The stress mechanism is indifferent to our notions of good and bad. A stressful job is stressful. Most of us will spot this clue. But a job promotion, even if desired, can cause a significant amount of temporary stress as we are getting used to the change. Change, even for the better, tends to be stressful. There are many potential sources of stress that are not obvious to the untrained eye.

response. Walking, from an intensity perspective, is a gentle form of exercise. Running a marathon is a lot more intense. Most of us could walk casually for two hours and suffer little to no stress response. The same is not true for running a marathon. A world-class marathon runner will finish a marathon in a bit more than two hours and suffer a huge stress response that will persist for weeks. In this case, it would not be exercising for two hours that is the issue; the issue is the relative intensity of what was done. Prolonging our exposure to something can turn an otherwise beneficial thing into something stressful. Increasing the intensity of something can also make something that might otherwise be benign, into a powerful stressor. Duration and intensity also interact. As something becomes more intense, we need to be more concerned with the duration. With less intense things, we can afford to prolong the duration a bit more. Let's return to exercise once again to illustrate this interaction.

Sprinting is more intense than jogging, which is more intense than walking. All are exercise, but are unequal in terms of their intensity. As a result, most of us could walk for a longer duration of time than we could jog, and we could jog for a longer amount of time compared with sprinting, before generating a stress response. If exercise is gentle, we can do it for longer periods of time before experiencing stress, but if it is extremely intense, it might cause a significant stress response in a matter of minutes. As we move up the intensity continuum—with anything—we need to scale back on the duration if we want to avoid having a detrimental stress response.

If our exposure to stimuli is prolonged, it is stressful. If stimuli are too intense, it is also stressful. The frequency of exposure also influences whether or not it is experienced as stress. Let's look at exercise once again to illustrate. Walking is a low intensity form of exercise. As long as we don't walk exceedingly long distances or for prolonged durations of time, most of us can go for a walk most days and it will improve our health. The same isn't true for more intense forms of exercise. If we were to participate in a much more demanding type of activity, such as long-distance running or weight training, unless we allow sufficient recovery time between bouts of exercise, we will experience *overtraining syndrome*. Overtraining is a stress syndrome. It negatively affects our physical, mental, and emotional health. Overtraining is in large part a frequency problem. We don't get faster or stronger because of running or lifting weights, respectively; we get faster and stronger because of the adaptations the body makes to running or weight training. Exercise is the stimulus. Adaptation is the response, but this response occurs during the rest period following hard training and takes time. If we train too frequently, failing to allow sufficient time for complete adaptation (recovery), performance eventually suffers. It suffers because the frequency is causing stress rather than improving fitness. As the duration lengthens, the intensity increases, and even more so if both of these factors apply, more downtime between bouts of exposures is needed to adapt and fully recover.

The more intense something is, the more likely that it will produce a stress response if our exposure to it is anything more than very brief. The more gentle something is, the more prolonged it can be before it is experienced as stress. But, and this is important, even mild stimuli will eventually produce a stress response if they are allowed to persist long enough. Noise illustrates this point. A jackhammer outside our window will usually be experienced as quite stressful almost immediately. It is such an intense sound we have little recourse physiologically. If we are near a freeway, we will be exposed to a far less intense sound—the low frequency drone of cars moving at fast speeds. This is a form of white noise or noise pollution. While we might not notice this as quickly as the noise of a jackhammer, or respond to it with as big a stress response, hour after hour of low frequency white noise is stressful.

HSI CLUE

To detect potential sources of stress it can be helpful to ask questions like, "What is really weighing me down?" or "What is burdening my heart?" These questions sometimes help us to identify mental, emotional, and social stressors that are contributing to our stress load (and perhaps our shape challenges).

How prepared we are for something, influences whether something is stressful and how stressful it might be. Let's return to exercise once again. Running a marathon is stressful. This is even true for elite athletes. But it would be far more stressful for an untrained, and hence, unprepared person. The same principle holds true for exercise of lesser intensity. An hour-long brisk walk could be enjoyable for a fit person, and yet highly stressful for a previously sedentary person. Complex adaptive intelligence tries to make best guesses about what things it might encounter. It tries to prepare itself for the things it expects. Unanticipated events or situations can catch it unprepared. It won't have had an opportunity to adapt, habituating itself to whatever the stimulus might be, and preparing itself for future exposure. Events and situations will be far more stressful when the body hasn't been allowed the opportunity to prepare itself. This is observed with sun exposure.

A fair skinned person from New York might experience severe sunburn from just fifteen minutes of direct sun in the tropics at midday during a winter vacation. The same person may be able to easily tolerate fifteen minutes of sun in New York in the springtime at noon. Duration, in both instances, is the same, but the sun's intensity causes very different responses. Now consider what might occur if complex adaptive intelligence were given an opportunity to better prepare itself for the intense sun exposure. If this person were allowed a chance to adapt to gradually increasing sun intensity— build up biological defenses (a tan)—they would be able to tolerate more sun exposure, in terms of duration, intensity, or both. They might even be able to tolerate fifteen minutes outside in the tropics. Whenever we introduce new situations or circumstances, it is imperative that we do so as gently as possible initially, and gradually increase duration and intensity. This gives complex adaptive intelligence a chance to prepare itself, and advance preparation tends to makes things less stressful.

Living things adapt to most new challenges in ways that allow them to perform better should the challenge reoccur. Without this capability, survival in a demanding and variable environment would be impossible. While living things have the capability to adjust to changes in their environment, taking a lab animal used to living at room temperature, and placing it in a frigid environment, is too big an adjustment for it to make; it's lethal. But if the animal is incrementally exposed to colder conditions in a step-wise fashion— habituated gradually to colder and colder conditions—it will survive cold temperatures that would otherwise have killed it. Many stressors are less stressful if we are given an opportunity to gradually adapt. This even applies to some potentially lethal substances.

The idea that humans can be conditioned to tolerate some stressors that might otherwise be lethal by exposing them to the stressor in small, incremental steps is not a new idea. In the book *The Count of Monte Cristo*, written by Alexandre Dumas and published in the 19th century, we see evidence of this idea. A murderer attempted to kill the character Old Monsieur Noirtier by poisoning him, yet Old

Monsieur Noirtier survives. He had been taking a medicine that contained small amounts of the poison, and as a result acquired some degree of resistance to the poison, which allowed him to survive a dose that otherwise, would have killed him. Since the poison was present in small amounts in his medication, complex adaptive intelligence had a chance to adapt and prepare itself. The practice of protecting oneself against a poison by gradually self-administering non-lethal amounts is called *Mithridatism;* being named after the historical king Mithridates VI, the King of Pontus, who so feared being poisoned that he regularly ingested small doses of poison, aiming to develop immunity. Some things, because of their nature, will always cause stress; poisons are an example. But even with poisons, preparation might make the difference between being sick and being dead. While the goal isn't to prepare ourselves against poisoning, or other unlikely circumstances, we do want to make sure we are doing our best to give our body every opportunity to gradually adapt to new demands or challenges.

Some things, like poisons, are always stressful. Other things will or won't produce stress depending upon how long they are ongoing, how intense they are, and how prepared we are to deal with them. Lighting conditions, discussed in chapter 12, illustrate the interaction of these three factors. Continuous lighting conditions cause stress because it is, well, continuous. In the *Cases of the Implanted Cancer* (chapter 12), it caused cancer to grow and be more lethal, as an example. Extremely bright lighting conditions, because of the intensity, can cause stress. Light at the wrong time in our day-night can be stressful; because from a body clock perspective we are prepared for light at some times and for darkness at others. These three factors—duration, intensity, and preparation—interact. We might only be able to tolerate extremely bright continuous lighting for a few hours in a row in the evening, before having a significant stress response. Yet we can readily tolerate naturalistic lighting conditions for a lifetime, even though, for brief periods every day around noon, the intensity of lighting conditions might be "off the charts". In nature, we don't ever have

---

HSI CLUE

In our investigations we have encountered many cases of "relationship stress"; unhappy marriages, abusive situations, lack of romance, etc. In some case, 25 to 30 pounds have vanished, without any effort whatsoever, within months of making and executing a decision to either (1) leave an unsatisfying relationship, or (2) remain in it but in a way that is satisfying. What are your relationships like? Could they be a tipping point for you?

to deal with lighting conditions that are being held constant—unchanging for prolonged durations of time. The only thing that is constant about naturalistic lighting is that it is constantly changing. It changes across the day and the year. Our eyes get to gradually adapt as we move from darkness to dawn to early morning to bright midday to late afternoon to dusk to darkness. While midday illumination can be brighter than most man-made light sources, it comes at a time when our body clock is ready for it—when we are physiologically prepared. We get to gradually habituate to higher intensity light as days lengthen and we move from the relatively low intensity light during winter months to the higher intensity sunlight of mid-summer. All of this makes a difference when it comes to whether the same external thing—light in this case—is easily tolerated or causes a big stress response.

HSI CLUE

Hans Selye was a pioneer in stress research. He said; "Survival depends largely on a correct balance of attack, retreat, and standing ones ground." How well are you doing creating this balance? Are there areas where you might be better served retreating, or standing your ground? Are there things worth fighting for rather than avoiding?

How long we are exposed to things, how much or how little they change during this time period, how intense they are, and how prepared we are, all matter. Sitting at a desk under fluorescent lights for four hours in a row looking at a computer might be very stressful. Sitting near an open window, doing a variety of work activities, with five to ten minute breaks every hour to stretch our legs probably won't be. The way we respond to four hours of work can be drastically influenced by the overall context—by things around us and by what we do or don't do. As you review the categories of stressors we list below, and as you search for stress clues at your health scene, please keep these principles in mind.

As a general rule, factors and situations are stressful because they:
1. Directly traumatize the body (injury, pain, extremes of temperature or exercise),
2. Disrupt the body's ability to function normally (calorie deprivation, lack of sleep, body clock stress, chemical and pollution exposure, alcohol intoxication, electromagnetic fields),
3. Are intense or prolonged sensory stimuli (loud noise, bright light, intense movies; prolonged white noise, continuous lighting, hours of TV watching or playing video games),

4. Require sustained attention or focus (hours of studying or work, extended computer use, long distance driving),

5. Represent new experiences or significant changes (starting college or a new job, ending a relationship, losing a job, going from being sedentary to exercising),

6. Are mentally or emotionally challenging (exams, working overtime, project deadlines, deaths, caring for a sick relative, loss of control over our circumstances or environment, financial pressures, marital unhappiness),

7. Place us under specific types of social pressure (subordinate social status, victimization, abuse, physical or emotional threats, conflict with others).

These examples are just some of the more common physical factors or psychosocial situations that can cause stress. Evidence strongly suggests that several of these types of stress contribute to worsening of shape. Others have yet to be investigated. Can you detect any of these at your health scene?

Key Point

Unresolved issues are stressful. Many of us have aspects of our lives that would cease being mentally and emotionally taxing if we made a decision—any decision. These chronic dilemmas place a constant weight on us; especially if family, close friends, a love relationship, or work is involved. A warning sign for unresolved stress is that we find ourselves thinking about something repeatedly and wondering what we should do. In some instances the solution to these situations is obvious but tremendously difficult. Often the best option is following the advice of Eleanor Roosevelt, "You must do the thing you think you cannot do." Or, as Holmes told Watson, "Any truth is better than indefinite doubt."

As you begin your investigation please keep one thing in mind. Stress is additive. All of the things in your life add up. Your stress load is the total of all of the interacting factors and situations. A person with one or two big stressors might be under a great deal of stress. This is usually easy to spot. But a person with no large sources of stress, yet many seemingly trivial ones might actually be under just as much, or even more, total stress, because all of these little things can be adding up to a heavy load.

The Solution: Playing the Camel Game

As a health scene investigator it is imperative that we be able to detect sources of stress in our lives. Once they are detected, the goal is to eliminate (or at least minimize) exposure to as many as possible. When it comes to stress, we want to lighten our load. There is also one other goal. We want to make ourselves as resilient to stress as possible. The analogy we use to explain solving stress problems in this dual manner is the *Camel Game*. Many different languages have proverbs that are akin to the English idiom, "The straw that broke the camel's back." This idiom is a way to point out that cataclysmic failure (a broken back) can occur from a seemingly inconsequential addition (a single straw). There is a limit to endurance. Everyone and everything has a breaking point. In 1966, Schaper's toys came out with a child's game based on this principle. The game was officially called *The Last Straw* and unofficially called the Camel Game (this vintage game can sometimes be found for sale on eBay). The game consisted of a plastic camel with two baskets that hung over its back. Players sequentially added straws of different colors, with each color having a different weight, to these baskets. There were heavy straws (yellow), medium weight straws (green and blue), and lightweight straws (red). At some point, the weight of the added straws would be too heavy and the camel's back would break.

HSI CLUE

Selye wrote; "It may be said for man, without hesitation, the most important stressors are emotional, especially those causing distress." He believed that situations that caused emotional stress were especially likely to cause health problems.

The Camel Game is a useful metaphor for real life stress. Every potential source of stress is like a straw that gets added to our basket. Some straws might be exceptionally heavy (such as divorce); others might be light (such as a scary movie); and still others will be somewhere in the middle. The Camel Game teaches us that there is no such thing as an unimportant straw. Each source of stress in our life—even ones which might seem trivial—adds to our stress load. While a few heavy straws will break the camel's back, it will still break eventually if the only straws added are lightweight. The same is true for stress. Big stressors like divorce, loss of a job, and the death of a loved one, occurring in rapid succession might cause the back to break in most of us. But how big a stress might be—its weight so to speak—isn't the only important consideration. Stress is additive. Given enough trivial sources of stress, we'll reach our breaking point—the point where health collapses—just as surely as we would if the only things in our basket were big sources of stress. Like the camel, we can carry a certain burden of stress before the back collapses. It doesn't matter if we reach this breaking point because of a few big sources of stress, many little ones, or some combination of both. Unfortunately, it's not easy in the game or in real life to always tell how close we are to this breaking point.

The Last Straw game teaches us that it is often difficult to tell how close we are to cataclysmic failure. Are we at the point where even a light straw will be too much, or can we add a few heavy ones with no worries? It's not always easy to make this determination in the game; imagine how much more difficult it is to make it in real life where many sources of stress are hard to detect, the relative "weight" of even obvious straws is essentially impossible to measure, and we each have vastly different carrying capacities when it comes to the stress loads we can support. Because of these and other complexities, typically, we won't know with certainty where we stand until after we have exceeded our limits; until we have passed our breaking points. We can keep adding straws— seemingly penalty free—until we can't. At this point, hindsight allows us to tell that we had too

> **HSI CLUE**
>
> Selye wrote; "It is especially true that the stressor effects depend not so much on what we do or what happens to us but on the way we take it." How are you taking things? Are you optimistic or pessimistic, self-responsible or a victim of circumstances? Are you solving problems or worrying about them?

many straws in our basket. Are you teetering at the edge, ready to collapse with even the tiniest new stressor? Do you have a lot of room to add more weight to your basket? Is there enough room in your basket for big life events? If a major life event were to occur will you be able to carry the extra weight or will it cause you to fly by your limit of endurance, causing you to collapse under the added weight? These questions aren't easy to answer. And life tends to dump heavy straws in our basket from time to time—often when we least expect it. We lose a job, a loved one gets sick or dies, a relationship ends. We want our basket to be as light as possible *before* these significant types of stress occur. Because of the inherent uncertainty, we believe the best solution is to keep our basket as empty of stressors as possible at all times. We accomplish this by building our awareness of what constitute stress and diligently reducing as many sources of it as possible.

Removing straws—sources of potential stress—is part one of the Camel Game. It can involve saying no more often, making decisions, resolving difficult issues, sharing stressful things with loved ones. It entails spending less time watching TV, using a computer, or listening to loud music, eliminating poor lifestyle habits, lessening our exposure to white noise, continuous lighting, or sources of pollution. It means doing our best to keep our baskets as light as possible when it comes to sources of stress. Every straw we identify and remove is, in a sense, insurance against catastrophic failure. We absolutely want to keep our stress baskets as empty as possible. But, at the same time, it makes a great deal of sense to maximize our ability to support a heavy load. This is part two of the Camel Game—building a stronger back, so to speak.

In *The Last Straw* game, the load the camel can support is a given. There really isn't anything we, as players, can do to change it. This is not the case in real life. Hans Selye, the originator of the modern idea of biological stress, had a vision for a new type of medicine. He felt that if we strengthened our body's defense against stress, we might prevent many diseases. These defenses are our ability to adapt to, cope with, and be resilient when faced with stressful things. These are positive capacities that influence our ability to deal with current stress. They also represent our ability to resist future stressful events in a way that will prevent our back from collapsing under the weight. Being well-rested, physically fit, and well-nourished; improving our self esteem and resourcefulness (feeling good about ourselves and believing that there are things we can do to alter our circumstances—being a survivor of, not a victim of, circumstances); cultivating connectedness and supportive social relationships with family and friends; being active in enlivening groups and organizations; spiritual beliefs; helping others; having hobbies that are relaxing and enjoyable; practicing relaxation techniques (like meditation or progressive relaxation); watching movies that make us laugh, cry (in a happy way), or feel hopeful; and paced breathing are among the best ways to strengthen the body's defenses against stress. So, part two of the Camel Game entails doing our best to include more of the above activities, practices and lifestyle habits into our health scene. We can't really know with certainty what load life might place on us. But we can always be doing things to be better prepared to tolerate this load.

Paced breathing is a specific cadence of breathing—six breaths per minute. Each inhalation is five seconds and each exhalation is five seconds. This breathing pace puts many aspects of our physiology in sync in ways that faster or slower breathing paces don't. We recommend that twice-daily people spend five to ten minutes practicing paced breathing.

When playing the real life Camel Game—the game aimed at removing straws and building a more resilient back—there are a few rules to keep in mind. Rule one is to be wary of "newness." When we start new things or have novel experiences there will be an initial period of greater stress while we are adapting. During this period, we want to avoid overdoing it. The goal is to be gentle at the beginning and to gradually, in a step-wise fashion, increase demands. This allows our body to tap into its potential for adaptation in the least stressful manner and to prepare itself adequately for the increased demands. As we adapt, we can tolerate a greater intensity of something whether the something is exercise, cold, noise, or some other stress. Rule two is that just because we might be able to adapt to something—to build tolerance to it—does not mean that we should subject ourselves to it in the first place. We can adapt to stress but only to a point. We can tolerate stress but only so much. It is better to underestimate our ability to tolerate stress rather than to overestimate it. It is better to never test our limits. Rule three is that we don't want to wear ourselves out unevenly. Think in terms of tires on a car. If they don't get rotated periodically, they wear out faster. The body is not designed to take too much stress always on the same part or system. This means it is not designed to do the same tasks for hours on end. To prevent a stress response we need what Selye called *deviation,* something that might be easiest to think of as variety. After spending all day sitting at a desk working, getting on our home computer doesn't add much variety; it stresses the same systems in the body. Going for a walk adds variety. Do your best to "rotate your tires," distributing wear and tear more evenly across all systems in your body. If you have spent hours doing one thing, make sure you do something completely different to relieve stress. Rule four is that we need to understand when deviation will help and when it won't. If we are completely exhausted or feel worn out, deviation is not a very effective strategy. What we really need when we are exhausted is rest. This is also true when general stress is excessive. At this point, we need a chance to recover. We can't afford a struggle anywhere. Deviation is not a productive strategy when we are worn out. Think of the soldiers from the *Case of the Army Rangers* from earlier in the chapter. After exposure to multiple stressors for weeks on end, they were having huge stress responses that persisted for weeks after the training period ended. Adding some variety into their routine won't help at this point. Rest and recovery is needed. Whenever possible, do not overwork any one part of your body or mind to the point of exhaustion. On any occasion you do, don't push yourself to do things that you think are going to be good for you. Unless the good thing entails rest, chances are it is going to be counter-productive. Rule five is that every "camel" is unique. No matter what our stress load (light or heavy), if it is beyond our individual ability to cope with it, we will collapse under the added weight. The load each of us can carry is different and is influenced by our genetics, our past and present lifestyle choices, our reserves for adaptation, and many other factors. It doesn't do much good to compare our load to someone else's. They might be able to carry much more or much less. Rule six is that if the camel's back collapses, it often takes removing much more than "the last straw" to fix the problem. More times than naught, recovery entails unburdening ourselves of many of the things we had in the basket before we collapsed under its weight. If we want to reverse the stress-induced changes, it might mean eliminating lots of straws. This might not seem fair. Nevertheless, it seems to be one of the rules of the game.

To win at the real life Camel Game requires putting efforts into removing straws and building a stronger back. After you have identified possible sources of modifiable stress, it will be your responsibility to take whatever steps are within your power to eliminate those that can be eliminated and to reduce your exposure to any which remain. Once stress is minimized we must learn to support the remaining stress load more effectively. If we do a better job managing stress, it is less likely Shape Intelligence will feel the need to get involved. Since Shape Intelligence seems to go about supporting us during stress by making our belly more substantial, we probably want to do our best to keep it from getting involved in the stress management business in the first place.

For further resources to assist your stress management skills, visit our website www.healthsceneinvestigation.com and click on: Stress Support.

Closing Dialogue

Health Scene Investigator: A table with thin legs collapsed when we placed weight on it. The same weight didn't cause a table with thicker, stouter legs to collapse. A more substantial table supported a weight that was, frankly, catastrophic for a less substantial one. These are verifiable facts. Now that we have examined details of stress and shape, do you understand why I mentioned that this might be a valuable clue to shape?

Apprentice: Yes, I believe I do. The details we examined indicate that stress and shape are not two independent phenomena.

Health Scene Investigator: Precisely so. We know that stress and shape are correlated. We also know that in many scientific experiments stress causes shape to change. This is our starting point. From here we can reason backwards and come up with plausible explanations. Would you use your scientific imagination and share with me one such explanation.

Apprentice: Sure. It would seem to me that an intelligent system might choose to adapt to added pressure placed upon it by becoming more substantial; by, in a manner of speaking, becoming a table with stouter legs.

Health Scene Investigator (laughing): Well said. Naturally, this is only a hypothesis; a possibility. Yet it seems to be a possibility supported by the details. Do you think there might be other examples of this intelligence adapting; making wise decisions when faced with certain details of our modern world?

Apprentice: I would imagine there might be. And my guess is that you do.

Health Scene Investigator: Well, now that you mention it, I just might. Which brings me to my next question, what do you know about chemical pollutants...chemical stress?

Chapter 15

Chemicals and Shape

"Might I trouble you to open the window, for chloroform vapor does not help the palate?"

Sherlock Holmes

Opening Dialogue

Health Scene Investigator: I have a question for you. Are you familiar with what occurs when oil is mixed with water?

Apprentice: Yes I am. They don't mix. The oil and water stay separate.

Health Scene Investigator: And if we had added a substance that dissolves in oil such as say, a fat-soluble nutrient like vitamin A or D, would it dissolve in the water, the oil or both?

Apprentice: It would dissolve in the oil but still stay separate from the water.

Health Scene Investigator: Exactly so. These are very important observations. In fact they inform us of an important relationship between chemical pollutants and body fat.

Apprentice: I am confused. How does the fact that oil and water don't mix teach us something about chemical pollutants and body fat?

Health Scene Investigator: Excellent question. Residues from things like pesticides, flame-retardants, and plastics are found in the body in fat tissue (pause)…you look confused.

Apprentice: I apologize but this is new to me. Do you mean to say that these chemical pollutants are inside our bodies?

Health Scene Investigator: Yes that is precisely what I mean to say.

Somebody Please Open the Window

Every year hundreds of billions of pounds of man-made chemicals are produced. They are used as biocides (pesticides, herbicides, anti-fouling agents), in consumer products (air fresheners, bedding, cosmetics, electronics, non-stick cookware, and toiletries), for industrial purposes (additives to gasoline and paints, dry cleaning solvents, making plastics and resins), and in many other applications. Many man-made chemicals persist in the environment, polluting it, and contaminating food, water, air, and household dust. We ingest and inhale them. Other chemicals are in things we apply directly to our skin; we absorb them. Chemicals have practical benefits; many of them also come with health-damaging side effects. Chemical exposure is an important health issue; it affects all of us.

If a chemical is found in the environment, odds are high it will be found inside living organisms, including humans, which live in that environment Three recent *biomonitoring* investigations illustrate this important point. The 2005 *European Family Biomonitoring Survey* analyzed blood samples from thirteen families in three generations (grandmothers, mothers, and children) from twelve different European countries. Blood was tested for 107 different chemical contaminants including organochlorine pesticides (like dichlorodiphenyltrichloroethane, better known as DDT), polychlorinated biphenyls (PCBs), brominated flame-retardants, perfluorinated chemicals (Teflon-like compounds used in "non-stick" cookware), bisphenol A (used in polycarbonate plastics and epoxy resins and abbreviated BPA), and several different man-made

> **HSI CLUE**
>
> Some of the factors with the strongest associations with a higher body burden of chemicals include (1) higher body fat, (2) increasing age, (3) sedentary lifestyles, (4) smoking (5) working in an occupation that involves chemical exposure, (6) living in proximity to sites with high chemical levels (examples include living near hazardous waste sites, in apartment buildings with dry cleaning stores, etc).

"scent" chemicals (used as fragrances in cleaning products, cosmetics, and toiletries). Brominated flame-retardants, organochlorine pesticides, PCBs, perfluorinated chemicals and scent chemicals were found in virtually every person tested, and BPA was found in one out of every four people. In 2009, the Environmental Working Group released the results of their investigation of umbilical cord blood from ten American infants. More than two hundred different chemicals were detected. Flame-retardants, perfluorinated chemicals, pesticide residues, gasoline additives, and BPA were found in almost every infant. The last piece of evidence comes from the *Fourth National Report on Human Exposure to Environmental Chemicals* released by United States Center for Disease Control and Prevention (CDC) in 2009. The CDC analyzed blood and urine of 8,000 Americans for 212 chemical contaminants. A few types of chemicals, including flame-retardants, perfluorinated chemicals, gasoline additives, and BPA, were found in all, or most, of the people tested. These investigations, and many others like them, indicate that having multiple chemical residues inside of us isn't the exception to the rule; it is the rule. Even newborn are, in essence, born polluted, exposed to multiple chemicals while in the womb. For almost all of us, the question won't be whether we have chemicals residues inside our body (we do); the questions will be a matter of which ones, how much, and the effects.

None of these questions is particularly easy to answer. Estimates suggest that an average person might routinely come in contact with as many as six thousand different chemicals. Trying to investigate for all of these chemicals would be prohibitively expensive. Even large government-sponsored studies, like the CDC study mentioned above, only investigate for a tiny fraction of man-made chemicals. Answering the question of *how much* is also difficult. Most man-made chemicals are *fat loving*; they accumulate in adipose and other fatty tissues. Investigating for, and detecting, chemicals in blood and urine gives a clue to their presence; it doesn't reveal actual body burden, much of which is below the surface, so to speak, hidden inside our tissues. Answering questions about *what* and *how much* are difficult enough; answering questions about the effects is downright daunting. Part of the reason for this is illustrated in the *Case of Chloroform*.

In the story *His Last Bow*, Holmes asks Watson if he could trouble him to open the window. He makes this request because he has been working with chloroform, which is toxic if inhaled. His solution was to ventilate, air out, the room. Taking steps to reduce his exposure to chloroform vapors was a sensible solution. While complete avoidance would have been even better, opening some windows was a step in the right direction. It would protect him against some, but not all, of the effects of chloroform, which like many substances, has acute and chronic effects.

HSI CLUE

Polychlorinated biphenyls (PCBs) were first made in the late 1800s. Exposure to a high dose of PCBs causes a skin condition called *chloracne.* This is easy to detect. Chronic effects took more time to detect. PCB makers fought back, publicly expressing skepticism about links to disease and sponsoring their own safety studies. Use of PCBs continued with few restraints up until 1977 when production was banned in the U.S. It's now 2009 and PCBs still persist in the environment; they're still found in our fat tissue.

In medicine and toxicology, the time scale of things is an important consideration. Some things have a fast time scale. They have an abrupt onset, last only a short time, or both. A cold, the flu, and the dizziness we might experience immediately after inhaling chloroform vapors would be examples of these fast time scale or *acute* phenomena. In acute situations we progress from good to bad rapidly and noticeably. Other things have slow time scales. Onset can be almost imperceptibly slow. The change from good to bad is very gradual; it might be occurring for months, years, or decades before it is large enough to be detected. This is an example of a *chronic* effect. In addition to slow onset, chronic things tend to persist. Arthritis, cancer, diabetes, osteoporosis, and sleep apnea are examples of chronic health conditions. Chronic problems, in most cases, occur because we get repeated exposure to whatever causes the problem. They are generally far more influenced by health damaging behaviors—lifestyle choices like smoking, sedentary habits, and poor food choices—and the environment. Whether something is considered acute or chronic is not a statement about its severity; it is a statement about its time scale. And time scale is a vitally important consideration when it comes to the science and art of detection. Things with a slow time scale are far more difficult to detect. This was the case with chloroform.

The acute effects of chloroform include dizziness, fatigue, headaches, and unconsciousness. These effects occur quickly, are easy to notice, and the last effect, unconsciousness, is the reason why it was used as an anesthetic from the mid-1800s to the early part of the 20th century. But the acute effects of breathing chloroform vapors don't end with unconsciousness. At a sufficient dose it can cause the heart to lose its rhythm, resulting in sudden death. This was eventually detected and chloroform's use in medicine was abandoned for safer alternatives. Chloroform's acute effects were easy to detect. People felt poorly soon enough after breathing the vapors that it was easy to put one and one together and pinpoint the culprit. The chronic effects weren't as easy to detect. Chloroform exposure is linked to cancer, miscarriage, birth defects, infertility, and liver and kidney damage. These illnesses aren't acute effects; they don't show up a few minutes after exposure and might not show up until years or decades later. They don't occur only because of one large inhalation, but can occur because of persistent exposure to doses of chloroform that are too low to cause detectable acute effects. Millions of people were exposed to chloroform before its chronic toxicity was detected. Up until 1976, when it was banned in consumer products in the United States, chloroform was in some toothpastes, cough syrups, ointments, and medications. The acute effects of chloroform were obvious by the 1850s. It took more than 120 years more before scientific consensus on the possible harm from exposure to low levels of chloroform was reached. For more than a century the less obvious chronic effects of low level exposure went unrecognized or ignored, and many individuals were routinely exposed to a something that was, in hindsight, harmful.

Answering questions about the effects of man-made chemicals is daunting because, like with chloroform, chronic effects might only occur with repeated exposure, can occur at doses far lower than those needed to produce acute effects, and often don't show up until far in the future. This is an important lesson. It applies to many chemicals we have been exposed to in the past, and which have since been banned. It likely applies to many of the chemicals we are being routinely exposed to today: Some of these substances might have health-damaging effects, but we won't know what these effects are until sometime in the future. In the meantime, many of us will be exposed repeatedly unless we reconsider our *default assumptions*.

Our default assumption is revealed in our behaviors: We often act as if things are safe until evidence proves otherwise. An example of this tendency is revealed in the *Case of Running Behind Mosquito Spray Trucks*. During the 1950s and 60s, it wasn't uncommon to see

HSI CLUE

When the World Trade Center towers collapsed thousands of tons of contaminants were instantly released into the air, creating a toxic cloud of dust and debris. First responders and volunteers rushed to help. Many of these people took almost no measures to protect themselves against this "wildly toxic" environment. The aftermath is "Ground Zero" illness, one of the syndromes suggesting that chemical stress can cause health to collapse.

children running behind trucks, which were spraying a mist to kill mosquitoes. The mist contained DDT; a now banned chemical pesticide. Exposure to DDT in childhood has been linked to, among other things, breast cancer in later life. With what we know now, using hindsight as our guide, running behind a truck that is spraying chemicals that kill insects appears foolish and risky. We might ask ourselves what the parents were thinking, allowing children to engage in this behavior. The answer isn't complicated; they didn't really know any better, so no one gave much thought to taking precautions. The same "after the fact" approach has been seen with many chemicals that have been banned during the past few decades; we used them, or products that contained them, taking little to no precautions, right up until sufficient information on their health-damaging effects was available to result in the ban. We did the equivalent of running behind mosquito trucks with some of these chemicals, and we are doing the same today— failing to take adequate precautions with today's man-made chemicals. When it comes to some chemical exposures, decades from now, people from the future will no doubt be looking back and wondering, what were they thinking? They might tell themselves that we didn't know any better. And we might not, but we should.

With banned chemicals, the story generally follows this script. Acute toxicity is observed, because, well, accidents happen, and some people handling the chemical get exposed to high doses. We are assured that, despite the acute toxicity, the chemical is safe at the lower levels of exposure that an average person would be expected to encounter. Eventually the potential for harm from chronic exposure becomes too difficult to ignore. The chemical gets banned. But this doesn't happen until after millions and millions of us have been exposed, with our roles being little different than that of guinea pigs. The chemical is legal to use right up until it isn't; during all of this time it is polluting our environment and each of us. This was the case with chloroform, DDT, and PCBs. This script is playing out today with BPA.

BPA is used in polycarbonate bottles and in epoxy resins (used to coat the inside of food and beverage cans). Estimates suggest that nine out of ten of us have detectable levels of BPA residues inside us. The chemical companies, which make this plastic chemical, assure the public that it's safe, while independent scientists claim it is harmful. As of July 2005, there were 11 published BPA studies that had been funded by the plastic industry. All reported it was safe. There were also 109 published government-funded studies reporting potential harm from low doses of BPA. Who should we believe, the companies that profits from BPA or independent scientists? In 2008, the National Toxicology Program (NTP) issued their findings, classifying BPA as a substance of "some concern" and noting that exposure during infancy might be detrimental to long-term health. During the same year, the United States Food and Drug Administration (FDA) essentially stated that BPA was safe. In January 2010 the FDA changed its mind, agreeing with the NTP assessment that there are some concerns about BPA exposure in infants and fetuses. Despite its new concerns, and its urging for Americans to take reasonable precautions to reduce their individual exposure, the FDA hasn't banned BPA, nor is it likely to anytime soon.

> **HSI CLUE**
>
> We have produced a world with a ubiquitous amount and variety of chemicals. Could being fatter, therefore having more capacity to store these chemicals, be an advantage in this world? Is it an intelligent response? Body fat acts as a chemical sump. It is a relatively safe storage place. Is it possible that the epidemic of overweight could, at least in part, be a response to the chemical world? And if this were the case, what might happen if we cleaned up the world?

With BPA, and other man-made chemicals, we can sit back and wait for the government to do things, or we can choose a *better safe than sorry* approach. It's up to each of us to decide what we will and won't do in terms of BPA exposure, whether we'll default to doing nothing, essentially placing a bet that BPA will be eventually found to be completely safe, or taking precautions to limit our exposure just in case. The same is true for other man-made chemicals. We can assume things are safe until proven harmful, as a society and individuals, or we can assume they might be harmful until proven safe. We believe that no matter what society chooses as a default option, the wisest course for individuals is the latter: It's better to be safe than sorry and to adjust our behaviors accordingly today.

HSI CLUE

Like dissolves and dilutes like. We can lower the toxicity of an oily chemical by diluting it with a large amount of another oily substance. Our body might take this dilution approach. A small amount of body fat and a large amount of chemicals would result in highly toxic fat. What would an intelligent solution to toxic fat be? One option would be to *water down* the chemicals by defending more body fat.

When it comes to man-made chemicals, especially many of the newer types of chemical compounds, there are lots of unanswered questions, and precious few reliable answers. But scientific evidence tells us several things with absolute certainty. We are being exposed to many man-made chemicals. This fact is indisputable. Some of the chemicals scientists detect in our body today were banned decades ago. Many man-made chemicals persist in the environment—in our food, water, soil, dust, and air—and in our bodies for decades. Things don't just magically get better after a chemical is banned. It takes time for the levels in the world outside of us, and in the world inside of us, to decrease. During this time, the chronic effects the chemical causes will remain an issue. This is also an indisputable scientific fact. The last thing we know with certainty is that we are being exposed to new generations of man-made chemicals; some of which are thought to disrupt our hormones (endocrine disrupters like BPA), might induce obesity (environmental obesogens), and in all likelihood have many other chronic effects that won't be entirely understood for quite some time. If the future is like the past, we will be told years, if not decades, from now that some of today's man-made chemicals are harmful. Are you comfortable waiting for this future news or would you rather be doing something to protect yourself now, just in case?

Holmes worked with many chemicals in addition to chloroform. We know this from Dr. Watson's comments about their first meeting in the story *A Study in Scarlet*. This meeting occurs in a laboratory in St. Bart's Hospital. Holmes's hands are discolored from chemicals and covered with the equivalent of bandages. During this meeting Holmes turns to Dr. Watson and with a smile states, "I have to be careful, for I dabble with poisons a good deal." Watson takes this revelation in stride. As a doctor he knows that working with chemicals invariably involves contact with chemicals and that this contact poses a risk. Taking precautions is essential. The effects of today's man-made chemicals on our future health and our current shape are a mystery that might not be definitively solved for decades. This is the bad news. The good news is that we don't need to wait for this mystery to be unraveled. We can start being more careful now. We might not be able to completely avoid chemical exposure. We can take precautions, finding and opening the windows in our lives.

Man-Made Chemicals and Shape

Much of our body burden of man-made chemicals won't be visible in blood or urine; it will be hidden in fatty tissues, especially in adipose tissue. Many man-made chemicals are fat-soluble and the safest place to store fat-soluble substances is adipose tissue. Even naturally occurring fatty substances, like vitamins A, D, or beta-carotene, are toxic at sufficiently high doses. It makes biological sense to put these, and other potentially harmful fat-soluble substances, someplace safe, and adipose tissue is a safer storage place than the brain, heart, or liver. All else being equal, a person with more body fat is likely to have greater amounts of chemicals in their body, in general, and in adipose tissue, specifically. This is circumstantial evidence. It doesn't mean the higher body burden is causing the increased fatness, per se. It might be; it might not be. It does mean that body fat amounts can be a clue to chemical body burden.

Circumstantial evidence links certain man-made chemicals with metabolic obesity—risk for diabetes, insulin resistance, blood sugar abnormalities, fatty liver disease, and polycystic ovaries. Direct evidence indicates that certain chemicals can actually cause these health problems. There is also direct evidence that several of these conditions improve when exposure to the chemical culprits ceases. An example of this evidence is the *Case of Fatty Liver Disease.* We mentioned liver fat in chapter 10. It is a pathological type of fat accumulation; a warning sign that we are traveling along a path that leads to poor health. In one study, 20 industrial workers, who were occupationally exposed to volatile petrochemicals, were identified as having a severe form of fatty liver. Their occupational exposure to chemicals was reduced by removing them from the workplace. Ten of the twenty had a spontaneous

HSI CLUE

Thirty-nine obese individuals dieted for 15 weeks. They lost weight. Before, during, and after the weight loss, blood and fat tissue samples were analyzed for 26 chemicals. When weight was lost, the amounts found in the blood increased to alarmingly high concentrations. Dieting displaced chemicals from a place of relative safety (adipose tissue) and resulted in far more toxic blood. This is one of many reasons why dieting is a poor choice.

improvement in their condition. Liver fat decreased and lab tests improved. In short, they got better by doing the equivalent of opening the windows. This is compelling evidence that at least some man-made chemicals have a causal relationship to aspects of shape self-regulation and to the health issues often mistakenly blamed on weight.

The clues do not end with this direct evidence. There is sufficient scientific evidence in support of man-made chemicals having an impact on shape self-regulation that not one, but two theories have been proposed as plausible explanations for why chemicals influence shape. One of these theories is the *Environmental Obesogen Hypothesis*. The other is the *Endocrine Disruptor Theory*. Environmental Obesogens are chemicals that (1) disrupt the normal developmental of fat cells and (2) negatively influence the self-regulation of shape and weight. Endocrine Disruptor chemicals have hormone-like actions in our body. They either have direct hormone actions or interfere with the actions of our hormones. These theories have some differences, but both hold that exposure to relatively small amounts of some chemical substances might lead directly to (1) the creation of new fat cells, and (2) the increase in size of existing fat cells. In other words, "fattening" is one of the chronic effects of some chemicals.

Based on existing scientific evidence chemicals of concern include:
- Atrazine: An herbicide used in agriculture
- Benzopyrenes: Byproduct of grilling foods, smoking, and burning of fossil fuels
- Bisphenol A: Used to make hard plastics and the epoxy resins
- Organobromides: Flame-retardants in electronics and textiles
- Organotins: Chemical anti-fouling agents
- Perfluoroalkyl compounds Used in stain repellents and nonstick cookware
- Phthalates: Used to make soft plastics and fragrance products
- Toluene: An industrial solvent

Some experts have hypothesized that exposure to Environmental Obesogens might be contributing to undesirable shape changes. One piece of evidence for this hypothesis comes from the *Case of Tributyltin Chloride*. Tributyltin chloride is used commercially as a biocide, a chemical ingredient designed to kill, or prevent the growth, of a wide range of living organisms (molds, algae, and fungal organisms). It is used in marine paints, pesticides, wood preservation, textiles, plastics (like shower curtains), industrial water systems, and breweries. Tributyltin chloride can leech out of products treated with this chemical and contaminate the local environment. Our exposure to tributyltin chloride is believed to occur largely through consumption of contaminated foods (shellfish and fish) and through direct contact with materials, air, or water that contain these biocidal chemicals (like bathroom air after we put up a new shower curtain that has been treated with tributyltin). In animal experiments, tributyltin chloride causes the animal to literally make new fat cells—resulting in an overall increase in body fatness. Scientific experiments have also observed that if a pregnant animal is exposed to tributyltin chloride there are striking elevations of body fat in the offspring of that animal. This chemical-induced fatness persists in the offspring into adulthood.

The second case from the Environmental Obesogen case files is the *Case of Benzo[a]pyrene*. Benzo[a]pyrene is formed from the combustion of wood, coal, diesel, tobacco, or food products. The biggest sources of human exposure are automobile exhaust fumes, tobacco smoke, charbroiled meats like steak, chicken, or hamburger, and charred foods (such as burnt toast or vegetables). Chronic exposure of mice to Benzo[a]pyrene results in the mice weighing 43 percent more. Almost all of this excess weight gain is body fat. The increase in fatness occurs with no detectable change in food intake. The mice are getting much fatter, not because they are eating more, but despite the fact that they aren't.

Now let's examine a case from the Endocrine Disruptor files—the *Case of Bisphenol A*. Global production of BPA is estimated to be approximately seven billion pounds every year. Much of this finds its way into hard plastic bottles and epoxy resins (used to coat cans). When we eat foods and drink beverages stored in BPA-containing cans, bottles, or food containers, we inadvertently ingest low amounts of this chemical. The industry that makes BPA would like us to believe that the levels we are ingesting are inconsequential. Independent scientists disagree. This disagreement was apparent at the 2007 annual meeting of the *American Association for the Advancement of Science,* a non-profit group of almost 120,000 scientists. In a session of this annual scientific conference titled "Obesity:

Are suspected Environmental Obesogens and Endocrine Disruptors making us fatter? What about the many other man-made chemicals—most of which have yet to be investigated for shape and body composition effects? Future research will give answers to these questions. Science marches forward. But this march can be slow. It took many decades after chloroform was widely used before the dangers of low-level exposure were understood. The same was true for PCBs. The same is likely to be true for newer generations of man-made chemicals. Any chronic shape and health effects they might be having on us will precede full scientific understanding of these effects, perhaps by decades. There is far too little evidence about far too few chemicals to arrive at any definitive conclusions.

What we do know with certainty is that chemicals banned decades ago and ones being producing today are routinely detected inside the body. We are being exposed to hundreds, perhaps thousands, of man-made chemicals and they are getting inside us. We can assume they are benign or we can assume that they are a form of chemical stress that might cause the body to adapt. We can sit back and do nothing or we can, in essence, play the Camel Game (discussed in chapter 14), removing chemical straws from our basket *before* the load becomes too much for us. A variety of syndromes have been linked to chemical stress: These include Ground Zero Illness, Gulf War Syndrome, Multiple Chemical Sensitivity, and Sick Building Syndrome. In these syndromes, in a real sense, the camel's back has collapsed and health suffers in a big and enduring way. The goal is to keep the camel's basket as empty as possible, removing any modifiable sources of stress. Chemicals are one of these modifiable stressors. Our individual exposure will be dictated in large part by what we do and don't do.

Using the Sense of Smell to Avoid Chemicals

The human body has evolved sophisticated senses that can help us to detect and avoid potentially harmful things. Eyes can see a poisonous plant or a poison symbol on a container. Taste buds can detect rancid compounds in foods. The nose can detect noxious odors. These are all part of a sensorial defense system. For our senses to protect us, three things must occur: The sense must be used to detect the thing in question, we must recognize it as harmful, and we must adjust our behaviors in health responsible manners.

One of our biggest allies, when it comes to avoiding chemicals, is our sense of smell. But it will only help protect us if we use it, recognize what it is trying to tell us, and alter our behaviors accordingly. For the sense of smell to work to its potential, it needs to be intentionally used to detect potentially noxious odors. It also needs to be, in a sense, educated. We need to become more skilled in knowing which smells are clues to the presence of chemicals. Lastly, we need to act on this information, adjusting our behaviors in ways that lessen our exposure whenever we detect these smells. This might mean opening windows (ventilation strategy), leaving the area (removing ourselves strategy), getting the thing out of the area where we will be (removing the source strategy), or a combination of all of these strategies. Let's look at the *Case of the New Car Smell* to illustrate these points and the three avoidance strategies.

HSI CLUE

Expectations influence what we see and what we think are important details. Toxicology testing has historically considered weight loss, not weight gain, as a toxic effect. According to Jerrold Heindel, of the National Institute of Environmental Health Sciences, a number of chemicals cause weight gain at low levels of exposure in older studies, yet this fact was typically overlooked.

The new car smell is caused by the dozens of chemicals that are off-gassed from the fabrics, upholstery, carpets, and hard plastics that fill the interiors of cars, as well as the adhesives, glues, sealants, etc. that hold all of these things together. Some of the chemicals that contribute to this smell—alkanes, aldehydes, benzene, styrene, toluene, xylene, phthalates, and polyvinyl chloride—have known or suspected toxicity. The levels of these chemicals in the air of a new car can be many times higher than what is considered safe. The air inside a brand new car can be so contaminated with volatile chemicals that it causes headaches, nausea, breathing problems and other acute symptoms in sensitive people. Some combination of opening windows and giving the car a chance to air out before getting in and driving, having windows open while we drive, and spending less time in new cars, will lessen our exposure. Almost every one of us can readily detect the new car smell. Our sense of smell does its job; it's up to us do ours. Some of us do a good job at practicing avoidance, while others don't.

Not only don't some of us follow strategies that will lessen exposure, we can intentionally increase exposure. The new car smell is so desirable that it has led to a booming market for car air fresheners and sprays that replicate this chemical odor. Rather than detecting the odor, recognizing that it might be harmful and avoiding it, we might be paying to expose ourselves to it.

HSI CLUE

Plastics, especially softer plastics, are chemically unstable. The chemicals and chemical additives in plastics migrate into whatever they contact, whether this is air, food, liquid, or our skin. Just as vapors from liquid chloroform migrated into, and contaminated, the air Holmes was breathing, chemicals in plastics migrate into whatever they contact.

The new car smell isn't an isolated example. There are many odors that should alert us to steer clear of the item giving off the smell, but we don't stay away. The problem isn't with our sense of smell; it's with recognizing that we should be avoiding the things giving off the smell. Another example of this is the *Case of a New Vinyl Shower Curtain.* Testing indicates that more than one hundred chemicals, including polyvinylchloride, phthalates, solvents and organotins can be off-gassed by a new vinyl shower curtain. Many of the chemicals detected have known or suspected toxicity. Bathrooms tend to be small and poorly ventilated. This combined with the high amounts of chemicals being released from the new shower curtain, results in high exposure in the first few weeks after hanging the curtain. The exposure is high enough to cause headaches, dizziness, and nausea for some. It can make us feel sick. We can readily detect the smell of noxious chemicals when the curtain is taken out of the package. The smell can be over-powering.

This should alert us to move into avoidance mode. The new shower curtain can be placed outside for a few days to air out. After it is hung, bathroom windows can be opened to ventilate the bathroom. We can spend as little time as possible in the bathroom. As long as we can detect the chemical smell, we want to be practicing avoidance.

[Note: An ideal solution would be to purchase natural fiber, eco-friendly, shower curtains that aren't off gassing chemicals.]

We observe the failure to use the sense of smell as a means to recognize noxious chemicals and a lack of health responsible behaviors at many health scenes. Not only aren't we avoiding things that have chemicals, in many instances we are seeking them out. The *Case of Fragrance Products* illustrates this point. Air fresheners are an example of a fragrance product. We buy them. We use them. Our default assumption is that they are safe, but are they? Most air fresheners do nothing to actually "freshen" the air. They don't remove odors nor do they eliminate them. They are designed to mask unpleasant odors by giving off strong chemical fragrances of their own. A household air freshener will release many chemicals into the air including the fragrance molecules intended to remind of us of something we consider safe and pleasant, usually scents of a flowers or spices. But this is only the tip of the chemical iceberg. Fragrance products including air fresheners, fabric softeners, and laundry detergents often contain dozens of chemicals including solvents, paint thinner compounds, and phthalates. Even Holmes's friend chloroform has been detected in some fabric softeners. Scientific evidence indicates that fragrance products like air fresheners aren't good for us. Air fresheners have reported links to diarrhea and earaches in infants, and headaches, depression and breathing problems in adults. We haven't learned to like air fresheners and other fragrance products because they are healthy or good for us. We like them because they smell pleasant, but this smell is a chemical smell and it masks the presence of other chemicals; often ones we are better avoiding than seeking out.

HSI CLUE

One rule of thumb to keep in mind is that scent is a clue to the presence of chemicals. Things that give off a strong scent usually do so because they are releasing chemicals into the air. Unless the item giving off a strong scent is a flower, spice, or other substance humans encountered as our genetics evolved, it might be best to minimize exposure to scented items and fragrance products.

The sense of smell (and other senses) helps us determine whether the environment is safe. When we encounter a novel odor, the brain is predisposed to assume it might be unsafe, so our olfactory system only lets part of the odor molecules in. It puts its toes in the water, so to speak. If nothing negative happens, with the next sniff, the olfactory system steps into the water a bit further, letting in more of the odor molecules. If things still appear safe, with the third sniff it dives in, letting most or all of the odor molecules in.

We can observe this gradated increase in the odor experience by sniffing a glass of wine three times with a short pause between each sniff. More odors will be unveiled with each sniff. As the brain becomes convinced that the wine poses less and less of a threat, the brain opens us up to experience more and more of it.

The wine smelling experiment teaches us two important things about our sensorial detection system. It is biased to protect us against novelty and it is a quick learner. It would take a lot of work if we started from scratch each time we detected an odor. The brain takes a short cut instead. It learns to associate certain odors with specific items, classifies these items as things it should avoid or consider safe, and then remembers the odor, and uses it as the clue to safety. This process is called *odor-associative learning.*

HSI CLUE

In 2007 the Natural Resources Defense Council released the results of a study of 14 common household air fresheners (scented sprays, gels, and plug-in air fresheners). Phthalates (a suspected endocrine disruptor) were found in 12 of the 14 air fresheners and weren't listed on the label of any of these products. They were even found in some products labeled as "all natural."

Let's assume for arguments sake that a jasmine flower is safe. We detect the scent of jasmine, nothing bad happens physiologically, so the brain learns that the flower and the scent are safe. Since we can detect smells of things we can't always see, the brain dedicates a significant amount of resources to detecting and remembering odors. In the future, anytime the jasmine scent is detected, the brain will be biased to assume safety because of its past experience with the scent. This goes for jasmine flowers (which are safe) and for fragrance products that have been scented to smell like jasmine (which may or may not be safe). The brain isn't as alert for the potential for harm if it detects scents that it has already learned are safe. Fragrance products use odor-associative learning to their advantage. They are designed to smell like things that the brain generally considers safe (flowers, spices, etc.).

Most of our responses to odors are learned from past experiences. We detect an odor, pair it with the item that produces it, and evaluate this information based on the *emotional context* in which the odor is detected. If we detect a new odor and we are having a positive emotional experience at that time, we learn to associate the odor with whatever is producing it and with these positive emotions. In a manner of speaking, the odor gets confused with the positive feelings. This results in a strong preference for the odor, and is the basis for the preference many people have to the new car smell. We don't like the new car smell because it is safe or pleasant; we like it because of the positive emotions that go with having a new car. In a conscious or unconscious attempt to duplicate these positive emotions, we might even purchase a fragrance product that gives off the new car smell. With air fresheners, and many other fragrance products, rather than protecting us, the sensorial defense system gets fooled. Our hope is that you will take steps to reeducate this system.

Start today and begin to use your sense of smell more consciously. Smell things. Wait a few seconds and take another whiff. Pause and repeat. Now spend a few moments paying attention to how you are feeling. What's your body telling you? Are there any subtle signs that continued exposure might not be such a great idea? Ask your body whether it really wants to be exposed to the product giving off the odor. What does your gut tell you when you ask this question? If you are like most people, you'll be surprised by the many strong aversions your body has to things you might have previously thought nothing about inhaling.
[Note: When it comes to odors, the emotional context matters. Do your best to be as emotionally neutral as possible when you educate your sense of smell.]

The Solution:
Avoidance, Elimination, and Systemic Detoxification

Toxicity isn't a new problem. It's an old problem that has been compounded by the introduction of thousands of man-made chemicals. The natural world has many substances that are toxic; poisons in plants and mushrooms, venoms from scorpions, spiders and snakes, and stings from stinging insects. Natural foods can contain substances that would be toxic if consumed in high amounts. A "safe" fat-soluble substance like vitamin A is an example. Like many things in the real world, it follows the *Goldilocks principle* mentioned in the last chapter. Too little results in deficiency disease, but too much is toxic and can cause serious illness. Human metabolism also produces compounds that, if allowed to accumulate, would poison us. Since some degree of exposure is a given, complex adaptive intelligence has evolved a variety of strategies to protect itself from potentially toxic substances. These strategies can be divided into two broad categories: (1) Avoidance Strategies (*before the fact* strategies intended to keep things outside of us), and (2) Damage Control Strategies (*after the fact* strategies intended to protect us from and clean up any mess already inside of us). Examples of the former include use of our senses to detect and avoid chemicals, and physical barriers like the skin, which prevent much, but not all of substances that we come in direct contact with from getting inside the body. Examples of the latter include the tendency to store chemical toxins in adipose tissue (bioaccumulation), converting toxins into forms that can be more easily eliminated (biotransformation), and using channels of elimination to remove toxins from the body (elimination). Biotransformation and elimination are typically referred to as detoxification.

Avoidance is the single most important solution for lessening chemical stress. The goal is to allow the body's detoxification capabilities to keep up with current chemical exposure, and even better, get around to dealing with old messes (bioaccumulated chemicals). This is hard to do if we are consistently being exposed to significant amounts of chemicals, but can occur spontaneously when the source of the chemical exposure is removed. This is illustrated in the *Case of Chloracne*. Chloracne is an acne-like eruption that is caused by over-exposure to a family of chemicals called chloracnegens. The first cases of chloracne were reported over one hundred years ago. Several large outbreaks occurred in workers, primarily in factories producing dioxin-based herbicides like Agent Orange, in the 1960s and 1970s. The primary medical approach to chloracne has been, and continues to be, removing the patient from the source of contamination. Chloracne improves, and, in many instances, resolves when the person avoids all chloracnegens.

The first step in practicing avoidance is to use the sense of smell to alert us to the presence of noxious chemicals. The second step is adjusting our behaviors to either air out the offending item, move it away from us, or remove ourselves from it. The next step is to improve our ability to detect and avoid the primary sources of chemical exposure. Some of these sources we will be able to smell; many we won't. While this list isn't all-inclusive, a good starting point for improving avoidance is reducing our exposure to, or use of, as many of the following as possible.

1. Products with Warning Labels: This includes cleaning products (carpet cleaners, drain cleaners, mold/mildew removers, oven cleaners, etc.), pesticides, herbicides, paints, paint thinners, gasoline and other products with labels warning of toxicity. If the label warns of toxicity, the best policy is avoidance. If these things are used, make sure they are used in well-ventilated areas, skin contact is avoided, and all label instructions are meticulously followed.

For almost all cleaning products, a "Green" option exists. In many instances, identifying the option is essentially an exercise in recall: What did our great-grandparents have available, before the modern chemical era, which served the same purpose? Some of the versatile cleaning products they used were baking soda and vinegar. Vinegar and baking soda, mixed with some water, can be used to clean almost anything. Dr. Bronner's soap is a great all-purpose soap and detergent. Eggshells can be crushed and used as scouring agents. Tips for creating a non-toxic cleaning kit can be found at the website Care2 (www.care2.com/greenliving/make-your-own-non-toxic-cleaning-kit.html#).

2. Fragrance products: These include air fresheners, scented detergents, and other scented consumer products. While not all scented products will contain man-made chemicals, some can contain dozens of man-made chemicals. The solution for fresher air is liberal use of plants (they actually do freshen the air unlike air fresheners), flowers and potpourri for pleasing scents, boiling spices like cinnamon in a pot of water, and opening windows to air things out. Baking soda is also a great air freshener. It can be sprinkled on carpets (then vacuumed up) and placed in areas where odor removal is desired. No matter where we live, outdoor air is likely to be less polluted than indoor air.

3. Personal care products: Soaps, shampoos, perfumes, skin care products, lipsticks, nail polish removers, hair dyes, etc. can contain many chemicals including phthalates, parabens, acrylamides, solvents and fragrance chemicals. Use of personal care products has been linked with body burden of phthalates as an example. Be very careful with things you place directly on your skin, since direct contact can result in some degree of absorption of many substances. The Environmental Working Group maintains a *Skin Deep Cosmetic Safety Database* (www.cosmeticsdatabase.com) and has a shopper's guide for cosmetics (www.ewg.org/files/EWG_cosmeticsguide.pdf). Natural alternatives for many personal care products can be found in health food stores, but just because something claims to be "natural" doesn't mean it is chemical-free. Read ingredients and do some homework. A general rule of thumb might be that if you would be comfortable putting all of the ingredients listed in something in your mouth, putting it on your skin would be fine. Traditional cultures often used naturally occurring substances for beauty—aloe, cocoa butter, coconut, olive oil, sesame oil, and shea butter. Using these

substances as stand-alone options for cosmetic purposes, rather than as part of a beauty product with many ingredients, is one way to lessen our exposure to man-made chemicals.

4. Non-stick cookware: Non-stick cookware contains perfluorinated chemicals. If the pan is scratched, the chemicals are released and can pass into foods cooked in the pan. But these chemicals migrate even when the pan hasn't been scratched. Perfluorinated chemicals vaporize with heat, migrate into kitchen air, and can be inhaled. Safer cooking options include stainless steel, ceramic and cast iron.

5. Plastics (this includes synthetic fibers): All plastics contain chemicals. Styrofoam contains polystyrene. BPA is in polycarbonate plastics and epoxy resins. Vinyl contains vinyl chloride. Plastic shopping bags are made from polyethylene. Polyester is made from polyethylene terephthalate. Soft plastics contain a plastic chemical and softeners like phthalates. Plastics, especially softer plastics, are chemically unstable. The chemicals, and chemical additives, in a plastic product migrate into whatever they contact, whether this is air, food, liquid, or our skin. In the case of children chewing on plastics, migration of plastic chemicals is directly into the mouth. We can reduce our exposure to plastics by buying fewer canned foods and beverages (they are lined with plastic containing resins), buying foods and beverages in glass containers, using glass as a storage container, using ceramic or glass mugs as drinking cups, and buying clothing and bedding made from natural fibers (cotton, silk, wool, etc.).

6. Dry Cleaned Garments: In instances where these products will be used, the goal is to follow Holmes's open the windows approach. We want to air things out, give things a chance to off-gas chemicals, and ventilate. A good rule of thumb is to put dry cleaned garments in areas of the home, or even better a garage if available, where we spend little time and which is as far away from rooms we spend lots of time in (like the bedroom) as possible.

7. New Furniture, Carpets, and Bedding: The new car smell was caused in part by off-gassing from glues and adhesives. Similar chemicals are used in new furniture, especially when made from pressed wood, and carpeting. These items are also usually treated with flame-retardant chemicals. With furniture a step in the right direction is buying furniture made from wood (either new or second

hand) rather than particleboard. Mattresses and pillows are often made using synthetic fibers and are treated with flame-retardants. Bedding made from natural fibers rather than synthetic fibers (which are in most cases plastics) are available. Because of regulatory requirements, finding bedding that hasn't been treated with flame-retardants can be challenging.

8. Charbroiled (Burnt) Foods: As was mentioned in the *Case of Benzo[a]pyrene,* a big source of exposure for this chemical is charbroiled meats like steak, chicken, or hamburger, and charred foods (such as burnt toast). Avoiding charred foods completely will decrease our exposure to Benzo[a]pyrene but we don't usually need to go to this extreme to significantly reduce our dietary intake. We can reduce our intake of Benzo[a]pyrene by cooking meats so they are not as well done, using marinades when we charbroil or grill meats and vegetables, removing any charred parts of our food—especially charred fat or skin and any areas of foods which appear to be burnt—while still enjoying foods which would otherwise contain high amounts of these chemical byproducts of high heat cooking.

9. Buy Organic Foods: The food chain is one of the biggest sources of exposure to man-made chemicals for an average person. Modern food production techniques are chemically intensive. Pesticides, herbicides, and fungicides are used to grow food crops. These foods are then used to make our food or fed to livestock, which might also be directly treated with one or more chemicals while being raised. These *conventionally produced* foods have been reported to have higher amounts of chemical residues than foods that have been grown following *organic standards.* This is understandable given the difference in how conventional and organic foods are produced. In order to be awarded a "Certified Organic" classification a food must be grown or raised on land that has not been sprayed with chemical pesticides and chemical fertilizers. It also can't be treated with chemical fungicides after it is produced. All else being equal, a food certified as organic would be expected to have lower amounts of chemical residues than would a comparable non-organic food.

Avoidance is part of the solution, but not the entire solution. The next part of the solution entails maximizing our body's capability to eliminate chemicals. Each of us has the capacity to eliminate chemicals. We might have certain strengths or weaknesses because of our genes, current lifestyle habits, or dietary choices. No matter what hand we are currently holding, the strategies we follow, starting today, will influence how our body actually performs when it comes to chemical detoxification. The most basic element of detoxification is improving the body's innate eliminative mechanisms. This starts with our digestive tract and bowel function.

HSI CLUE

Create one or more "Clean Rooms" in your home. The bedroom is a great starting place. This entails (1) opening bedroom windows for at least a bit of time every day, (2) placing more plants in the room, (3) removing anything that is scented, (4) storing dry cleaned garments in closets elsewhere in the home, and (5) choosing furniture and bedding that is less chemically treated or has had ample time to off gas.

Food is a big source of exposure to man-made chemicals. The first contact ingested chemicals have with our body occurs in our digestive tract. If a food we eat has chemical residues—most do, though organic foods generally have less—these residues will either be captured and eliminated or absorbed into our body. The goal is to tilt the balance strongly in favor of capturing and elimination. We do this by eating foods that help to bind chemical residues (directly or indirectly), and foods that promote healthy, regular bowel movements. The two most important types of foods for these purposes are high fiber foods and fermented foods.

Fiber is important for both capturing—binding—compounds in our digestive tract and for supporting better bowel habits. We can increase our fiber intake significantly by eating more fruits, vegetables, nuts, seeds, beans, lentils, and whole grains. Fermented foods are foods that are made using some type of a starter culture (safe, beneficial microorganism). In the case of yogurt, the starter culture is bacteria, like lactobacillus and bifidobacteria. In the case of the Japanese fermented foods miso, traditionally fermented soy sauce, and amazake, the starter culture is usually koji. The presence of a starter culture in the ingredients is the clue that informs us whether a food is actually fermented—like traditionally made soy sauce—or not—like most of the commercially available soy sauce. Fermented foods improve gut barrier function (making the gut wall a better physical barrier against chemicals), capture chemical residues, and promote better bowel elimination.

Bowel function is an important aspect of the body's ability to eliminate toxic waste products, whether from food, metabolism, or man-made chemicals. It isn't the only channel of elimination.

Chemicals can be inhaled, consumed, and absorbed through our skin. They can also be eliminated through these same routes, as well as through our kidneys in urine. Elimination through these routes can be improved by following certain strategies. Many different approaches exist for systemic detoxification. Most of them have in common strategies that promote better bowel elimination, as well as improving elimination via the kidneys, skin and lungs. Many approaches also recommend specific dietary supplements. It is beyond the scope of this chapter to detail all the aspects of these approaches, but there are a few key things to keep in mind when it comes to detoxification.

First and foremost, rapid weight loss does not improve detoxification; it can hinder it. Preventing the body from absorbing chemicals requires metabolic work. Detoxification also requires metabolic work. But rapid weight loss, which would result in a person being below natural weight, slows metabolism. The result is that we don't get rid of bioaccumulated toxins when we diet, and we tend to absorb even higher amounts of the ones we are still being exposed to. The net effect is usually for the worse. Rapid weight loss also mobilizes chemicals from fat cells (a place of relative safety) and places them in the blood where they can be redistributed to other tissues like the brain and nervous system (places of lower safety). Unless steps are being taken to protect these more sensitive tissues, and to open channels of elimination, rapid weight loss is going to cause more toxicity problems than it solves because the blood gets more contaminated with toxins when weight is lost rapidly. While detoxification has not received anywhere near the degree of scientific investigation it merits, the limited investigations to date suggest that it is better to discourage weight loss—maintain our current weight—while actively detoxifying the body. Second, when it comes to detoxification, faster is not better; it is worse. If we are following a detoxification program and start to feel sick or poorly, this is usually a sign that we are going way too fast, dumping more toxins into the blood than our body can comfortably eliminate. If detoxification is making us feel worse, it's a sign to back-off, to slow down. Third, there are safe things we can do for ourselves to promote better systemic detoxification. The safest of these include (1) low intensity exercise, (2) deep breathing, (3) exposure to fresh air, (4) drinking more pure water, (5) skin brushing, (6) low temperature saunas and steam rooms, and (7) application of natural oils (like coconut oil, cocoa butter, or olive oil) to the skin.

Closing Dialogue

Health Scene Investigator: Have I cleared up your confusion?

Apprentice: Yes, you have. I had no idea that so many chemicals were found in our body. Or, that they accumulated in fat tissue. I also had never heard that some of these chemicals had such direct links to shape. You have really opened my eyes.

Health Scene Investigator: Good, good. Now that they are open, will you see your way clear to begin to make improvements in this area?

Apprentice: I will, I most certainly will.

Health Scene Investigator: Wonderful news. Now, let's turn our attention to a special category of chemical substances—medications.

Chapter 16

Medications and Shape

In solving a problem of this sort, the grand thing is to be able to reason backward.

Sherlock Holmes

Opening Dialogue

Health Scene Investigator: If a person complained of weight gain after starting a medication, what would you advise them?

Apprentice: I would recommend that they ask their doctor, or perhaps a pharmacist, whether the drug can cause weight gain.

Health Scene Investigator: And what if the doctor or pharmacist assures them that their weight gain is not related to their medication: What would you do next?

Apprentice: I would investigate their health scene for other causes of weight gain.

Health Scene Investigator: Ah, not so fast…if a medicine is known to have weight gain as a side effect, we can always rule it in as a possible suspect. But just because the side effect is unknown does not necessarily mean we should rule it out.

Reasoning Backwards

On a given day in North America, a scene similar to the following will play out in countless medical offices. A patient comes in for their appointment. They tell their doctor that they have gained weight since starting a new medication and ask if it could be because of the medication. The doctor checks, notes that weight gain isn't a listed side effect, and assures the patient that the medication is not the cause. The doctor might then advise the patient that, if they are concerned, they should watch what they are eating and exercise more. In the above scene, who is reasoning correctly? One answer to this question is that they both are. The doctor can be correct—weight gain isn't listed as a side effect. The patient, who is in essence, reasoning backward, can also be correct; the medication is causing this *individual* to gain weight. Both persons can be reasoning correctly and come to different conclusions because of issues with the ways medications are investigated and how side effects are reported, and because of limited understanding of complex adaptive individuality.

HSI CLUE

In the period between 1995-6 and 2002-3 medication usage in the United States increased an average of 46 percent. During this same time span the use of antidepressants doubled, allergy medications increased by 73 percent, blood pressure medications doubled, cholesterol medications more than doubled, diabetes medications doubled, and ulcer and reflux medications increased by 60 percent. As a society we are taking more medications and many of the ones we are taking have shape side effects.

Before a new medication is approved years of research are required to determine its safety, efficacy and side effects. Side effects, including weight gain, will be noted during this pre-approval time period, if the clinicians conducting the trials detect them. Like the reporting of other side effects, weight is an incidental finding, not an intentional focus of the research efforts for most medications. There is no requirement to monitor weight, never mind more vital shape clues, during the pre-approval process. Despite the huge effort in time and money during the approval process, the long-term consequences of most medications aren't completely known until years after the medication is being extensively used in the population. The net result is that many side effects, including adverse effects on shape, aren't discovered until *after* a medication is widely used. The system for exploring the effects of drugs before they are approved for sale is far from perfect; many side effects are missed. The system for noting, reporting, and disseminating information on side effects, after a drug is approved and sold to the public, is also imperfect. A drug can have long-term, subtle, or rare side effects that might go unreported for years.

There are numerous reasons why many side effects escape detection during the approval process of medications. One of these reasons is *complex individuality*. Every human is different from every other human. Even identical twins can be different from each other in subtle ways. Medication trials are far more limited in terms of the number of participants they can include compared with the total population of all persons who might *eventually* take the medication. It is a virtual certainty that there will be more variance in the general public taking the medication than there was in the study population. And with greater variance, the odds of someone experiencing unintended consequences increases.

Polypharmacy, taking several medications at the same time, is another reason that side effects can escape detection. Side effects can occur when two or more medications are combined that would not occur if only one of the medications was used. There are many issues with the pre-approval and post-marketing process for single drugs. There is absolutely no system in place whatsoever for understanding how two or more medications interact. This is an important consideration. More people are taking medications, and many people are taking multiple medications. The annual report by the United States National Center for Health Statistics indicates that almost half the population over age 18 takes at least one prescription medicine; one in every six of us is taking three or more medications. These statistics don't include the use of over-the counter medications. With every additional medication a person takes the risk for side effects increases and the ability to predict what these side effects might be decreases.

Time is another reason for the failure to detect shape changes in pre-approval studies. Side effects can occur shortly after starting a medication but they don't always occur this quickly. Sometimes side effects won't occur until weeks, months, or even years of continued use. With some medications, the longer it is used, the more likely that the user will experience a side effect, and often these side effects are different than those that occur early on. The effect medications have on the population using them isn't always constant. Over short periods of time one thing might happen, but over longer periods very different things can occur. Intelligent organisms adapt, but adaptation takes time and shape is an adaptive process. Many drug approval studies are relatively short-term. A medication might not cause detectable weight gain during the first few months of use. This doesn't mean it won't cause weight gains over longer periods of time. Sometimes it takes many months to adapt, and a medication will cause gains in weight over one year, even when it had no effect on weight during the first few months. This is a big problem because many drug trials are of far shorter duration compared with the amount of time a person is expected to take the medication.

HSI CLUE

Two patients were given Risperidone alone for three months. No increases in body weight were detected. When a combination of Paroxetine and Risperidone were given weight increased by about 30 pounds in each of them over a four to five month period. Medicine has essentially no scientific understanding of how several drugs might interact to affect shape even in groups of people (never mind in complex individuals). This is a problem because many people take two or more drugs.

There is one other reason why shape side effects escape detection. As we discussed in cases from earlier chapters—the *Cases of Hormone Replacement therapy (HRT), Tamoxifen,* and *Insulin*—weight can be a misleading clue. Even if weight is assessed and the medication is studied over a long period of time, weight can be unchanged while a lens that allows us to observe the finer details of shape, body composition, and body fat types and distributions might be detecting worsening shape, an increase in body fat, a decrease in muscle, or increases in visceral and liver fat.

It is difficult to predict with certainty—it might be argued that it is impossible—how a single medication will interact with a given individual's unique genetics, diet, lifestyle habits, and environment. Humans are complex; we adapt in highly individualized manners. The *Case of Overfeeding Identical Twins* (Chapter 5) indicated that all humans don't respond in an identical manner to something as seemingly straightforward as massive overfeeding. Would we expect our response to medications to be any less varied? This dual complication—adaptation over time and complex individuality—makes any effort to predict the long-term side effects of even a single medication for a given individual a very daunting proposition. Now imagine how difficult it is to predict what will occur when people are combining two, three, four or at times as many as ten different medications. Making guesses about the side effects of these "medication stews" is a lot like trying to predict the weather a month from now. It can't be done with anything resembling scientific certainty. The only things we can state with certainty are:

1. Individuals can experience highly unique side effects.
2. Side effects often occur immediately but sometimes don't occur until long after a medication is used.
3. Combining more medications together increases the chance of unintended effects.
4. Medications can worsen aspects of shape even when they aren't causing weight gain.

Health sciences have not yet begun to think of the body as a complex adaptive system or to realize the implications this new science has for how we view the body and its response to things. Intelligent adaptation isn't the exception; it's the rule. Health science also has trouble with individualized medicine. Large studies are designed to determine what occurs in a group of people; they are not as reliable when it comes to predicting what will or won't happen to any single individual in the larger population. Humans vary in many important ways that result in highly individualized responses. Complexity informs us that things can be more than the sum of their parts. The side effects caused by taking three medications can't always be accurately predicted by looking at what each medication does on its own when taken as a single substance. These complexity issues have caused medicine to fail to appreciate the inherent uncertainty that exists with medications. The issues that arise from complexity also cause medicine to vastly under-recognize the role medications can play in shape.

> **HSI CLUE**
>
> Protease Inhibitors are antiviral medications used in the treatment of HIV. These drugs can cause shape changes even when weight stays the same. The most common shape change is an increase in fat in the belly, trunk fat, and upper back (buffalo hump), which can occur with or without losses in fat from the face, arms, legs and buttocks. With these and other medications, weight isn't always a reliable clue.

Reliable information about the shape effects of single medicines is woefully inadequate. Information about the shape effects from taking combinations of many medications is, in most instances, non-existent. Complexity issues make applying the limited existing information a guess, of sorts, that might correctly identify what occurred in the group studied, but which can fail to accurately predict what will occur to all of the individuals in a larger population. These and other issues create a problem when it comes to investigating individual health scenes. The solution to this problem resides in individual self-experimentation, using what Holmes mentions in *A Study in Scarlet* as our guide: "In solving a problem of this sort, the grand thing is to be able to reason backward." We won't always be able to rely upon a drug maker, and the drug information they provide, to accurately predict whether a medication will or won't be a tipping point for shape in an individual. In many cases, it will be up to the individual to reason backwards.

Investigations into Medications and Shape

Some medications produce such a large change in weight so quickly that the effect they have is obvious. Even when this is the case, some doctors can be unaware of this side effect. Others will be aware of it, but consider it to be an acceptable trade-off for the presumed benefits the medication might provide. Some of these latter doctors naively assume that advice to eat less can somehow overcome the complex interaction the medication is having with Shape Intelligence. As bad as this situation sounds, medications that fall into this category are the easy ones to pinpoint at a health scene. Other medications can have much more subtle, variable, or distant effects on shape. Still other medications can profoundly influence shape while the effect on weight is far less apparent. These medications can be much more difficult to spot. Let's explore a few cases to highlight each of these issues.

Certain medications cause such rapid or significant weight gain that it is a well-known side effect. The *Case of Risperidone* illustrates an example of this type of medication. Risperidone (brand names Belivon®, Rispen®, Risperdal®) is a type of medication classified as an atypical antipsychotic drug. It's primarily used to treat schizophrenia, forms of bipolar disorder, psychotic depression, obsessive-compulsive disorder and other types of mental health issues. It is a relatively new drug, granted approval by the Food and Drug Administration (FDA) in 1993. Despite the relative brief time on the market, it is the most commonly prescribed antipsychotic medication in the United States. Many of the people taking Risperidone will experience weight gain, often staggering amounts of weight gain. Average adult weight gain is ten to twenty pounds during the first two years. Some individuals will gain in excess of fifty pounds. Risperidone is not an isolated example; many antipsychotic medications are capable of causing significant weight gain, with some promoting faster and greater gains in weight than Risperidone.

Certain antidepressant medications are well known for causing weight gain. An example is the *Case of Amitriptyline*. Amitriptyline (brand name Elavil) is a special type of antidepressant called a *tricyclic*. It is used to treat severe depression, prevent migraines, and help people with insomnia. It is expected that people will gradually and progressively gain weight once they begin using this medication. An "average" person might gain between five and nine pounds in the first year of treatment; less fortunate individuals can gain thirty five to forty pounds within just the first few months of treatment! Similar to the *Case of Risperidone*, since noticeable weight gain occurs early on, typically within six weeks of starting the medication, in a large number of people, Amitriptyline is known to have weight gain as a side effect.

Some medications have pronounced effects on shape and these effects occur quickly. Other drugs have somewhat more subtle or slower developing effects. The *Case of Beta Blockers* is an example. Beta blockers are a family of medications that are designed to block beta receptors on tissues. Blocking this receptor decreases pulse rate and blood pressure, leading to these medications being widely prescribed for cardiovascular purposes, especially hypertension. Because these same receptors are found on muscle and fat tissue, blocking them also slows metabolism, can make exercising more difficult, and can slow the release of fat from adipose tissue. Unsurprisingly, weight gain and fatigue are commonly reported side effects, and tend to worsen over time as the medications continue to be used. A review of trials on beta blockers suggested that the average weight gain over a period of about six months is two and one half to three pounds. This amount of weight gain might sound trivial; it isn't to most people. This *average* weight response is also misleading because it fails to account for the *variance* in response. Beta blockers don't cause weight gain

---

HSI CLUE

Antipsychotic medications can cause large amounts of weight gain. Estimates indicated that about 9 out of every 1000 children were taking an antipsychotic drug in 1995-96. By 2001-02 this had increased to 40 out of every 1000. Is it possible that this increase, and the increase in other medications being prescribed to children, might be contributing to the growing childhood obesity problem?

equally among all users. They have a fairly wide variance when it comes to weight gain. Some people don't gain any weight; many of those who do gain weight gain more than the average. The study that reported a two and one half to three pound average weight gain, also reported that weight changes varied from a loss of about one pound to gains of almost eight. Other evidence has suggested that certain beta blockers can cause as much as a ten to twenty percent increase in weight in a modest amount of people. The average weight change beta blockers cause in a group of people isn't particularly large, but the effect they have on certain individuals in that group can be very large.

HSI CLUE

During several months of Gabapentin use 10 patients gained more than 10 percent of their initial weight, 15 gained 5 to 10 percent, 16 had no weight change, and 3 lost 5 to 10 percent of their initial weight. Weight gain for the group was relatively modest when this data was averaged. But this average is misleading. Almost 1 out of every 4 subjects gained massive amounts of weight, and another 1 out of 3 persons gained significant amounts of weight. This fact is obscured by the average response.

This difference between the average response and the variance of response is a commonly missed clue in studies of all types, as well as in many real world situations. While the average helps us to predict what we might expect in a large group as a whole, or when something is done many times, the variance—the distribution of the data—provides valuable information about what we can expect with specific individuals or in isolated incidents. The *Case of the Four Yard Run* illustrates this point. Year after year, running plays in the National Football League (NFL) average close to four yards. But on any given run, a player might lose yardage, gain no yardage, gain a few yards, gain exactly four yards, gain a bit more than average, or run for as many yards as there are from where the ball is spotted to the end zone (the longest run in NFL history is 99 yards). In the NFL, the most common occurrence on a running play isn't running for four yards, it is running for one yard or less (including losing yards), which occurs roughly on one out of every four running plays. On a handful of plays every year, a team will have runs of greater than thirty yards. These runs are outliers; they are not a common occurrence but they are a possible occurrence. In this instance, the average paints a very different picture than the most likely result, and an even more distorted picture of outlier results. This same data distribution issue arises with many medications.

There is a large variance in shape responses to beta blockers, antipsychotic drugs like Risperidone, and many other medications. For people who happen to be the outliers, the average can drastically misrepresent the dramatic shape changes that can occur.

It's difficult to spot medications that have a subtle effect on shape; it's also difficult to detect distant effects. A fundamental realization in the science of complex adaptive systems is that these intelligent systems can, and often do, respond differently over the course of many months than is apparent in the first several months as they learn and adapt. If we are not watchful for this very real property of complex adaptive systems, we will misinterpret evidence. We might miss the distant effects—effects that occur after a sufficient amount of time has passed to allow for the complex adaptive intelligence to solve a novel problem. This is illustrated in the *Case of SSRI*.

In 1988, a brand new type of antidepressant medication arrived on the scene in North America. Its generic name was fluoxetine. Most people know it better by its brand name—Prozac. Prozac is a selective serotonin reuptake inhibitor (SSRI). It expanded the antidepressant market faster and further than any antidepressant before or since. It is now just one of many SSRI medications. Most medications are initially studied for relatively short periods of time. If they appear to be helpful longer studies are conducted. SSRI were no different. The initial short-term data indicated that SSRI medications reduced appetite and were associated with weight loss in some people. This led to a widespread, but premature, belief that SSRI help people lose weight; a belief that still persists to an extent today. In fact, based on this mistaken belief, SSRI were even marketed as anti-obesity drugs. They are still prescribed for weight loss by some physicians today. But the distant effect of SSRI is often weight gain. In fact, for a large number of people prescribed these medications it is substantial weight gain.

The initial short-term data indicated that SSRI reduced appetite and were associated with weight loss *in some people*. In the exuberance that followed, an important early clue was overlooked. Some people were not losing weight and others were gaining weight. Just like with beta blockers there was a variance in the response to SSRI. Research published just two years after the introduction of Prozac in North America gave an insight into who might get which short-term response. Depressed individuals were divided into underweight, ideal weight, and overweight groups, and started on Prozac. The overweight group experienced an average weight loss of 3.3 lbs during the first two months. The underweight individuals showed no consistent trends—some lost weight, some gained weight, and some remained the same. The ideal weight individuals gained an average of 4.4 lbs during the first four months on Prozac. This evidence suggests that weight changes in the first few months after beginning Prozac could vary from significant weight loss to significant weight gain. It also suggests that a person's initial body weight might influence the direction weight would change. This variability of response would not be the only missed clue.

HSI CLUE

Nine obese volunteers were given Prozac to help with weight loss. After seven weeks it appeared to be working, some weight had been lost. By week sixteen, the lost weight had been regained. In this study, Prozac worked until it didn't. Prozac isn't alone; many "weight loss" medications stop working over time as the body adapts to them.

After SSRI became available on the market longer studies were conducted. These longer studies indicated that weight gain, not weight loss, was the most likely long-term effect. Approximately one out of three people prescribed an SSRI lost weight during the first three months, but by month six most people who had lost weight initially, regained all of it. Other less fortunate people experienced significant weight gains over the same six months. As studies began to look further and further out into the distance, greater and greater amounts of weight gain were observed in more and more people. While different brands of SSRI medications have been associated with slightly different degrees of weight gain, approximately one out of four persons prescribed an SSRI gains at least seven per cent of their body weight within a year. That's about 9 pounds for a 130-pound person or 14 pounds for a 200-pound person. Some people gain much, much more than this amount. Because this weight gain is hidden by time—a distant effect—it was originally missed. Do you think it is possible that we might be missing undesirable shape changes caused by other medications because they too take time to develop?

There are hundreds of different categories of medications. Some have been studied for their short-term effects on weight. Fewer have been investigated for their long-term effects on weight. Even fewer have been investigated to determine whether they are affecting something more vital than weight—shape, body composition, and body fat distribution. This is even true for many of the drugs known to cause weight gain. The *Case of Oral Hypoglycemic Agents* provides an example of why it is important for science to begin to systematically investigate medications for their effects on these more vital clues. Oral hypoglycemic agents are used to control blood sugar in persons with type 2 Diabetes. Weight gain is a common side effect. It is caused, at least in part, by the medications doing precisely what they are intended to do; lowering blood sugar, which is accomplished in part by moving sugar molecules from the blood into fat and muscle, causing gains in weight as a direct result. Generally speaking, these medications are only as effective in lowering blood sugar as they are in causing weight to be gained. Without the latter, we don't get much of the former.

There are several different types of oral hypoglycemic agents. One type, called Glitazones, work by sensitizing the body to insulin. Another type, called Sulfonylureas, work by causing the body to secrete more insulin. Both lower blood sugar. Both are associated with weight gain. But do both cause identical changes in shape, body composition, and body fat distribution patterns? A study published in May 2006 in the journal *Diabetes Care* suggests that Glitazones and Sulfonylureas have very different effects. In this particular study the Glitazone medication studied was Pioglitazone (trade name Actos) and the Sulfonylurea medication used was Glipizide (trade name Metaglip). Nineteen persons with type 2 Diabetes were randomly assigned to one of the two medications for twelve weeks. While blood sugar control was essentially the same with both drugs, the effects on shape, body composition, body fat, and weight couldn't have been more different. The average weight gain for the group receiving Pioglitazone was just less than seven pounds. For the group receiving Glipizide it was a bit over one pound. With this limited bit of information Glipizide appears to be the clear winner; causing far less average weight gain. The researchers also assessed changes in body fat. The average fat gain for people taking Pioglitazone was two pounds. Users of Glipizide lost, on average, a small amount of fat. Judging by changes in weight and fat amounts, so far, Glipizide looks to be the better choice. In this study, changes in belly fat

> **HSI CLUE**
>
> Glitazones tend to cause increases in weight but much of this weight (perhaps as much as 75%) is water. These medications also are associated with fat gain and with redistribution of body fat (increases in subcutaneous fat at the expense of visceral fat).

(including visceral adipose) were also assessed. One medication decreased belly fat. The other increased it. Which medication would you guess did which?

Since Pioglitazone caused more weight and fat gain than Glipizide, it makes intuitively sense that it would have been the medication that worsened belly fat. It wasn't; it decreased belly fat. Glipizide, despite slightly decreasing body fat, increased belly fat. When amounts of weight and fat are viewed in isolation Glipizide appears to be a better choice, but when the location of fat is considered the picture shifts. Glipizide no longer appears to be the obvious better choice. Do you think it might be possible that other medications might affect shape in complex ways that can be missed when the only thing assessed in drug trials is weight?

The Case of Drugs in our Drinking Water

In 1998, scientists investigated drinking water for the presence of medications. They detected them. In 2000, they investigated again, and, once again, medications were detected. In 2008, medications were detected in the drinking water in 24 major metropolitan areas. When scientists have tested for the presence of medications in our drinking water, unfortunately for us, they find them. Drinking water in many places is contaminated with low amounts of several to many medications. Some of the medications detected in drinking water supplies include drugs with shape side effects—antibiotics, beta-blockers, chemotherapeutic agents, mood stabilizers, oral contraceptives and seizure medications. This is an established scientific fact. Could this be one of the *little things* contributing to the current epidemic of shape issues?

Many of us are consistently being exposed to prescription medications, not because we need them, but despite the fact that we don't. We can be exposed to them in tap water; beverages made from tap water; and in bottled or canned beverage made using unpurified water. The question that must be answered, and which to date has not been, is whether chronic exposure to trace amounts of these medications is capable of having a biological effect. This issue has not been investigated at all. No one can say for sure whether the levels of drugs present in drinking water have or don't have biological effects, including shape effects, until this is investigated scientifically. Any expert who claims they have no effect—which some have—is guilty of theorizing in advance of evidence.

Are any of these medications capable of affecting our shape or having other unintended consequences when we are chronically exposed to low doses? This is an important question; it is not the only question. Many medications have been found in drinking water. Pharmacology teaches us that effects cascade when multiple agents act together. Rather than the effects being additive, they can multiply. Could the trace amounts of medications be adding together, or even worse, acting synergistically to create unintended side effects? Despite the low levels of any one medication, could the presence of low levels of many medications be causing a problem? Are some of us more susceptible? Even if contaminated drinking water were safe for an average adult, would the same be true for a pregnant woman, a developing fetus, a newborn infant, or a child? We don't have answers to these questions. No one does. What we do know is that the levels of medications in our drinking water are very low, but they are detectable. We also know that some medications, like synthetic hormones, are biologically active even in trace amounts. The rest is conjecture and veiled in uncertainty. What should we do when things are scientifically uncertain?

When an area is scientifically uncertain there are generally two broad camps that form. One camp—usually the one with an interest (financial or otherwise)—takes a position that things are safe and the status quo is fine. To support their side, they point to the fact that there is no evidence of harm. They are correct. There isn't but how can there be if no one has been investigating? The other camp takes the opposite tack; they believe it is wiser to presume the worst until evidence to the contrary exists. They advocate using the *precautionary principle*. The precautionary principle is an approach to areas of scientific uncertainty. It takes a default position that public health and the environment should be protected against things that have uncertain effects. Rather than assuming something is safe until proven otherwise, advocates of this position believe the opposite approach is wiser: We should presume something might be unsafe until safety is proven. They also believe that the burden of proof of safety should fall on the shoulders of those responsible for profiting from, or the advocates of continuing, the uncertain practice. If there is no scientific consensus about the safety of something—in this case the presence of medications in the water supply—the precautionary principle informs us that we should not use that as an excuse to do nothing. The wiser course is to take precautionary measures now.

If you want to take an approach that is more like the precautionary principle, what should you do? Current evidence is that boiling tap water does not eliminate medications but that some water purification steps might. Purification using activated charcoal and reverse osmosis are each believed to remove some medications. Your municipal water supply might be taking these or other steps to remove medications. Ask them what they are doing. If they are not doing anything, the burden will fall on your shoulders. One thing you can do, should this be the case, is to purchase a water purification system for your home. This system should be capable of removing medications from tap water. This will take care of your home drinking water but not things made from water that you buy outside your home. When it comes to bottled or canned beverages, including bottled drinking water, don't assume they are medication-free. Many will be; some won't. Ask vendors what they are doing to purify and test the water they are using in the products they are selling. The same holds true for beverages or things like soups made with water at restaurants, coffee shops, etc; some will use purified water and some won't. Ask. If you are concerned about being exposed to low levels of medications in water, the most prudent step is to be more informed about what you are drinking and to take reasonable steps to at least minimize any unwanted exposure to potentially contaminated water and products made using it.

Investigate—Learn More About Your Medication(s)

The evidence is overwhelming that at least certain medications can contribute to one or all of (1) gains in weight, (2) shifts in body composition (decreases in lean mass, increases in fat mass, changes in fluid status), and (3) changes in the types and distribution patterns of body fat. We can also infer from existing evidence that, when it comes to shape, we don't all respond in an identical way when taking the same medication. Some of us might gain weight; others might not. Some of us might gain just a bit of weight; others might gain massive amounts. Some of us will experience a worsening shape and the composition of our weight that coincides with gains in weight; others might experience a worsening of shape and the quality of their weight even though their actual weight is staying the same.

Some of us might experience relatively quick deleterious shifts in our shape; for others it might be months into the future before any noticeable effect occurs. The way medications interact with our complex individuality is, well, complex and highly individualized.

When we consider our complex individuality and the relative scarcity of long-term shape and body composition data that exists for many medications, it leaves those of us who are taking one or more medications in an unenviable position. A medication we are taking might be (1) worsening our shape and the quality or composition of our weight, and (2) preventing us from enjoying the shape benefits from other diet, lifestyle, and environmental changes we have been making. Both of these issues are wildly under-recognized issues. We have discussed the first issue. Let's highlight this second one by investigating two cases.

The first is the *Case of Medications Possibly Preventing Weight Loss*. This case looked at medication use in 90 individuals participating in a 20-week weight management program. It found that the average number of medications being taken by the people in this study was four. While some people weren't taking any medications, one was taking fifteen different ones. Forty-eight percent of the individuals were taking at least one medication that has been associated with weight gain. These people weighed more at the beginning of the weight management program—the drugs might have already been causing weight gain—and were less likely to lose weight during the program. The *Case of Oral Contraceptives* also highlights this problem. Public perception is that oral contraceptives cause weight gain. Many doctors view this perception as inaccurate. They claim that while the original, higher dose, versions of "the Pill" did cause weight gain, the modern lower dose versions of "the Pill" don't. At least on average, in a large group of women, studies report that those taking "the Pill" are no more likely to gain weight than those who don't take it. There are problems when using this type of group study as the sole basis of predicting how an individual's shape might respond. But this is not what we really want to discuss at this point. We want to share the evidence from a study of 73 young

---

H S I   C L U E

Antibiotics have been used in livestock operations to fatten animals. Some medications used to treat manic depression can cause massive weight gain. Hormonally active substances like estrogens and contraceptive agents can affect shape. Beta blockers have weight gain as a side effect. All of these medication types have been detected in some municipal water supplies.

women who participated in a 10-week weight-training program. About half the women were taking "the Pill"; about half weren't. Did this influence how they responded to the weight-training program? Yes, it did. The women taking oral contraceptives built much less muscle, responding poorly compared to the women who were not taking oral contraceptives. What can we infer from the evidence in these two cases? We can infer that some medications might be an obstacle to achieving our desired shape outcomes even when we are doing things that might otherwise be working. It's not bad enough that some medications can make things worse with respect to shape, they might also prevent us from fully enjoying the benefits of the efforts we are putting into things that otherwise would improve our shape. Because of this, and the cases investigated earlier in this chapter, it is important that we become better investigators when it comes to medications.

HSI CLUE

Our individuality interacts in complex ways with medications. This and can result in a big variance in what happens when we take the medication compared with others. This is illustrated in the *Case of Lithium*. In one year long study just under half the women taking lithium gained weight. Fewer than one out of five men did. Gender, which is just one aspect of our complex individuality, strongly influenced weight gain.

The first step in this investigation process is to identify whether you are taking a medication that has a known shape or weight affect. You can check the information sheet that comes with your medication, or ask the doctor who prescribed it or the pharmacist who filled the prescription. While we recommend this as your first step, we don't think it is wise to stop with this step for the many reasons we have mentioned in this chapter. The next step in this investigation is to use the Internet to find out whether other users are reporting shape changes with the drug. This can be done in one of two non-mutually exclusive manners—doing a broad search or looking for answers at dedicated patient sites. The first option can be accomplished by using a search engine like Google or Yahoo. Type in the name of the medication, the word *forum*, and the phrase (in quotes) *weight gain*. If other people are noticing weight gain with the medication, this search will typically return a list of message boards where patients have asked if others have noticed something similar. The second area of Internet investigation can be done by going to a dedicated patient site. These are websites where the individuals taking medications are sharing their personal experiences (askapatient.com is one such site). The third step in your investigation is to visit our website (healthsceneinvestigation.com). While the scientific investigations into the shape and body composition effects of medications is far from where it would be in an ideal world, there is far more known currently than we can do justice to in a single book chapter. Our website is a far better resource for getting information about known effects than this book can be, and has the advantage that it can be updated as new information is discovered. There is also something you can do to help us and help others. Bearing in mind the axiom that *We are smarter than Me,* we invite you to visit us online and share your experiences directly with the health scene investigation community in our forums. Use the available message boards to ask questions, and share your observations and real world experiences. We might be holding our breath for a long time if we wait for drug companies and independent studies to find the answers for us when it comes to medication-shape interactions. In the meantime, we can help ourselves and others tremendously by, as Holmes might say, "reasoning backwards" in our own cases, and by then sharing these observations with others. By collaborating on the massive scale that the Internet allows, we will be able to more effectively help ourselves by helping each other.

> **HSI CLUE**
>
> Proton Pump Inhibitors (PPI) are used to treat ulcers. Weight gain is not listed as a side effect. Yet Internet searches reveal complaints of weight gain, occasionally massive weight gain, after starting a PPI. There are even complaints of weight gain by people who claim to be doing their best to exercise and eat healthy. These patients are *reasoning backwards.* Complex individuality informs us that they might also be reasoning correctly.

Identifying a medication-induced shift in shape can be challenging, because of the examples we discussed in this chapter. It can be challenging because each of us are in a sense an *experiment of one.* If you experience a shift in your shape after starting a medication, "reasoning backwards" and questioning whether the medication might be a contributing factor is warranted. Investigation might lead to evidence that the medication has produced what you are experiencing in others. It might not. Complexity science teaches us that each of us is unique in terms of the way our particular diet, lifestyle and environment interact with our genetics to create a highly individualized human. The manner any person responds when a medication is added into this incredibly complex situation is ultimately an individual experiment. No amount of data from other people can predict with perfect certainty what we will experience.

Because of this, investigation also entails getting as comprehensive a baseline shape, body composition, and fat distribution assessment as is possible *before* starting new medications. If you are already taking a medication, get a baseline of where you are now and monitor for changes moving forward.

Taking a medication is a form of self-experimentation. You will be conducting an experiment, in collaboration with your doctor, to determine whether the medication is helping for whatever its intended therapeutic purpose might be. You will also be running an individual self-experiment in terms of adverse effects, including shape side effects. These vital clues should be monitored periodically, preferably at least monthly. Tracking our individual response is the only way to objectively observe what is occurring within our body. Watch for changes and take steps early if you note a trend for worsening shape. Once unwanted shifts in shape have occurred, they can sometimes be difficult to reverse, and even when they can be reversed, it might take a long time. If a medication is causing Shape Intelligence to adjust its best guess about what shape to defend, it's better to catch this as early on in the process as possible.

Solution: It's Complicated

Once you have identified a medication that might be an obstacle to improving your shape what do you do? We wish we could give you a cookie cutter answer. Unfortunately, there isn't one. Individual needs, risks and benefits of medications, are a complex matter. Suddenly stopping a medication might cause or contribute to a significant worsening of an existing health problem. It is rarely a good idea to abruptly cease taking a medication, and never a good idea to stop a medication without consulting with the physician who prescribed it. We recommend you discuss the risks and benefits of the medication and what other therapeutic options might be available for your unique situation with your physician prior to making any decisions about stopping or changing the dose of a medication.

In some instances, another medication option might exist which has a better track record in terms of its effects on shape. An example of this is contraceptives. While the effects oral contraceptives have on shape is open to debate, any effect they might have pales in comparison to the effects of injectable (so called "depot" or "depo") contraceptives. Depot contraceptives, on average, cause massive gains in weight and body fat, as well as more pronounced shifts to an apple shape, compared to oral contraceptives. And these shape changes don't appear to go away quickly once depot contraceptives are stopped. In one study, depot contraceptives resulted in an average gain of 12 pounds of weight and 9 pounds of fat over three years. This shape change did not magically disappear after depot contraceptives were stopped. If a woman switched to a non-hormonal contraceptive method, she lost an average of about 1 pound in six months. If she switched to oral contraceptives, she continued to gain, on average, 1 pound over the next six months. If concerns about shape are an issue, and they are with most women who would be using contraceptives, oral contraceptives are a wiser choice than depot contraceptives.

In instances where no other, or better, medication option exists, the benefits of the medication might outweigh potential interactions it is having with your shape. Only you, in consultation with your physician, when the two of you work together to take into consideration your health history, goals, and uniqueness, can make this determination. In many instances, the wisest short-term course of action will be remaining on the medication. But just because we are continuing to take a medication today, doesn't mean we will always need it. We might need to remain on it, but could do some things that would allow us to lower the dose, perhaps eventually tapering off it completely. We might be able to get off it completely if our overall health improves sufficiently over time: And there are always things we can be doing to improve our health whether or not we are taking medications. Following some of the suggested solutions in other chapters—sleeping more, improving body clock function, reducing stress, minimizing chemical exposure, exercising more effectively, and eating better—can build health, and as a result, can indirectly influence the need for and reliance on medications over time.

Closing Dialogue

Health Scene Investigator: Let's return to our starting question. If a person complained of weight gain after starting a medication, what would you advise them?

Apprentice: My advice would vary depending on the medication they are taking.

Health Scene Investigator: How so?

Apprentice: If they are taking a medication with weight gain or shape changes as a known side effect, than I would advise them about these facts.

Health Scene Investigator: Go on...

Apprentice: If shape and weight changes have not been reported as a side effect, I would not dismiss their complaint. It strikes me that we know far too little with most drugs to ever declare with certainty that a medication would be "guilt-free". While it might not be a usual suspect, it is possible that for this individual, the medication is contributing in some way.

Health Scene Investigator: Well put. It is far better to have an open mind, approaching the complaint from a perspective that there might be an element of truth in the person's "reasoning backward" even if the drug maker assures us otherwise.

Chapter 17

Movement and Shape

We hastened onward at such a pace that my sedentary life began to tell upon me, and I was compelled to fall behind. Holmes, however, was always in training...his springy step never slowed.

Dr. Watson

Opening Dialogue

Health Scene Investigator: Do you remember the cases we discussed which included exercise....the *Case of the Conserved Calories* and the *Case of Swimming*?

Apprentice: Yes I do. I had believed that the only reason that exercise helped with shape and weight was because we burn calories while we exercise. The evidence in these cases provided exceptions to this obvious fact.

Health Scene Investigator: Very good. Our axiom that an exception disproves the rule means that these exceptions disprove the conventional wisdom about why exercise improves shape. But the fact still remains that appropriate exercise is one of the most consistent methods to improve our shape. Why does it do this?

Apprentice: I must admit that I do not have a theory to explain the facts.

Health Scene Investigator: Not to worry. I think if we look at the evidence in more detail and then use our Scientific Imagination, we will be able to come up with a theory that best explains the real reasons exercise shifts our shapes.

The Case for Movement

Watson informs us, in the *Adventure of the Solitary Cyclist,* that he had difficulty keeping pace with Holmes. Watson correctly infers that his sedentary life is responsible. If we had an opportunity to investigate Watson's health scene, it is extremely likely that this would not be the only area where his lack of movement was "telling upon" him. A sedentary lifestyle takes a predictable toll on the body: Shape worsens, quality of life suffers, health deteriorates, and we age at an accelerated rate. If it were not already the case, sooner or later, Watson's sedentary lifestyle would take a toll in these areas. As long as he chooses to remain sedentary, we would expect him to "fail to keep pace" when it comes to shape and health compared to a more active person. The only way to keep up—improve his shape and his health—is to move. The same is true for us: When it comes to our shape and health, the choice boils down to move it, or lose them. The *Case of Remaining Sedentary* highlights this fact.

HSI CLUE

Fitness trumps fatness. We are predisposed to assume that if someone is overweight or obese based on current standards, that they are less healthy than thinner people. Studies disprove this assumption. A physically fit heavy person is at essentially the same heath risk as a physically fit leaner one. And a fit heavy person is at a far lower risk of death and disease than a sedentary thin or "normal" weight person.

The STRRIDE study was conducted by scientists at Duke University Medical Center. It entailed assessing body fat amounts and locations in a group of previously sedentary, overweight men and women at the beginning and end of a six-month period. Some of the volunteers remained sedentary throughout the study period; others began activity programs. The fat stored around internal abdominal organs—visceral fat—increased by almost 9 percent in the volunteers who remained sedentary. The increase in belly fat was completely prevented, and in some cases reversed, by becoming active. Belly fat is among the riskiest types of fat tissue. It also results in a less appealing shape. The *Case of Remaining Sedentary* provides compelling evidence that a choice to remain sedentary is in effect a decision to gain more and more belly fat and to increase our risk for illness. Remaining sedentary for just six months caused these individuals to fall noticeably behind similar individuals who became active. This is not an isolated case. The evidence of the shape and health consequences of sedentary lifestyles, and the benefits of active lifestyles, is overwhelming. This is true for people of all sizes and shapes, both genders, and across the lifespan. When we combine the proven consequences of a sedentary lifestyle with evidence that we are in the midst of an epidemic of inactivity, as a society we have reached activity levels that might be the all-time low for the human species, is it any wonder we are experiencing an epidemic of shape problems? Is it any wonder that our health is suffering?

Our options are simple. If, like Watson, we find ourselves falling behind, we can continue to fall further behind or we can do something about it. The choice is ours. We can remain sedentary: Odds are shape will progressively worsen (and we'll become less healthy). We can engage in a bare minimum amount of walking or similar activity and keep our shape about the same. Or, we can become active enough as individuals, and as a society, to improve our shape. If we do make the choice to be more active (and we hope you will), what specifically should we do? What types of activity produce the best results? How much activity do we need? How often? These are some of the important questions when it comes to movement-related exercise. Before we investigate these questions, let's turn our attention to a vitally important area: How exactly does movement influence Shape Intelligence?

Exercise Activity and Shape Intelligence

Evidence is overwhelming that exercise can improve shape, build muscle, reduce body fat, and favorably shift the distribution of the remaining body fat. When done appropriately, exercise produces these changes spontaneously; they occur without the need to restrict calories. Rather than investigating all of the evidence that leads to these inferences, a more important question is why do these shape changes occur; in other words, how does exercise really work?

The conventional wisdom, when it comes to exercise and weight, goes something like this. If we want to lose weight, we need to create a calorie deficit. To lose one pound of fat a week, we must expend 3500 more calories through exercise and metabolism than we consume. So, in theory, exercise helps us control our weight because, when we exercise we use up, or burn, calories that would otherwise be stored as fat. There are lots of facts that don't fit with this theory. We have discussed some of them in other chapters. Just sticking with the exercise part of the energy balance equation, we have already mentioned two examples where things start to fall to pieces. One example was the *Case of Swimming* (Chapter 7). Swimming did not produce the same shape and weight response as running or bicycling did. It shouldn't matter what type of exercise we do; burning the calories should be the only important thing. Yet evidence exists where this is simply not the case. It also shouldn't matter if we are at, below, or above our natural weight.

H S I C L U E

Data from the National Weight Control Registry—a database of more than 2000 individuals who have been able to maintain significant weight reductions for at least one year—indicate that more than 90 percent of successful individuals report exercise as a key element in their success.

If we exercise a certain amount, we should burn the amount of calories needed to move that weight. But the *Case of Conserved Calories* (Chapter 6) indicated this might not be what occurs in the real world. In this case, as a person lost weight through dieting—moved below their natural weight—they burned fewer calories while exercising than expected: The body became thrifty with its use of energy. Exercise does not seem to work the same way when we are below our body's defended weight as it does when we are at it. Any athlete who has cut weight to compete can attest to this. As we move further below natural weight, proportionately greater and greater feats of exercise are needed to lose incrementally less and less weight.

Another case to consider is the *Case of More Isn't Better*. The two most common pieces of advice people who want to lose weight receive are: (1) Eat less; and (2) Exercise more. We have explored in past chapters why advice to *eat less* doesn't work long-term, and can even produce an unwanted shape consequence—body fat overshoot; a regain of more fat once the diet is broken than was lost by dieting. While advice to move from being sedentary to active is sound advice, implying that a person can have any desired shape by taking exercise to extremes appears to be fatally flawed. We observe evidence of this in experiments of forced activity in animals. Sedentary rats are fatter and die faster than active rats. When allowed to run in a wheel for a few minutes a day, lab rats lose a slight amount of fat and eat a bit less than normal—natural weight and appetite both decrease. At an hour a day or so of wheel running a rat's body fat reaches a minimum, and as it happens so does food intake, while longevity reaches a maximum. But if the rat is forced to run for significantly more than an hour daily, body fat does not decrease below the amounts observed with an hour of exercise because the rats eat more to compensate for the extra physical activity. And if forced to run more than six hours daily, rats are literally and figuratively run ragged. Shape tends to worsen and the rats die even faster than sedentary rats. In one study, forced wheel running resulted in five times as many lab rats dying during the study period compared to the rats allowed to exercise voluntarily. Even compared to the sedentary rats, forced activity doubled the death rate. As if this were not enough, the rats that were forced to run for extended durations of time ended up being almost as fat as the sedentary rats. While under most circumstances exercise is a beneficial thing, too much exercise in this instance was catastrophic. It was a form of severe stress. If we approach exercise in a way similar to forced activity in animals, using it as a means to try to reduce our scale weight by doing hours of it daily, exercise doesn't tend to improve shape in the long-term, and it can be as damaging to health and shape as other types of stress.

These three cases are only the tip of the iceberg. In studies where an identical caloric deficit has been sustained over months, but, in some people, it's been done by dieting alone, and in others exercise is used in combination with dieting to produce an equal calorie deficit, the shape results consistently differ. Even when similar weight loss is achieved, the people who also exercise (1) deplete more fat, (2) preserve more muscle, (3) eliminate more belly fat, and (4) don't experience the same degree of "slowing of metabolism". If it's only a matter of calories, why does the same caloric deficit, achieved in different ways, produce such different shape and metabolic responses? This is just one of many questions without a tidy answer when we view exercise as solely a way to burn calories. Others include:

- Why does weight loss caused exclusively by dieting result in an increase in appetite, yet weight loss achieved through consistent moderate exercise, with no restriction of calories, doesn't?
- Why does spontaneous physical activity decrease, and lethargy increase, when weight is lost through calorie restriction?
- Why does a moderate amount of daily exercise (an hour or less) tend to decrease appetite, while many hours of daily

exercise increases it? In other words, why doesn't appetite compensate for the calories burned with moderate exercise but does seem to compensate for calories burned with excessive exercise?

- Why do walking, jogging, aerobics, and weight lifting cause such different shape outcomes even if done in ways that allow similar amounts of calories to be burned?
- How is it that some activities—weight lifting or brief bouts of intense exercise—produce shape benefits far out of proportion to the calories used to perform the activity?
- How do we explain adaptation to exercise or the overtraining syndromes that arise when we push ourselves too much?

There are many facts that don't fit a theory that proposes exercise is solely about calories burned. If we were to approach exercise with a blank mind, which as Holmes tells us is a distinct advantage in the art of detection, what explanation could we come up with to better fit the actual facts?

In Chapter 7 we mentioned a new type of science—a science of complex adaptive systems called Complexity. This scientific model proposes that when a complex adaptive system encounters a novel challenge, it (1) learns, (2) store this knowledge, and (3) updates its best guesses about the future. In short, it adapts; changing the rules of the game as the game is being played. This is precisely what seems to occur with exercise. Exercise is a challenge that causes Shape Intelligence to make intelligent adaptations. A muscle that is trained with weights will become bigger and stronger. If we are sedentary and go for a one-mile walk, we might find ourselves struggling, breathing heavily and feeling exhausted. Yet if we consistently walk a mile, in no time we find ourselves covering the same distance while breathing easily and feeling invigorated. Our body adapts to the challenge and improves our walking fitness.

While weight training and walking produce very different shape responses, in both instances, the results can be explained by the following process: The body (1) encounters something new, (2) realizes it is ill-equipped to deal with it, (3) guesses that the same situation is likely to occur again, and (4) decides it is going to be better prepared next time. It then makes the necessary adaptations to be better prepared. The adaptations in our muscles, fitness, and other systems are highly specific depending on which exercise we do. We believe this same principle—the body adapts in an intelligent manner to new challenges—should guide how we view the way exercise influences shape. Rather than asking how many calories we might burn doing a certain type and amount of exercise, we might be far better off if we asked ourselves what our body is likely to learn from and how is it going to adapt to this experience.

When applied to exercise this means we should ask questions like:

- Are all types of exercise the same when it comes to producing shape adaptations?
- If I do this specific exercise in this exact way, what would an intelligent adaptation be to this situation?
- If I want my shape to improve in this area (or these several areas) is there a best way to approach exercising that would be most likely to convince Shape Intelligence to build more muscle or reduce fat in these places?
- Are there things I can do before, during, or after exercise that will help Shape Intelligence adapt more successfully?

On Intensity and Frequency

In the *Adventures of Black Peter* Holmes tells Watson, "There can be no question, my dear Watson, of the value of exercise before breakfast." We agree with his statement. Getting some activity before breakfast is a wonderful way to start the day; it can be a tipping point to improve both shape and health. Let's explore some of the other important tipping points for how Shape Intelligence adapts to the challenge of exercise. Let's begin this investigation with *intensity*.

Exercise can be divided into 3 broad categories based on how intense it is—Low, Medium, and High. The intensity of exercise causes different adaptations. If you were to go into a gym, you would observe some people participating in high intensity activities such as weight

HSI CLUE

One group of volunteers ate 25 percent fewer calories for six months. Another group got to the same calorie deficit by reducing calories by 12.5 percent and increasing exercise to burn an additional 12.5 percent of calories. Six months later both groups had decreased their weight by about 10 percent, but metabolism was much slower in the group that lost weight by calorie restriction alone. In the other group, metabolism was essentially unchanged. Why, when both created the same energy deficit, was the metabolic response different?

training. Others would be participating in activities such as walking on a treadmill or using an exercise bike at a pace that would qualify as low intensity. Still others would be participating in medium intensity activities. You would also notice that some of the people invest time participating in exercises that fall in two or more of these intensity categories—they might weight train and ride on a stationary bike. Our experience is that the people who get the best shape results from the time they invest in exercise will be those from this latter group. Even more specifically, they will be the people who combine low and high intensity exercise but do each in a *just right* way. This chapter will focus on the low intensity part of this shape solution; high intensity will be discussed in the next chapter.

HSI CLUE

Prolonged endurance training and weight training produce extremely different and distinct adaptations. At a superficial level this is obvious in both overall body shape and muscle size and shape. But the adaptations are far more than skin deep. A body exposed to long distance running will adapt its muscles and metabolism in highly specific ways that best prepare it to run long distances. A body exposed to lifting heavy weights will adapt in entirely different ways; ways that best prepare it to meet this challenge.

Low-intensity exercise means that we are continuously active or moving but are not exercising at a level of intensity that would cause us to experience shortness of breath. When we are exercising more intensely than this, but not intensely enough to be considered high intensity, we are doing medium intensity exercise. Walking, bicycling, Pilates, yoga, tai chi, and most types of dancing would be examples of low intensity exercise. Medium intensity exercise is a continuous exercise or movement such as running, spinning, or an aerobics class, which is done at a level where it would be difficult, or impossible, for us to carry on a conversation: We are breathing too heavily. The key to determining whether some type of continuous exercise is low or medium intensity is our breathing, not the type of exercise. Many people think that improving shape requires a commitment to aerobics classes, jogging, or some other relatively vigorous type of sustained activity. By our definition, these vigorous activities, especially for individuals whose fitness levels are below average, are almost without exception considered medium intensity. While medium intensity activities certainly offer some shape and health benefits, a strong case can be made that low intensity activity—something as simple as daily walking—can produce even better results and is safer for the long haul.

The goal is to move enough, and in ways, that provide the stimulus for Shape Intelligence to adapt in desired ways, without moving so much, or in ways, that produce unnecessary wear and tear. Put another way, we want to improve shape without undermining health in either the short or long-term. We accomplish this "low wear and tear result" by putting most of our efforts into types of activities that are, because of their intensity and biomechanics, low wear and tear activities. Walking is an example. Most people will be able to go for a gentle walk, something akin to ambling or a stroll, every day for a lifetime without wearing out the ability to walk.

It can be tempting to view an activity like walking as being inadequate. Exercise charts inform us that we burn more calories during an hour of doing aerobics or jogging than we do if we walk for an hour. This is true. But the goal isn't to use exercise as a means to try and control energy balance— forcing our body to burn more calories because we want to lose weight faster. Shape Intelligence, not us, controls the internal processes related to energy balance. We don't want to use exercise to simply reduce scale weight; we want to use it as a way to reduce our natural weight. The goal is to find the minimum stimulus needed to create this adaptation; it isn't to use exercise as a form of dieting. If, because of how much a person is exercising and how little they are eating, a sufficient negative energy balance is created to push a person below natural weight, Shape Intelligence appears to respond in much the same manner we have discussed in the cases of underfeeding. We observe similar changes in hormones, appetite, and metabolism as we observe during energy restriction by dieting. We might even see fewer calories burned for a given activity than we anticipate similar to what we discussed in the *Case of the Conserved Calories*.

And why shouldn't we? After all, from the perspective of Shape Intelligence, why should it matter how we got to be below natural weight? We are in essence teaching it the same thing—available

---

HSI CLUE

Volunteers wore devices for seven days that were designed to detect and measure all movement. For the group as a whole, breaks from being sedentary were short, averaging about five minutes. The number of breaks was associated with shape: Individuals who spontaneously took more breaks to interrupt sedentary routines had better shapes. This does not *prove* that taking more breaks *causes* a leaner shape. It is circumstantial evidence, but it is circumstantial evidence that warrants further investigation.

calories are insufficient. Its predictions about how much fat to defend and where to store it must be updated accordingly. This usually looks like defending less muscle, more fat, and shifting some fat to our abdominal region. This response by Shape Intelligence becomes particularly evident if an injury, illness, or some other factor prevents a person from exercising. In these situations we often observe a catch-up fat gain that is very similar to what would be observed in the period after coming off a low calorie diet.

HSI CLUE

Two hundred and two previously sedentary men and women were divided into two groups and followed for one year. One group was encouraged to do 60 minutes of physical activity a day, six days a week; the other was given no specific exercise advice. The persons, who actually exercised 60 minutes daily, six days a week, lost 10 to 15 percent of their total body fat, decreased belly fat between 10 to 20 percent, and got both of these results without losing muscle.

If Shape Intelligence only made its decisions based upon the calories burned while exercising, medium intensity activity—an aerobics class or a long run—would indeed be the preferred exercise type. However, based upon the actual evidence, we don't think this is what drives its decisions. In fact, we believe that the only time calories burned becomes a significant factor in Shape Intelligence's decision making process is when exercise is used as a form of dieting. The critical factor Shape Intelligence uses to determine how much weight, and more specifically, fat to defend, and where to locate it, is our *need for mobility*. While this is just one of the many considerations that ultimately determines how Shape Intelligence solves our individual diet/lifestyle/environment learning situations, frequency of movement—how often we move—appears to be a vital factor that is *weighed* in the decision making process. The analogy we use to describe this dynamic is: If you were going to move from one home to another a few times in the next year, what makes the most sense?

A. Collecting more and more stuff.
B. Keeping the same amount of stuff.
C. Getting rid of stuff you no longer need.

Sensible people tend to eventually opt for answer C and get rid of stuff they no longer need. In our experience, Shape Intelligence is extremely sensible. It seems to use a very similar strategy as part of its considerations when deciding upon a preferred shape.

When it comes to considering frequency of movement, if we are sedentary the decision is easy. There is no penalty for accumulating more stuff—body fat—so we get fatter. If we are active two to three times a week, we might convince Shape Intelligence it should not accumulate any more stuff, and might even cause it to decide to get rid of a small amount of stuff. But, in our experience, the real magic comes when we hit four plus days a week of movement. In most cases, this frequency of movement absolutely convinces Shape Intelligence to get rid of any non-essential stuff. This theory means that Shape Intelligence won't learn the same thing if we walk two days a week no matter how long or far we walk on those days as it would if we go for a walk on four plus days a week. Walking for six hours, by walking for three hours on Saturday and three hours on Sunday, isn't the same thing as walking for six hours by walking an hour a day on six different weekdays. These are very different experiences and cause different adaptations. When it comes to improving shape, it's not about how many hours we exercised over a week (and how many calories we burned during these hours); it's about how many days in a week we are moving

How Much? How Often?

We seem to respond to exercise according to the *Goldilocks principle*. If we get too little, our shape worsens, we defend more fat, and our longevity might suffer. But more isn't necessarily better: Excessive exercise is a form of stress. Because of this the goal is to move a *just right* amount. In our experience, the just right amount of daily movement is about one hour. With one hour of gentle movement activity, body fat usually reaches a minimum level (at least with respect to what is achievable and *sustainable* though exercise) and health benefits are maximized. Moving for significantly more than one hour a day rarely provides any significant additional shape advantages because our appetite usually increases to directly compensate for the extra energy being used to exercise this much. And if we exercise excessively or force ourselves to exercise in amounts that are far beyond what Shape Intelligence would consider appropriate, based upon our nutrition, rest, recovery, stress levels, and other factors, there can be significant costs and consequence to both shape and health. In terms of how much activity, the general rule of thumb is that the goal for most days should be to move for somewhere between 20 to 60 minutes daily.

Walkable environments have strong associations with leaner shapes. The same is also true for walking to work and for occupations that entail being more active verse those that entail being sedentary. These are forms of circumstantial evidence. They don't *prove* that being active is *causing* the observed leanness. But ample direct evidence does prove that walking improves shape. A walking program consisting of as little as 30 minutes of walking on most days of the week, significantly improves shape over six months to a year.

Shape Intelligence appears to place a premium on the frequency of movement. We think this is because survival requires that the need for mobility be balanced against the need for contingency plans against future time periods of low food supply. Moving more frequently appears to *shift* this balance in favor of mobility so the contingency plan against a period of low food availability—body fat—becomes less important and is sacrificed in favor of changes that make mobility easier. This theory explains a frequent observation in health scenes we have investigated. This observation can be simply stated as; "weekend warriors", no matter how much they move on weekends, rarely experience the same degree of shape benefits as do people who move most days of the week. We have consistently observed that people who participate in movement types of exercise five to six times weekly have far superior shape results than do people who move only two to three times weekly. As amazing as it might sound, the rate at which body fat declines can be as much as two times faster when a person is active for 60 minutes or so a day, four times a week rather than three times a week. So, from our perspective, the magic number is four days a week of activity. While moving on five or six days during the week usually produces even better results, the big shift happens when we go from being active three or fewer days a week, to at least four. This means that if we were to engage in movement exercises five hours each week, we would expect to benefit more, if we moved an hour a day on five separate days, than we would if we did the same five hours of activity in just two days. In terms of how often, the general rule of thumb is that a minimum of four days of movement each week is the goal, but that the best results occur when we move on most days.

The power of taking a 20 to 60 minute, most days approach to movement, is illustrated in the *Case of Gradually Increasing Walking Duration*. Grant Gwinup from the University of California, Irvine, asked a group of overweight people to forget about controlling what they ate and to begin a program of physical activity. The amount of activity was carefully adjusted to the capacity of each individual. For most people this meant they began by walking for ten to fifteen minutes daily. Extremely unfit individuals started with as little as five minutes of walking a day. As people adapted to this low level of exertion, they extended the amount of time they walked. Anyone who reached a point of walking briskly for at least thirty minutes five times a week began to lose weight spontaneously—virtually exclusively as body fat—without dieting or controlling food intake. A year and a half after starting, the eleven women who had continued daily walking had reduced body fat by an average of 22 pounds. There are very few things that a person can do that will result in a reduction of 22 pounds of fat. The few interventions that might do this are either high risk, like weight loss surgeries or medications, or unsustainable, like dieting. Walking not only carries minimal risks, its side effects include better health, more energy, improved mood, and prevention of disease. And unlike dieting, which gets more and more difficult with each passing week, walking gets easier over time because we adapt to it by becoming fitter and fitter.

We want to share one more case with you—the *Case of the Dog Walkers.* The people in this case were sedentary, economically disadvantaged adults with multiple chronic illnesses. They were asked to walk loaner dogs and started by walking the dogs for ten minutes three times per week. Eventually the participants walked up to twenty minutes per day five days per week. After 50 weeks—a bit less than a year—these dog walkers had lost an average of 14 pounds. They had improved their flexibility, balance and ability to walk. And equally as important, they felt better about themselves. Despite the barriers of poor habits, economic disadvantage, and long-term illness, these people faced at the outset, they made a sustainable change—they walked dogs for just twenty minutes a day on most days—and look what they received. They looked and felt better. What will taking more steps each day do for you?

HSI CLUE

Rodents given access to an exercise wheel will exercise shortly after waking. They get into this ritual and stay with it. Getting in a morning exercise routine might also be good for us. Circadian research indicates that people who consistently exercise in the morning *teach* their body to be ready for exercise at that time of day. As a result, they tend to feel like exercising. Morning exercisers also tend to be more consistent exercisers. Perhaps this is because of body clock issues, but perhaps it is simply because they exercise before anything else has a chance to interrupt this habit.

On Varying Our Pace

Experts believe that our ancient ancestors experienced punctuated exercise. A hunter-gatherer might go on long walks in search of food, but might randomly need to sprint for quick bursts to capture prey or elude dangers. Punctuated exercise—hour-long walks with intermittent bursts of higher intensity exercise such as a sprint or a walk up steep stairs—might be a way to duplicate this more naturalistic activity. By varying our pace at intentional intervals, or in a random manner, throughout a longer walk, we might send very different messages to Shape Intelligence than would be the case if we walked at a steady pace the entire time. The theory of punctuating exercise in this manner as a means to improve shape is currently based more on anecdotal evidence than hard scientific fact. That said, existing evidence suggests that we might get better health results from varying our pace while walking than we would if we walked at a constant pace. This is illustrated in the *Case of Varying Our Pace*. Elderly participants were placed in one of the following three groups:

1. No walking
2. Walking at a constant pace
3. Walking while repetitively varying the pace

The no walking group was asked to maintain a sedentary lifestyle. The constant pace group was instructed to walk at a steady, moderate pace for more than 8,000 steps a day. The varied pace group was told to walk for two to three minutes at a slow pace, pick up the pace to a very brisk walking pace for the next three minutes, and to repeat this cycle five times on four or more days each week. Five months later scientists investigated the effects of the three different programs. Not surprisingly, members of the no walking group gained weight. Members of the two other groups had lost weight; with the people who had followed the programs most consistently losing the most weight. While walking at a constant pace and at a varied pace both produced weight loss, the results in several areas were vastly better in the varied pace group. This exercise program produced the biggest increases in thigh muscle strength and peak aerobic capacity. The decrease in blood pressure was also approximately three-times greater than that observed in the constant pace group. This study detected much greater improvements in health and fitness when people walked and repetitively varied their pace during a walking period. Shape, body composition, and body fat types and distribution were not studied, so drawing inferences in these areas would be premature.

Please don't wait for studies on punctuated exercise and shape to take place before trying this approach to walking. Instead, we encourage you to experiment with varying your pace while walking and test for yourself whether it is meets the most important real world test—the response in your body. There are several options for practicing punctuated exercise. The participants in the above study walked for two to three minutes at a moderate pace, increased to a brisk pace for the next two to three minutes, slowed again to a moderate pace for two to three minutes, and then repeated this cycle up to five times. A punctuated walk that followed this approach would take between twenty to thirty minutes to complete. This would be a regimented approach. Its opposite would be to take a more random approach. This could be accomplished by suddenly, at fairly random time intervals, sprinting for five to ten seconds several times during a long walk. Between these two extremes of regimentation and randomness, there are many options, limited only by our imagination, on how something as simple as a walk can be turned into punctuated exercise.

HSI CLUE

In July 2007, a press release titled "Breaking up workouts may burn fat faster" described a study which suggested that men might use more fat to exercise if they exercise for two 30-minute periods, taking a 20-minute rest break in between, than if they exercise continuously for 60-minutes, and then rested afterward. While more study is needed in this area, there is currently little reason to believe that all of our daily movement must be continuous, occurring all in one dedicated time chunk.

Turning Our Movement Goals into Reality

How do we make our movement goal a reality? Let us share three quick stories with you.

1. People were asked to submit a report within 48 hours and then divided into two groups. The first group was asked to do one thing and the second group was not. Three out of four of the people in the first group handed the report in on time. Only one out of three in the second group did.
2. Women were asked to begin breast self-exams and then divided into two groups. The first group was asked to do one thing and the second group was not. Nearly 100 percent of women in the first group completed the self-exams compared with only about 50 percent of the second group.

3. People were given information on how to exercise and then divided into two groups. The first group was asked to do one thing and the second group was not. Nine out of ten people in the first group adhered to the exercise program. About four out of ten in the second group did.

The *one thing* in each of these three cases was the same. In each case the little thing that made the big difference was writing down where and when they would complete the activity. This simple, yet powerful step causes us to look into the future and find a time and place where the new activity will fit into our lives. Once we have accomplished this step, the chances we follow through go up dramatically. To turn your movement goals into reality your first responsibility is to write down today where and when you will go for a walk, or participate in some other form of movement activity, on at least five of the next seven days.

HSI CLUE

Individuals who join a fitness program with a spouse are more likely to be active a year later. People who make activity commitments with friends are more likely to become and remain active. We are social creatures. Use this tendency towards socialization to your advantage when it comes to becoming and staying more active.

When we are trying to improve any area of our lives, one of the most valuable gifts we can receive is accurate feedback. This holds true for movement. One way to get feedback on how much we are actually moving would be to time each period of movement we have in a day, write these numbers down, and add them up. If we consistently reach our target of moving for between thirty to sixty minutes daily, we will objectively be meeting our movement goal. Unfortunately, this method fails to capture the smaller and subtler movement activity most of us also get—things like walking from our car to our office, or to lunch, or around our home. When it comes to shifting our shape, all movement matters so we want you to get feedback on this movement as well. A simple, direct and inexpensive method to achieve this feedback is to wear a pedometer (a device the size of a watch that you wear on your belt). Use this pedometer to keep track of the total amount of steps taken in a day. Some experts recommend 10,000 steps as a daily goal. We believe that this is a very useful target but want you to realize that even 5,000 steps every day will carry you a long way on your journey to a better shape. With every additional one thousand steps a day above and beyond 5000 steps, the probability that your shape will improve increases.

The Movement Solution

Let's summarize. Shifting your shape can be as easy as:

1. Moving continuously,
2. Starting slowly with just five minutes,
3. Building to thirty to sixty minutes per day, gradually as we become more fit,
4. Either all at one time, or in smaller fifteen minute segments,
5. On most days of the week.

It may seem obvious, but simple steps like taking the stairs, parking your car a few blocks away from your destination, getting off public transit early, taking a brief walk at mid-morning or afternoon coffee break, are all easy ways to incorporate more daily movement activity into your life. All activity over the day accumulates, so these modest changes in lifestyle toward more movement can act as tipping points and make a difference.

It is critical that we realize what we are and aren't trying to accomplish through low intensity activity. We are not concerned with how many calories we are burning. We are concerned with convincing Shape Intelligence that it will need to adjust its solution to our diet/lifestyle/environment learning situations, in favor of a need for mobility. This requires moving consistently. It also may require time and patience. We have investigated cases in which Shape Intelligence has responded to new input—to changes in diet, lifestyle or environment—quickly. We have also investigated cases in which it has taken months before new input creates big shifts. Quite often, movement falls more into this latter category. Shape Intelligence may sit back and observe for a while, making sure you are truly serious about this new movement habit, before deciding to defend less fat. Once it makes this decision, assuming you continue to be active, pounds begin to vanish and shape shifts. For some people, Shape Intelligence makes this decision quickly—within weeks of making and demonstrating a commitment to daily movement; for others it might take months. If you fall into the latter group, the only advice we can give is to persevere. It will be worth it. Your Shape Intelligence will eventually decide you are serious about being more active and will update its shape predictions accordingly.

To qualify as low intensity activity we must be able to pass the *talk test* (the exception would be during the brisk walking or sprinting phases if we decide to go for a varied pace walk). If the pace we are going at is sufficiently brisk that we are breathing hard and would find it challenging to carry on a conversation, it is a virtual certainty that we have moved into a medium intensity activity level. Medium intensity activity is more stressful on our body, creates a higher risk for over training and injury, and generally produces more wear and tear. So, if you find yourself feeling out of breath, slow your pace. In the long run you will be better served by exercising at a pace that will allow you to take long, slow breaths (ideally about six per minute) than you will be if you go at a faster pace. We refer to taking six breaths a minute (five second inhalation and five second exhalation) as *paced breathing*. We have found this pace of breathing to be fantastic as a stress management technique and as a good check and balance to make sure we are walking at a pace our body can handle without it causing stress. As we become adapted to exercise, we will be able to gradually increase our rate and duration of walking while still being able to breathe slowly. A well-conditioned athlete will be able to run, ride a bike, or walk briskly for prolonged periods of time and still easily maintain this pace of breathing. Because of this, sixty minutes of activity would be easy for them. This is not the case for someone who has been sedentary. A person who has been sedentary for months or years might only be able to sustain this type of breathing for a few minutes while walking at even a moderate pace before breathing becomes labored. This is fine. When this is the case, a gradual approach to exercise is preferred. In other words, stop at this point. The way to build fitness is to nudge it up from below. There is not a problem with only being able to walk comfortably for five to ten minutes. The problem is when you go past this point. If you are consistent, five minutes becomes ten minutes, ten becomes fifteen, fifteen becomes twenty, and, eventually, you will be able to walk for prolonged periods at a comfortable pace.

Other factors, unrelated to movement, might strongly influence the shape results we experience from exercise. Evidence for this inference comes from many areas including the *Case of Exercise and Fish Oil.* The study divided obese volunteers into four groups. One group took six grams of sunflower oil every day. Another group took sunflower oil daily and was asked to walk briskly or jog for 45 minutes three times a week. A third group took six grams of fish oil every day. The last group took fish oil daily and was also asked to walk briskly or jog for 45 minutes three times a week. Twelve weeks later the researchers measured what had happened with shape. Only one group experienced a reduction in weight. The same group was the only group to deplete body fat. Which group experienced these benefits? It was the group of people who were taking fish oil and exercising. The people in this group reduced their weight by an average of about four and one half pounds and depleted almost three and one half pounds of body fat. And they did this while eating anything they wanted.

It's important to remember that Shape Intelligence is learning from and adapting to *everything* in our life. What we eat, and when we eat it, influences the shape results we get from exercising. The same is true for aspects of our lifestyle (like sleep, light exposure, and stress). The body is a complex system. Things don't occur in isolation, everything interacts, with each thing capable of influencing our responses to other things. Because of this, we absolutely don't want to make exercise into something that is doing more to add stress than it is to convince Shape Intelligence to defend a lower natural weight. Rather than forcing ourselves to participate in a dreaded aerobics class that leaves us feeling drained, it would make more sense to go for a stroll that leaves us feeling recharged.

The last thing to keep in mind is what we refer to as the *itch to move.* As we have mentioned in previous chapters, appetite seems to emerge out of nowhere when a person diets. It becomes like an itch that won't be soothed until a dieter eats more food and replenishes depleted fat stores. We have witnessed cases where an itch to move, for lack of a better description, seems to occur spontaneously. This itch won't be satisfied until movement occurs. Movement often contributes to a desire to move even more, so

---

HSI CLUE

What does the *Case of Exercise and Fish Oil* mean for you? It means that exercise and fish oil appear to help each other, and hence, help you, when it comes to positively shifting your shape. If you want to get the most shape benefits from your walking or other low intensity exercise program one thing you can do is supplement your diet with low amounts of fish oil.

beginning (and sticking with) a low intensity exercise program can contribute to this movement itch. Other things at the margins of our life—things seemingly unrelated to movement—can also have a big impact on our desire to move. A commitment to meeting our sleep needs, reducing stress, improving body clock function, or eating higher quality foods might produce this movement itch. Also be aware of times when the itch to move goes away. This can be a clue that we might not be meeting some other important need. We might need to get more sleep, exercise differently or at a different time of the day, get more daylight, or adjust some other area of our diet, lifestyle, or environment.

Closing Dialogue

Health Scene Investigator: Now that we have examined the evidence, do you have a clearer understanding of why appropriate exercise shifts our shape?

Apprentice: Yes I think I do. Exercise is one of the things Shape Intelligence considers when deciding how much fat to carry. If we are sedentary, there is no penalty for getting fatter. We carry more fat. But if we move frequently, extra fat would be a burden, so Shape Intelligence decides to carry less.

Health Scene Investigator: Very well said. Do you recall what else, besides reducing body fat and changing where the remaining body fat is located, is vital for shape?

Apprentice: Yes. The amount and distribution of our muscle is vital for our shape.

Health Scene Investigator: Your memory is excellent. Let us now discuss how exercise can be used to shift this vital area.

Chapter 18

Resistance (Weight) Training
and Shape

*Few men [referring to Holmes] were capable of greater
muscular effort, and he was undoubtedly one of the finest
boxers of his weight that I have ever seen.*

Dr. Watson

Opening Dialogue

Health Scene Investigator: I promised to begin our next discussion
with exercise's effects on the amount and distribution of our muscle.
Let's begin. Do you recall my mentioning in an earlier discussion
why the amount of muscle and its location are vital for our shape?

Apprentice: Yes, I do. I recall you saying that if we want to turn a
stone into a statue, so to speak, it often requires reducing body fat
and adding muscle.

Health Scene Investigator: Exactly so. In most cases, in order to
improve our overall shape, we must also get our muscles in shape.
Based on what you know, do you have any thoughts as to how we
accomplish this task?

Apprentice: If I understand Shape Intelligence correctly, we would
need to challenge it in ways that would cause it to think that having
bigger and more shapely muscles would be an intelligent adaptation.

Health Scene Investigator: Very well said. You have come quite a
ways in your mastery of this material. Now let us discuss how we
accomplish this task in more practical terms.

The Case for Muscular Fitness

Holmes was ahead of his time in many ways, one of which,
according to Watson, was his dedication to muscular fitness.
Muscular fitness pays big dividends. When we train our muscles in
the right types of ways, we:

- Look and feel more youthful
- Become more attractive and shapely
- Slow and even reverse parts of the aging process
- Lower our risk for diseases like heart disease, osteoporosis,
  and cancer

If any, or all, of these are things you desire, one of the surest paths
to success is training our muscles in ways that cause them to, literally
and figuratively, get in shape.

We mentioned in Chapter 8 that losing weight won't necessarily turn
a stone into a statue. It might, but it might only create a less heavy
stone. To turn a stone into a statue requires changing its shape;
sculpting, removing weight in just the right places. Changing our
shape is no different. It involves more than simply removing weight.
Our shape is influenced by how much, what type, and what
distribution of *fat* and *muscle* we have. It is also influenced by muscle
tone. If the shape of our muscles leaves a great deal to be desired,
we can lose weight and be left with a body that is still less visually
attractive than most of us desire. Calorie restriction serves as a
cautionary example. It temporarily depletes body fat reserves, but
doesn't improve the amount, location, and tone of muscles. In fact,
it has been known for decades that dieting causes us to lose muscle
tissue. When our willpower gives out and we break the diet, we
regain lost weight, but, as we discussed earlier in the book, the
weight gain is often characterized by proportionately large gains in
body fat. Phrases such as "dieting-induced adiposity" and "body fat
overshoot" describe this frequently observed phenomenon. The
result for many dieters is that, after dieting ends and the lost weight
is regained, they have not become more statuesque; they have
become more stone-like, with more fat and less muscle than before.
To get a different result we must engage in activities that create
shapelier muscles. If we create shapely muscles *and* we deplete fat,

we create a much more visually appealing body than would be created by doing just one or the other. The right approach to exercise can accomplish both of these goals. Low intensity activities, like walking, can convince Shape Intelligence to defend lower amounts of body fat. High intensity activities, like resistance training, can convince Shape Intelligence to defend less fat and to improve the amount and tone of muscles. The combination of both will, in almost all cases, do a far better job in producing an appealing shape than either would when relied on alone.

When it comes to improving the contour and definition of our muscles, the composition of our body, our overall shape, and how we feel about our shape, nothing produces the degree of improvement as quickly and reliably as high intensity exercise; especially when the activity includes resistance training. And if we want to turn back the clock on aging, countering the health declines and the unwanted shape changes that accompany the passing years, there is no better exercise investment.

High Intensity Activity and Complex Adaptive Intelligence

Complex adaptive systems, like our body, learn from and adapt to experiences we give them, demonstrate intelligence, and have good memories. We see this with activities that use quick bursts of muscle activity. There is little doubt that muscle size, shape, and distribution is internally self-regulated. We can't simply wish for big muscles and have them show up. Nor can we significantly increase the size, or change the shape of our muscles by just eating more protein (any more than we can permanently change our shape by restricting calories). Muscles only get bigger and better shaped when the body has a *reason* to have bigger or better-shaped muscles. If we provide the reason by doing the right types of exercise activities, and we allow sufficient time for the body to completely adapt, it does the rest, with the result being more shapely muscles.

A common, and as it happens incorrect way many people think about resistance training, is that our muscles get bigger and stronger *during* the time we are lifting weights. There are several reasons for this mistaken belief. One of these is that our muscles seem to get pumped up when they are used intensely. But a pumped up muscle should not be confused with a bigger and stronger muscle. A muscle is weaker after an intense workout than it was before the workout. Muscles get weaker while they are being used, not stronger. The apparent increase in size is also an illusion. It is an acute response caused by working the muscle, but it is a fleeting, not permanent response. The lasting effects from weight training aren't the temporary responses we detect during a workout; they are the ones that occur after the body has an opportunity to adapt to and recover completely from it.

HSI CLUE

To improve muscle shape, we must convince Shape Intelligence that there is a need to do so. This requires *stimulus* and *recovery*. Each bout of exercise is a challenge to our body. It is a stimulus for adaptation. The actual adaptation occurs during the recovery periods between exercise sessions. New exercisers usually do a good to great job on the exercise part. Where they often slip-up is in failing to allow enough time for recovery.

Lifting weights is a form of stress on our muscles. It tears them down. It represents a challenge. Our muscles get bigger and stronger, not because of this challenge, but in *response* to it. To understand this important distinction pause and think about taking an exam. If we haven't prepared for an exam, we aren't likely to do very well. Taking an exam without having studied doesn't make us any smarter; it just causes stress. We might make this mistake once, but most of us will learn from this experience and be better prepared *next time*. It is during our efforts to be better prepared next time, not during the exam, that we get smarter. This being better prepared next time effect is a characteristic of good students; it is also a hallmark of complex adaptive intelligence. It is during the time periods between the exercise sessions that getting smarter occurs; with getting smarter in this instance, as it is with all challenges, being a process of learning and adapting in ways that result in being better prepared just in case the challenge occurs again. This *just in case game* involves (1) figuring out what just happened, (2) making best guesses about how to be better prepared next time, and (3) adapting in ways to execute on these best guesses. This is precisely what occurs when we participate in resistance training. The end result of this game is that our body creates bigger and stronger muscles, not so much because we lifted weights a few days ago, but because complex adaptive intelligence is concerned that we might lift weights again in the future The body learned and adapted, muscles got bigger and stronger, because it's the smartest thing to do in order to be better prepared next time. While the weight training session was the stimulus that got the ball rolling, the adaptations that lead to bigger and stronger muscles occur in the recovery period after the weight training session.

In the most general sense, resistance training causes the body to adapt in ways that result in muscles getting bigger and stronger. Intricate adaptations are also occurring inside muscles. Some existing fast twitch muscle fibers get bigger, new fast twitch muscle fibers might be created, and existing muscle fibers might be converted into fast twitch muscle fibers. Tendons, cartilage and bones are remodeled to support stronger muscles that can lift heavier weights. The nervous system learns and adapts to allow us to better perform the exercise. Blood supply will be altered to better support the muscle's needs. The muscles, and everything needed to support them, reshape themselves from the inside out just in case we encounter a similar challenge again. All of the adaptations made are finely tuned depending on which muscles we use and the specific way we use them. This specificity is evident in the *Case of Eccentric and Concentric Muscle Activity*.

In exercise physiology, there is a difference between a movement that lengthens a muscle and one that shortens it. Lengthening is an *eccentric* movement. Shortening is a *concentric* one. We can do the same movement, use the same amount of weight, but we will produce different adaptations if we work the muscle as it is lengthening verse shortening. If we focus our efforts into the time when a muscle is lengthening, it will get a lot stronger in a way that allows us to better perform muscular movements that require lengthening strength. If we focus our efforts into the shortening muscle action, we get a big gain in strength tasks that require shortening the muscle. In both cases, the adaptation is specific and intelligent.

Another specific adaptation is what occurs with intermuscular fat—muscle marbling. We discussed intermuscular fat in the *Cases of Marbled Steak and Foie Gras* in Chapter 10. As general rules, marbling of muscles increases with (1) lack of use, (2) poor diet, and (3) aging.

Unless we take steps to avoid it, we marble. When science has investigated marbling of muscles, it becomes apparent, once again, how specific Shape Intelligence can be in its adaptations. This specificity is in evidence in the *Case of Disuse and Use*. A common example of disuse of a muscle, or group of muscles, is a broken bone placed in a cast.

HSI CLUE

Two groups of young women were placed on strength-training programs for nine weeks. Both groups did the same exercises, with similar amounts of weights, for the same amounts of time. One group lifted the weights in 2 seconds and lowered them in 6 seconds. The other group did the opposite, lifting for 6 seconds and lowering for 2. Better muscle fiber adaptations were detected in the latter group. Lifting weights causes muscular adaptations, but these adaptations differ depending upon *how* we lift and lower the weights.

When the cast is taken off we notice that the muscle has atrophied. But this is only part of the picture. If we had a lens that allowed us to look inside the muscle we would also observe a localized increase in marbling that is specific to the *unused* muscles. These muscles and only these muscles will have marbled. It doesn't require something as significant as a broken limb to cause muscle atrophy and marbling. All it takes is a period of disuse of a muscle, and independent of what is going on at the level of our whole body, the unused muscles will be atrophying and marbling. Use of specific muscles is the flip-side of disuse. It creates highly localized adaptations in the other direction—muscle fibers increase and marbling usually decreases.

Adaptation is highly specific. If we only challenge our lower body (leg muscles) with weight training, only these muscles will adapt by increasing size and strength (and decreasing marbling). If we get even more specific and only use one leg, while resting the other, it will only be the muscles in this leg that reshape themselves. Shape Intelligence is capable of highly intricate local regulation of muscle and fat and uses this capability when specific muscles are used or not used. It doesn't take long for these adaptations to be evident. Within a period of a few weeks to a month, muscles can dramatically reshape themselves from the inside out because of disuse or use. The shape change in different muscles we each produce over the next month to months will be dependent on whether or not, as well as how, we are using them. If we start sprinting, our body will adapt in ways that improve sprinting performance, including adaptations to the muscles used to sprint. If we swim, muscles adapt to make swimming easier, but won't necessarily adapt in ways that significantly improve sprinting. If we train with weights, the specific muscles used to lift and lower the weights will adapt, but we won't necessarily perform better sprinting or swimming. Adaptation tends to be task specific.

Complex adaptive systems have great memories when it comes to remembering past adaptations. This can be witnessed in the *Case of Muscle Memory*. Our muscles learn when they encounter a new task. Part of the learning process includes the neuromuscular system memorizing motor skills. This is evident in the process of learning to ride a bike. Many different muscle groups must learn to work together in coordinated ways so that we can peddle while keeping our balance. Fortunately for us, complex adaptive intelligence is a great learner; in no time we move from a starting place of never having ridden a bicycle to being skilled cyclists. Increasing our levels of task accuracy through repetition is one facet of muscle memory. Another facet is long-term memory. The neuromuscular system will remember how to execute previously mastered tasks for long periods of time even if we are no longer performing them. We might not have been on a bike for years, but as the cliché "it's just like riding a bike" reminds us, once we have learned to ride a bike, riding one again is simply an exercise in recall. Muscle memory allows us to ride a bike even if it has been years since our last ride. This same principle of muscle memory applies to other muscular tasks that we learned through training and repetition. But even this long-term memory might not be where muscle memory ends.

The concept of muscle memory is also used to describe a frequently observed phenomenon in weight training. When we train with weights, muscles adapt by getting bigger and stronger. When we cease weight training, this adaptation is no longer necessary, so muscles shrink (and marble). Training causes one adaptation and detraining causes another. Both make sense given what is being done or not done, respectively. Now imagine that we have two people of the same size and shape, with comparable muscle size and strength. One of these people trained with weights previously, but hasn't lifted a weight for years. In the past, when they were lifting weights, their muscles were a lot bigger and stronger than they are now. The other person has never lifted a weight. Their muscles have never been bigger and stronger than they are now. What do you think will happen over the next few months if both individuals begin and follow an identical weight-training program? Since both individuals have a similar starting point—untrained and with similar muscle size—and are doing the same thing, we might expect them to get similar results. Is this what we actually observe? Anecdotal evidence suggests the answer is often no. A common observation in weight training circles is that the person, whose muscles had been bigger and stronger in the past, will experience quicker gains in muscle size and strength. In a relatively short amount of time, they are back where they were before they stopped training. Meanwhile, the person who has never weight trained before, while doing an identical weight lifting routine, will have far more modest gains in size and strength. This observation—it seems to be much easier for our muscles to return to their previous size and strength than it was to get there the first time around—is another example of muscle memory. Complexity science informs us to expect this type of unequal response.

An assumption within complexity science is that living systems are *history dependent*. Our current responses to anything will be influenced by things we have done, or that have been done to us, in the past. Because the history of these two individuals, when it comes to weight training, isn't the same, complexity science predicts that the same thing now—weight training—might lead to different responses. History dependence prepares us to expect that the way muscles respond to current challenge will be dictated, in part, by what these muscles have experienced in the past, perhaps even the distant past. It shouldn't be a surprise that muscles, which adapted to a certain stimulus in the past, would remember when presented with the same stimulus again. As soon as this stimulus is present again, the solution to the challenge—the intelligent adaptation—is just a matter of recall.

When it comes to the size and shape of our muscles, Shape Intelligence has a great memory and is capable of highly specific adaptations. This is great news for us when it comes to altering the shape of individual muscles or the shape of our body. If we give Shape Intelligence the correct types of learning situations, allow sufficient recovery time for adaptation to occur, and provide it the resources it requires to reshape muscles, this intelligence will take care of the rest. One question then becomes, what types of learning situations convince Shape Intelligence that we need better shaped muscle?

Remembering that Shape Intelligence is constantly adapting and making new predictions about what it needs for the future, the answer is, as Holmes might say, elementary. A primary role of our skeletal muscle is to contract, which, when done in combination with our skeletal structure, produces power. In physics, power means the rate at which work is performed. If we walk at a modest pace for 30 minutes we might do a great deal of leg muscle work, but we are spreading it over a relatively long time period. We don't need powerful leg muscles to accomplish this task; we need leg muscles that have endurance, the ability to sustain work over longer amounts of time. Since endurance doesn't require lots of power, there's little reason for Shape Intelligence to make our leg muscles more powerful even if we walk every day. Intense efforts in a brief amount of time result in adaptations that favor power. Imagine doing an all out sprint for ten seconds or lifting a very heavy object six times in succession. These types of efforts require a great deal of muscle power—high amounts of work squeezed into a brief time. When we consistently challenge our body with these types of high intensity, brief duration efforts, it adapts. The result of this adaptation is muscles that are better prepared—bigger and stronger—to complete the task the next time it's encountered. In a sense we are convincing Shape Intelligence that its future predictions better include an ability to do tasks that require high amounts of muscle power. It does the rest and reshapes our muscles. As it happens, more powerful muscles are usually more shapely, having better size, tone, and definition.

HSI CLUE

If we use our muscles to perform endurance or aerobic exercises, they adapt in completely different manners than if we train with weights. These differences in adaptation are seen in the obvious (muscle size, shape, coordination, and sport-specific performance) and the less obvious (fiber types, muscular metabolism, energy sources used, and the degree of marbling,). Running a long distance and lifting a heavy weight are vastly different activities. They require different adaptive strategies. And, as a result, they produce vastly different shapes.

A Study in Resistance (Weight) Training

While high intensity activity includes a variety of exercise types, the most studied type is *resistance training*. In the context it is being used in this chapter, resistance training means any exercise done using some form of resistance, whether free weight or machine, that opposes muscle contraction (strength training and weight training are synonymous). Resistance training has been studied in people whose ages range from children to the elderly, in both males and females, and in persons of different shapes and weights. Irrespective of age, sex or starting body shape and weight, it consistently produces exceptional shape results.

<table>
<tr><td>

HSI CLUE

Resistance training is the most reliable way to shape and tone muscle tissue. It is also the most reliable way to change the way we feel about our shape. But estimates suggest that only one in five of us regularly engage in resistance training. Many people, especially women, choose to do other types of exercise that offer less in both of these areas. As a result they do not re-shape their bodies, or their satisfaction with it, to the degree they desire, despite spending ample time exercising.

</td><td>

The shape benefits of resistance training cannot be judged by weight changes measured on a scale. As discussed in Chapters 8, 9, and 10, weight is an incidental fact. Shape, body composition, and fat types and distribution patterns are vital. The same is true when it comes to muscle distribution and tone; they are more vital clues. This is evident when we review the clues left by resistance training. There are cases in which individuals reduce their weight significantly. There are also cases in which weight will remain relatively unchanged, or even increase, but shape will have changed dramatically for the better. When we participate in resistance training, Shape Intelligence almost always decides to add muscle while it is depleting body fat. Some of the fat being depleted is visible; much of it is invisible to the naked eye (marbling, liver and internal belly fat). If Shape Intelligence adds muscle at roughly the same rate that it's depleting fat, weight will stay about the same, despite the fact that we are figuratively sculpting ourselves into a statue from the inside out. Resistance training also tones our muscles; it creates contour and definition. These appealing changes are invisible on a scale, but become readily apparent when we observe ourselves in a mirror or when friends or family observe the way our body is changing.

</td></tr>
</table>

Shape Intelligence typically decides to defend less body fat in people of all sizes, shapes and weights when they participate in resistance training. This occurs without a need to restrict calories or food intake and is true whether someone's weight would be currently judged as low, normal, overweight, or obese. Shape Intelligence usually redistributes some of the remaining fat. The result of this redistribution is that we tend to make shape improvements in the specific areas many of us view as problem areas. In men and post-menopausal women, this is often the area around the waist and trunk. In younger women it might be the area around the thighs and hips. The types of changes that occur with resistance training— depleting fat from these areas while toning and shaping the underlying muscles—make it among the most reliable methods for improving our satisfaction with how these areas, and our entire body, look. Research observations indicate that, as a general rule, exercise will improve self-esteem and body satisfaction. But of all types of exercise studied, resistance training is clearly the most effective for delivering the goods in these important areas. The *Cases of Body Image Satisfaction* illustrates this point.

In the first case, women in their mid-40s participated in either a fifteen-week weight training or walking program. Weight training did a better job increasing muscle size and strength. Walking did a better job in building endurance. Both programs depleted body fat. But only the women who trained with weights *felt* significantly better about how they looked. In the second case, college-aged men and women participated in a six-week weight-training program. In stark contrast to subjects who did not participate, these young men and women thought their bodies had become significantly more appealing and became much more satisfied with how they looked. We might lose weight, improve our shape, or both, but if what we accomplish does not also change how we *feel* about how we look, we have, in our own realities, gained little.

The last important thing about resistance training is the relative speed with which the body responds to it. Within weeks after starting a resistance exercise program, muscles will have already started to significantly remodel themselves in their attempts to adapt to the unique type of challenge this type of exercise presents. Weight training done in a just right way, with a time commitment of as little as twenty minutes, once a week, can produce noticeable changes in how we look within a few months. In comparison, low intensity and medium intensity (aerobic) activities almost always take a greater daily time commitment, more days a week of participation, and a more prolonged duration of following the program before shape changes become obvious.

While low and medium intensity activities are important and can be useful for depleting fat, decades of evidence indicates that they are not nearly as valuable in building and toning muscles; for giving our body the *shape appeal* we want. They also are less likely to significantly alter the way we feel about the way we look. And neither typically produces the shifts in our shape as quickly as we will experience when we participate in resistance training or other high intensity activities.

A Study in Start-Stop Exercise

When it comes to exercise, less might be more, and bursts of high intensity activity followed by complete rest or light activity, might be better than steady-state continuous activity. An example of evidence leading to this inference was mentioned in Chapter 17—the *Case of Varying Our Pace*. Varying our pace while walking, produced greater fitness and health benefits than walking for greater durations of time at a constant pace. We also mentioned that long ambling strolls punctuated by brief sprints would be another way to approach exercise.

HSI CLUE

Whole body vibration uses a specialized platform that sends mild vibratory impulses through whatever is in contact with the platform (feet, hands, etc.) and into the rest of the body. When resistance exercises are done on this platform, the resistance exercise and the vibration challenge the body. Shape Intelligence has to adapt to both. Evidence suggests that adapting to both might result in better overall shape changes than might be experienced by resistance exercise on its own.

These are examples of what might be considered *naturalistic* activity, something more analogous to what human hunter-gatherer ancestors experienced, how children tend to play, and how animals in the wild generally move. When we watch young children play outside, many of their games and social interactions are characterized by brief bursts of activity followed by relative rest. Duck, duck goose is an example. A child will go from being motionless to moving all out for a short burst and then back to being motionless. This start-stop pattern of movement will repeat over and over again. We see a similar dynamic in nature. In the animal kingdom, while it is common to see animals engage in start-stop activities, we would be hard pressed to find animals that did the equivalent of human jogging. We might see a hare sprinting but we would never see it out for an afternoon jog. We have been conditioned to believe that to count as exercise we need to move continuously for thirty to sixty minutes at a time. But what if this idea were wrong? What if, just like with children and animals, adult bodies were meant for explosive bursts of movement followed by relative rest? What would happen if we actually trained this way? A growing body of evidence is answering this last question.

In June of 2005, *Science Daily* had a press release titled "A Few 30 Second Sprints As Beneficial As Hour Long Jog". They were reporting on results of a study that found that as little as six minutes a week of time spent doing high intensity bursts of activity could be as effective as an hour of daily moderate continuous exercise for improving aspects of fitness. The training program consisted of between four and seven 30-second bursts of all out cycling with each burst followed by four minutes of recovery. This start-stop, high intensity-exercise protocol was done three times a week. In this study, an exercise session lasted between 14 to 28 minutes (depending on how many repetitions of the all out cycling were done in a session) but almost all of this time was spent *recovering* from the bout of high intensity sprint-like activity. The total time spent in exertion was as little as two minutes and no more than three and a half minutes.

In May 2007, *The New York Times* had an article titled "A Healthy Mix of Rest and Motion", which also supported the benefits of start-stop activity. While commenting on the same research from the above press release, this article also goes on to comment about a newer research study that appeared in the *Journal of Applied Physiology* in 2007. Eight women in their early 20s did ten sets of four minutes of hard cycling with each set followed by two minutes of rest. Over two weeks, they completed seven of these interval workouts. Bursts of hard exercise, followed by rest, not only improved cardiovascular fitness but also the body's tendency to use fat for energy needs.

Other studies of start-stop approaches to high intensity exercise have observed positive changes in fitness and aspects of health. These improvements include:
- Increased cardiovascular fitness
- Improvements in blood pressure
- Improved blood sugar regulation
- Improved insulin sensitivity
- Better moods

HSI CLUE

Men sprinted for 30 seconds, rested for 4 minutes, and then repeated this cycle 3 to 5 more times. It took 17 to 26 minutes to finish a session, but only 2 to 3 minutes of this time was spent in exertion. Blood sugar and insulin levels improved significantly after only 6 session of this start-stop exercise program. How do we account for such a positive change with so little actual exercise? What other changes might occur if we incorporated sprint-type start-stop activities into our life regularly?

Start-stop high intensity exercise is one of, if not the most time-efficient type of exercise activity. With a time commitment of as little as 14 minutes, four sprint-type bursts can be completed with four-minute rest breaks between each. Seven pulses of exertion-rest can be completed in less than 30 minutes. This type of activity doesn't require much in terms of specialized equipment. While we could do the burst of activity on an exercise bike or using a jump rope, we could also find an open space outside or some stairs (inside or outside) and use these as our opportunity to do a sprint-like burst of activity. If you decide to experiment with start-stop activity we recommend the following:

- Keep the exertion phase short (10 to 30 seconds) but go all out during it.
- Make sure the rest phase is long enough to fully recover (two minutes is the bare minimum and up to four is often better).
- During the rest phase feel free to sit down or lie down. The goal is to rest and recover for the next burst of activity.
- For people who are already physically fit a target range of four to seven pulses of exertion-rest are recommended. More is not necessarily better so unless you are training for a particular task or event, we recommend keeping to a maximum of seven pulses.
- For people who are not in "sprint" shape, be gentle on yourself. Overdoing things at the beginning is a recipe for injury. While you are working yourself into sprint shape, take a more measured approach (don't go all out), do fewer pulses (even one or two is a good start), and feel free to take more rest time between pulses.
- Don't overdo things. The more intense the activity, the more recovery time we need for the body to completely recover from it. Integrating some start-stop activity, even once a week, into an overall activity program is a good start.

Remember it is not the type of activity that will determine whether it is high intensity; it is how we do it. In order to get the best response, we need to really go for it during the brief bursts of exertion. We need to be like a cheetah bursting after its prey and then we need to come back to a more resting physiology before we go all out again. A few repetitions of starting and stopping, with enough rest between bursts, can be a springboard for rejuvenating our health.

What to Do and How to Do It

Resistance training is the preferred stimulus for challenging the body in ways that lead to muscular reshaping. Sprinting, jumping rope, climbing stairs, doing push-ups and pull-ups, or doing some other burst-like activity are other ways to approach high intensity activity. In our experience, these are all excellent options; however, because adaptation is highly specific, the best whole body shape results occur when *all* of the body's muscles are involved. If we only sprint, the muscles used to perform this movement will adapt to perform better, becoming shapelier as they do, but uninvolved muscles won't. Whether we decide to use resistance training or another form of high intensity exercise, we want to involve all major muscles. In resistance training this can be accomplished by doing three of more complex exercises that involve leg muscles, upper body pulling muscles, and upper body pushing muscles. If we weren't using resistance training, doing sprints, pull-ups, and push-ups would be a way to involve most major muscles.

There are several reasons why we have a preference for resistance training. The most important is that it lends itself perfectly to progressively challenging the body. Muscles get bigger, stronger, and better toned because some stimulus gives Shape Intelligence a reason to believe that these are intelligent adaptations. If we were to lift the same amount of weight, in the same ways, week after week, at some point the body will have completely adapted to this challenge. Since the challenge isn't getting more difficult, there will be no need for further adaptations. We will reach a plateau in performance and in terms of shape changes. In order to make continued progress at this point, we need to do something to make things a bit more challenging. This can be accomplished by (1) altering an existing routine to one that our body is unaccustomed to, (2) following a similar routine but progressively working a bit harder during each subsequent exercise session, or (3) combining elements of both of the above. Resistance training is perfectly suited to provide an ever-evolving challenge. Every six to eight weeks, we can alter our routine by varying the types of exercise we do, the machines we use, or the emphasis we place on our muscles. We can progressively work harder by adding a bit more weight, doing one more repetition, or working the muscle for a slightly longer amount of time. Progressive adaptation requires progressively challenging the body in new or more demanding ways.

There are three areas that should be the focus when beginning a new exercise program. These are safety, correct form, and providing the *minimum* stimulus needed for adaptation to occur. Injuries are more likely to occur (1) when initiating a high intensity program, and (2) if the activity is performed incorrectly. The first few resistance training sessions should focus on building the foundation for future gains, not on trying to get years worth of gains within a few weeks. There is a very real tendency, both on the part of the exerciser and many personal trainers, to overdo things in the beginning. This is a mistake. It increases the chance of injury. And if we are still trying to do more repetitions after muscles are already fatigued, we tend to cheat, recruiting other muscles to help with the effort. Form breaks down and poor habits can be created that will persist. The goal is to provide the body a safe and effective challenge that will result in it adapting. When we are new to any form of exercise it takes very little to accomplish this goal. Overdoing things is a form of trauma and trauma is stress. For those new to high intensity exercise we recommend taking it easy at the beginning and progressively working a bit harder only *after* your muscles have had a few weeks to habituate and adapt to the movements. The initial focus should be almost entirely on doing the movement correctly while maintaining the proper posture. After this acclimation period, once the neuromuscular adaptations have been made through repetition, the intensity can be gradually increased. The important thing at the beginning is keeping within the limits of your current capabilities, not trying to keep pace with someone who has been doing resistance training for many months or years. As you adapt, your capabilities will gradually increase, and you can safely do more.

There are many variations on resistance training. One could train with free weights, machines, or both. There are dozens and dozens of different types of exercise movements. A few repetitions of a movement can be done using heavier weights, or more repetitions can be done with lighter weights. Multiple sets can be done in sequence, progressively adding weight, or one set can be done to muscular failure. Resistance exercise can be done several times a week, or just once weekly. In a sense, resistance training is like a menu at a restaurant. These are many options to choose from, and everyone isn't in agreement on which one is the best. Some people prefer one thing, others like something very different. This can make it a bit disconcerting for beginners. Who should they listen to and what advice should they follow?

When trying to answer this question keep in mind the concepts of complex individuality and complex adaptive intelligence. It's highly unlikely that there is any one right way that is perfect for everyone, and what is right today might no longer be six months from now. We don't need to get too bogged down in trying to figure out which advice is the best for us when beginning to resistance train, because almost anything we do will produce gains when we encounter a novel challenge. Whether a lot is done, or a little, no matter how we do it, progress tends to come relatively easily at the beginning. With that in mind, there are a few useful principles worth committing to memory. One of these is that, at any given point in time, there is going to be a *minimum* amount of stimulus needed to trigger adaptation. We don't get more adaptation by doing more than this amount. Adaptation is a form of learning. There are limits to how much we can learn in one setting. If we continue to force feed ourselves information past this cut-off point,

> **HSI CLUE**
>
> If we settle into a routine where we do not progressively challenge ourselves to work a bit differently or harder each week, there is little reason for Shape Intelligence to continually add incrementally to the size, strength, or tone of our muscles. We need to be progressively challenging ourselves, if we want the adaptation process to be ongoing.

we don't continue to learn, we become saturated, or even worse, confused and stressed. How much we can learn in any one lesson is finite. Resistance training is a form of learning for muscles. Each time we exercise is a lesson. The goal is to keep lessons manageable, performing the minimum amount needed to trigger adaptation. If we do much less than this amount, little to no adaptation will occur. If we do more, entirely new problems emerge. Efforts put into resistance exercise after we have exceeded this minimum adaptive threshold, (1) waste time, (2) increase the risk of injury, and (3) in some instances can be counter-productive. More isn't always better; sometimes it's just more—more time, more wasted efforts, and more risk for injury.

Adaptations that lead to stronger muscles occur because muscles are used in ways that significantly weaken them, temporarily. If we were to do a leg press ten times against sufficient resistance, we will get to a point where we can no longer lift it. The muscles involved will have been worked to exhaustion and will be much weaker now than they were before performing leg presses. Feeling too weak to complete a task is a tremendous stimulus for adaptation. In response to it, complex adaptive intelligence will take steps to ensure that more can be done next time. So, the goal is to perform resistance exercise activities in ways that work a muscle to the point where the weight can no longer be moved. Once we have gotten to this point, we are done. There is no need to rest for a few minutes and then do another set. The goal isn't to profoundly weaken a muscle multiple times during a resistance exercise session; it is to significantly weaken it once. Significant weakening doesn't occur by simply moving a weight from point A to point B; it occurs because of how the weight is moved.

The general rule of thumb, when it comes to anything, including exercise, is that intensity is inversely proportional to duration. The higher the intensity, the quicker it will produce both adaptation *and* trauma. The bigger the stress, the less time we can be exposed to it before experiencing a stress-related breakdown. Mid-day summer sun exposure will cause sunburn far faster than late afternoon sun. With exercise, the application of this principle is that the greater the effort we put into a specific resistance training exercise, such as a leg press with heavier weights, the less time we *can* do it, and the less time we *need* to do it to trigger adaptation. One of the best ways to increase the intensity is to put a muscle under a continuous load with higher weight for brief periods of time. The key points to remember are (1) heavier, (2) slower, and (3) constant effort. Doing resistance exercise, while applying these three points, will get muscles to the point of failure quickly.

Traditionally, resistance training has followed a formula similar to the following. Sufficient resistance is used so that the person is able to complete three sets each consisting of eight to ten repetitions. Rather than rapidly lifting and lowering, and using momentum to help with subsequent lifts, the resistance is lifted for two seconds and lowered for four seconds. There is no magic to this formula. It is a useful approach but not necessarily the best approach. And its most important element is its emphasis on both *lifting* and *lowering* the weight using a six-second *time under load* (also called *time under tension*). The newest evidence indicates that time under load, not the number of repetitions or number of sets, is the critical variable for working a muscle to the point of complete exhaustion—the trigger for adaptation.

Time under load is the amount of time the muscle is actively working against the resistance. If ten repetitions were done against sufficient resistance, and the weight was lifted and lowered rapidly (one second for each movement), the total time under load would be twenty seconds. If the weights were lifted for two seconds and lowered for four seconds, time under load would be 60 seconds. Fatiguing the specific muscle fibers required for the most positive muscular shape adaptations requires a time under load of somewhere in the range of 45 to 90 seconds. The emphasis should not be on the number of repetitions and number of sets, it should be on working the muscle from the start in a way that puts it under *immediate* load and keeps it under *constant tension* for the entire duration of the specific resistance exercise. This entails using heavier weights and moving them *slowly* while lifting them *and* lowering them. This slow cadence lifting and lowering produces more muscular fatigue in much less time. Studies also indicate that controlled slow lifting and lowering is safe (even for elderly individuals) and effective (producing toned and bigger muscles quickly). One set done in this way will take less than 90 seconds to complete and can replace multiple sets, which typically have several minutes of rest between each.

> **H S I   C L U E**
>
> A single bout of resistance exercise measurably increased metabolic rate for the next two days. Studies have shown lasting increases in metabolic rate with consistent resistance exercise. The metabolic benefits of resistance training aren't limited to the time spent training; they are a lasting gift because of the adaptations the body makes to this challenge.

An ideal exercise program will include some form of resistance training. The training will be done in a way that is safe and time efficient. Sufficient weight will be used to allow the source of resistance to be moved slowly for between 45 to 90 seconds. If the weight is too heavy, exhaustion will arrive too quickly, and at the next exercise session, weight should be removed. If the muscles aren't fatigued by 90 seconds, the resistance is too light, and more resistance should be added the next session. The emphasis during each exercise is on working the muscles through the entirety of the movements; it is on the *process* of the lifting and lowering, not on the amount of weight or the number of repetitions.

The Importance of Recovery

The goal of resistance training is to provide the stimulus for adaptation. Once a muscle has been significantly weakened, by working it to the point of fatigue, this stimulus has been created. There is no need to continue to work the muscle. Nor is there a need to work it again until Shape Intelligence has been given a chance to completely learn from, and adapt to this stimulus. Resistance training is a challenge; it is a form of stress. If a muscle is worked to the point of fatigue, significant trauma occurs on the inside. Healing from this trauma takes time. Rebuilding the muscle so that it will be more capable *next time* can take even more time. During this recovery period, a muscle shouldn't be re-traumatized or placed under high stress again. Rest is the priority.

As mentioned earlier in the chapter, the downfall of many people when it comes to resistance training isn't lack of effort; it's inattention to recovery. If we don't allow sufficient time for the adaptive processes to be fully complete, we end up short-changing ourselves, running in place so to speak. We might put in tremendous efforts, but we won't gain as much from them as we would if we allowed more recovery time. The more intense something is, the more time is required for recovery from it. If we go for a gentle stroll for an hour, we might be fully recovered and ready for another stroll the next day. If we perform an intense resistance exercise session, not only won't we be completely recovered the next day, we might not be fully recovered until next week. The more intensely the muscles are made to contract, the more trauma takes place at a cellular level and the longer the amount of time it will take to heal. If you can still detect any muscle soreness or fatigue in a group of muscles from your last workout, it's too soon to work out these muscles again. A good general rule of thumb is, if you have worked

---

HSI CLUE

Several popular books in the past six years focus on slow cadence resistance training: *Body by Science* by Little and McDuff, *The 12 Second Sequence* by Jorge Cruise, *The Power of 10* by Zickerman and Schley, and *The Slow Burn Fitness Revolution* by Hahn, Eades, and Eades. While these books don't agree on all points, they do agree that workouts should be kept brief, weights should be lifted and lowered slowly, and that there should be plenty of recovery time between workouts.

muscles to point of failure, allow one full week for them to fully recover before challenging them in an intense manner again.

Solution: The Program

There are four core elements to designing an efficient resistance-training program:

- Selecting exercises that will engage all major muscle groups.
- Using enough weight so that lifting and lowering movements, when done in a slow and controlled manner, will result in muscle failure in 45 to 90 seconds.
- Lifting and lowering the resistance with sustained focus and effort throughout the entire time engaged in the specific exercise (no pauses, rests or locking out of the joint between repetitions).
- Allowing sufficient recovery time before the muscles are challenged in a similar manner again.

Our suggested approach to the above is as follows. We recommend that beginners use machines instead of free weights. Nautilus® and MedX are based on the work of Arthur Jones. These machines have had the most extensive scientific testing, are designed to match the body's biomechanics, maintain more even resistance throughout the entire motion, and allow for safe and effective movements. Other machines, such as Hammer Strength, are good options should these machines be unavailable. The goal in the beginning is to choose a few foundational exercises that each works multiple muscle groups. In the book *Body By Science: A Research Based Program to Get the Results You Want in 12 Minutes a Week,* authors John Little and Doug McGuff, M.D., recommend what they refer to as the Big 3—leg press, pulldown, and chest press. Each of these movements is a compound movement, exercising multiple muscle groups. When all three are done properly, all major muscle groups in the body are worked. These authors also suggest that adding an overhead press and a seated row form a Big 5 of resistance exercises. They recommended working out once a week, doing three to five of these foundational exercises till muscle failure during this one workout, and then allowing one week to fully adapt. This is a far more streamlined program than most gyms, personal trainers, or muscle magazines typically recommend. We highly recommend reading this excellent book to find more information on why they prefer these exercises, as well as details on how to perform them.

Video instructions for completing these exercises can be found on our website. In our experience, a streamlined program like they describe is safe, effective, and takes a minimum amount of time, all of which are important considerations for beginners. Our recommendation is to spend the first six to eight weeks focusing on learning to do these few exercises correctly.

When doing these resistance exercises, or any others that you choose to do, we recommend focusing your efforts on completing the movements in as slow a manner as you can comfortably execute. A good starting place is to lift for four to six seconds and lower for four to six seconds, matching breathing to this cadence. Lift and lower as many times as you are able for a total of 45 to 90 seconds. The amount of resistance selected should be sufficient to produce muscle failure—an inability to lift the weight one more time after the last lowering—in less than one and one half minutes of slow controlled lifting and lowering. Finding this just right amount of weight is often a process of trial and error. We advise clients to start with less than they think they can lift in this manner, working up if needed. Do each exercise one time. Rest 30 to 60 seconds as you move to and adjust the next machine. Now complete the next resistance exercise. After completing the last of these three to five foundational exercises its time to go home and recover until next week. The total amount of time spent lifting and lowering against resistance will be between two and one half to seven and one half minutes. The total amount of time spent in the gym can be as little as fifteen minutes. Next time add a bit more weight, lift and lower for a bit more time, or both.

Over time, as your body adapts to these exercises, they may cease to be as challenging. Gains may slow or plateau. This is a normal facet of complex adaptation. We need progressive challenges to stimulate positive adaptations. We also need variety. Spending a bit more time dedicated to recovery or taking a week off is one way to introduce variety. Adding or dropping exercises is another way. Performing the exercises differently, which might consist of simply using a different type of machine, is a third way. As your muscles become bigger and stronger, finding new ways to challenge them to grow is a bit of a problem, but there are many solutions to this problem. This is a problem that only occurs over time, so this is a good problem to have. It means you have been sticking with the program, and by the time this problem occurs, you will have noticed significant changes in your shape. Little and McDuff offer some of the best solutions to this problem that we are aware of in *Body By Science*.

The last piece of advice we have for you is to *track your progress*. Convincing Shape Intelligence to build bigger and stronger muscles requires creating progressively more demanding challenges. We do this by adding more weight, spending more time under load, or finding other ways to give it something more challenging. While we could trust our memory for this, we haven't found this to be a particularly effective strategy. Writing down precisely what we do in each exercise session is far more reliable. The best results we have individually experienced, as well as the best results we have seen with clients we have coached, have occurred when a written record is being kept of resistance training workouts. A sample form for tracking your progress is available as a PDF on our website and can be printed and used for your workouts.

While climbing stairs rapidly for brief periods of time, sprinting, or jumping rope are great forms of high intensity activity, we encourage people to do at least some type of resistance training exercises even if they are doing these other pulsed high intensity exercises. We also want to remind you of the importance of frequent movement: Find more opportunities to walk and move in low intensity ways. High intensity activities don't replace frequent low intensity movement; they synergize with it.

Closing Dialogue

Health Scene Investigator: In response to my question about how we might go about getting muscles in shape, you answered that we would need to convince Shape Intelligence that having more shapely muscles is necessary. Do you have a better understanding of how we can do this convincing?

Apprentice: Yes, I do. Progressively challenging Shape Intelligence with resistance types of exercises would be one way to convince it to adapt in ways that produce more shapely muscles.

Health Scene Investigator: Well said. Now let's turn our attention to another important area—what we eat.

Chapter 19

Cases of Diet-Induced Fatness and Leanness

We must look for consistency. Where there is want of it we must suspect deception.

Sherlock Holmes

Opening Dialogue

Health Scene Investigator: Food is an important element when it comes to shape. Why?

Apprentice: Prior to our investigation, I was certain about many things, almost all of which are, as it turns out, wrong. Calories were one of these things. I was sure that people got fat because they ate too many of them. Now I'm not only unsure of whether this is the case, but I am fairly confident that there will be far more to the story than I had previously believed.

Health Scene Investigator: Well said. Most people presume that when it comes to food, the important factor is "how much". But is this an *obvious fact* or an actual fact? Is it a case of *theorizing in advance of the evidence* or does the evidence support this presumption?

Apprentice: Is this your way of hinting that I should approach this topic with a *blank mind*?

Health Scene Investigator: Precisely so. It is a tremendous advantage. With this mindset we are free to observe the clues and to draw inferences from them. Let's proceed.

Inconsistencies and Deceptions

When it comes to shape, one area fraught with a great deal of inconsistency is what we are advised to eat. Some experts tell us that a calorie is a calorie. In terms of the contribution food makes to shape, the thing that matters is how many of them we eat; their source is irrelevant. Other experts inform us that it's not simply a matter of calories; it's the type of calories. One diet might tell us to avoid calories from fats and eat carbohydrates. Another informs us we should avoid carbohydrates and eat fats. This advice is mutually exclusive; it is inconsistent. Yet diets based on these two conflicting premises have cycled in and out of popularity for decades. There are disagreements over specific ingredients. Some experts tell us we should eat according to the glycemic index of a food (a ranking of the effect a food has on blood sugar). This theory leads to advice to use fructose instead of sugar as a sweetener because fructose has a lower glycemic score. Other experts assure us that fructose is more fattening than sugar. There are disagreements on specific foods. A baked potato scores poorly on a glycemic index. According to the satiety index (a rating of how well or poorly foods keep us feeling full and satisfied), baked potatoes are one of the better foods we can eat because they keep us feeling full far longer than do most other sources of carbohydrates. One theory advises us to avoid baked potatoes and another to eat them.

There's inconsistency in dietary advice. There's also inconsistency in what we have been eating that has roughly paralleled the expansion of our waistlines. In 1890, the principle fats we ate were, in descending order of market share, lard, beef fat, chicken fat, butter, olive oil, and *unrefined* tropical oils (coconut and palm). By 1990, these "old fats" had been replaced by soybean oil, canola oil, cottonseed oil, peanut oil, corn oil, and *refined* tropical oils. The source of fat is not where the inconsistency ends. In 1890, fats were essentially unprocessed. The vegetable oils that are the primary source of calories from fats in the food supply today can be heated, solvent extracted, degummed, bleached, deodorized, refined, hydrogenated, fractionated, and/or interesterified.

Fats and oils are not the only dietary shift that has coincided with bigger waistlines. According to the latest *USDA Dietary Assessment of Major Trends in U.S. Food Consumption report* our consumption of high fructose corn syrup changed to a far greater extent than any other food or food group during the 25-year period from 1970 to 2005; increasing a staggering 10,673 percent (consumption of table sugar declined by 38 percent during the same time period). Estimates suggest that an average person consumes 40 to 59 pounds of high fructose corn syrup each year. Prior to 1967, we didn't eat any.

New oils and sweeteners are two of many big changes in our food supply. Processed foods contain many ingredients that humans never ate—artificial (non-caloric) sweeteners, fat substitutes, texture enhancers, flavor enhancers, flavoring agents, preservatives, and food colorings. Food production methods have also changed dramatically over the past century. Issues including genetic modification, food irradiation, chemical-intensive agriculture, the presence of antibiotic, chemical, and hormone residues in foods, and more, are new issues. When shape and food are studied thoughtfully we find inconsistencies in how we are told food effects shape, inconsistencies in what we are told to do, and inconsistencies in what we are eating today compared with what leaner generations consumed. There is a strong cultural and medical bias that seeks to explain body fatness as primarily a consequence of how much is eaten. How much we eat is treated as if it occurs in a vacuum, unrelated to anything else. But in complex systems, everything is interrelated. There is little doubt that food has a powerful effect on shape. But does it influence shape because of how much of it we eat, or are there other less obvious reasons?

Can Food Alter Natural Weight?
We have made a case for the defense of specific amounts and locations of body fat and muscle. These variables are constantly being intelligently adjusted based on how our unique genetics interact with the lifestyles we lead and the environments we live in.

HSI CLUE
If the source of the calorie does not matter, we should be able to eat any two foods with an equal amount of calories and get identical shape responses. Do we? As Holmes teaches us in *The Sign of Four*, exceptions disprove the rule. If we can find instances where the same amount of calories from different sources produces different shape results, we can, in principal, falsify this theory. As you will discover in this chapter, coming up with these instances is elementary.

They are not a fixed amount; they're changeable. They vary in an intelligent manner. While we are not the ones in charge of directly changing them, specific changes in aspects of lifestyle or the environment will cause amounts and locations of fat and muscle to be adjusted for us. The same is true for diet; specific ingredients and foods influence natural weight. Adding or subtracting items from the diet changes the shape being defended.

HSI CLUE

One might think that if Peck dieted the fat rats down to their pre-vegetable shortening weight, they would be content at this "normal" weight. After all, this weight was "normal" for them in the past. This was not the case. They acted as if they were starving when they were dieted down to their old weight. Having weighed some amount in the past does not make this weight our current natural weight. Natural weight isn't what we once weighed; it is the weight Shape Intelligence is *currently* defending.

Jeffrey W. Peck, in the *Case of Peck's Rats,* instead of focusing solely on *how much* was being eaten, hypothesized that natural weight might be influenced by *what* is being eaten. He fed one group of rats standard rat chow mixed with hydrogenated vegetable oil (vegetable shortening). These rats got fatter. The next group received the usual fare for rats. Their weights remained normal. He added quinine to the rat chow of the third group. These rats became somewhat lighter than normal. After a brief period on these diets the rats stabilized at their new weights. When compared to a standard rat chow diet, adding hydrogenated vegetable oil increased weight. Adding quinine decreased it. An increase or decrease in weight is an important finding, but the key aspect in identifying whether something has changed natural weight is a *defense* of the change. After Peck succeeded in altering the weights of his rats, he tested whether the new weights were defended.

Peck manipulated aspects of the diet and environment to observe whether his animals held to their new weights or reverted to their previous (pre-hydrogenated vegetable oil or quinine) weights. When he gave the rats less food than they would eat left to their own devices, all of Peck's animals clearly behaved as though they were starving. It did not matter if he dieted thin (quinine fed), normal weight (standard rat chow), or fat rats (hydrogenated vegetable oil fed); they all pushed back against losing weight. He replaced large amounts of food with eggnog. He made alterations to the environment. He tried many ways to test what weight they defended. No matter what variable he manipulated, the rats responded by eating the precise amount of food needed to defend their new natural weights. He had succeeded in increasing natural weight by adding vegetable shortening to the diet and decreasing it by adding quinine. He then decided to try and change things back. Peck placed the fat and thin rats back on standard rat chow diets. Over time, both the heavier and lighter rats reverted to, and defended, weights typical of rats that had been eating standard rat chow all along.

Peck's work illustrates a key lesson. Hunger, food intake, and ultimately shape are not based on some arbitrary notion of "normal" scale weight. This was the case even when this "normal" weight was the rats old scale weight. It was based upon whether the rats were, from the perspective of their Shape Intelligence, at or below the weight that was being defended; a natural weight that thanks to the addition of vegetable shortening to the diet, was much higher. In Peck's experiment, vegetable shortening increased natural weight. Quinine decreased it. An unbiased investigation into food and shape reveals similar cases; where adding specific ingredients into the diet changes natural weight. The *Case of the Fat Sand Rat* indicates that dropping a habitual food out of the diet can also shift natural weight.

Psammomys obesus (Sand Rat) is a mammal from the gerbil subfamily. It is found in desert environments in North Africa and the Middle East. In their natural habitat sand rats eat large quantities of a plant called saltbush and remain lean. In lab environments, when fed standard rat chow, they become obese. When saltbush is added to a lab chow diet, body fatness decrease in direct proportion to the amount added. Something about dropping saltbush from the diet of sand rats is fattening. Eating large quantities of it is slimming. Dropping saltbush from the diet of a sand rat is as detrimental to their shape as adding vegetable shortening was to the shape of Peck's rats. What sand rats eat influences how much they eat, and ultimately, the shape they defend.

Are All Calories the Same? Cases of Fats and Oils

It seems obvious that we'll get fat if we eat fat. It's easy to imagine that if we eat the visible fat that was stored on an animal, it will wind up in the same place on us. It's also common knowledge that, gram-for-gram, fat has more calories than carbohydrates or protein. It follows logically that something with more calories should cause greater weight gain. It seems equally sensible that if we eat less fat that shape should improve in direct proportion. Could this be a case of being misled by an *obvious fact*, oversimplifying a complex issue?

HSI CLUE

In 1930 average per person butter and margarine intake in the U.S. was about 18 lbs and 2 lbs, respectively. By the end of the 20th century, these averages had flip-flopped. We were eating far less butter (about 4 pounds yearly) and much more margarine (about 8 pounds yearly). Up until recently, hard margarines were 25 to 45 percent trans fats. The swap of butter for margarine resulted in big societal increases in trans fats. Stick with what humans have eaten for centuries. Be suspicious of new food science inventions.

Are all fats and oils equal when it comes to the affects they have on shape? In Chapter 10 an HSI clue mentioned research where rats were fed diets containing similar amounts of calories for six months. Some rats were fed lard, others corn oil, and still others fish oil. At no time during these six months did the weights of the rats fed different types of fats differ, but shapes and body compositions did: Fish oil resulted in less total and visceral fat than did lard or corn oil. This is not the only instance we have mentioned where the type of oil consumed produced different shape responses. In the *Case of Exercise and Fish Oil* (Chapter 17) two groups of obese individuals exercised and added an equal amount of oil to their diets. One group took six grams of sunflower oil every day and was asked to walk briskly or jog for 45 minutes three times a week. Another group was asked to follow an identical exercise program but took six grams of fish oil daily. Persons in both groups were allowed to eat anything else they wanted. In theory, if the only thing that matters is the amount of calories, not the source of those calories, the expected results should have been identical whether sunflower or fish oil was the source of the added fat calories. These theoretical results were not what were observed. Persons in the fish oil and exercise group reduced their weight by an average of 4.4 pounds and depleted 3.5 pounds of fat. There was no improvement in weight or loss of fat in the persons who exercised and added a similar number of calories as sunflower oil. This isn't an isolated case; other types of fat can have shape effects that are not predicted by caloric content alone.

Partially hydrogenated vegetable oils eventually displaced fats like butter and lard in food applications, most notably in the fast food, snack food, fried food and baked goods industries. The end result has been a big increase in our intake of trans-fats. In 2003 the United States Food and Drug Administration (FDA) estimated that the average American was consuming 5.8 grams of trans-fat every day, almost all of which was from partially hydrogenated vegetable oils (more specifically the margarines, vegetable shortenings, baked goods, and processed foods that contain these chemically altered oils). Circumstantial and direct evidence indicates that this increase has been fattening.

The Health Professionals Follow-up Study tracked more than 16,000 doctors and nurses for nine years. After analyzing the data statistically, scientists concluded that a two percent increase in the percentage of calories from trans-fats, when substituted for the same number of calories from either polyunsaturated fats or carbohydrates, was associated with a 0.77 cm increase in waist circumference. Scientists looking at the population of the Nurses' Health Study concluded that every one percent increase in percent of calories from trans-fats was associated with 1.7 pounds of weight gain. Compared with all other categories of fats (including saturated fats), trans-fats had the greatest association with weight gain. Neither of these studies proves a causal relationship; they simply point to the presence of some relationship between trans-fats and shape. The *Case of the African Green Monkeys* proves that, at least in these primates, the relationship is causal.

Scientists placed 51 African green monkeys on a subsistence diet, intended to provide an amount of calories that would prevent any weight gain, for six years. The monkeys were divided into two groups; both were fed an identical amount of total calories and calories of fat. The only thing that differed was the sources for part of the fat calories. One group of monkeys was fed eight percent of their food as trans-fats. The other group ate monounsaturated fats in place of trans-fats. If the only thing that mattered was how many calories were eaten, not the source of the calories, since both groups

---

H S I   C L U E

A 2002 study found that the major sources of trans-fats in the diet of pregnant women in Canada were bakery foods (33% of trans-fat intake), fast foods (12%), breads (10%), snacks (10%), and, margarines or shortenings (8%). Trans-fats are in many non-obvious foods and can even be disguised in foods that claim to have no trans-fats. If the ingredients include vegetable shortening, hydrogenated or partially hydrogenated oils, or mono- and/or diglycerides, trans-fats are likely to be present.

consumed an identical amount of calories, and even an identical amount of dietary fat, shape responses should have been the same. They weren't. After six years, weight increased by 1.8 percent in the monkeys fed monounsaturated fat but by 7.2 percent in those fed trans-fats. In a human weighing 160 pounds this would be the difference between gaining less than 3 pounds and gaining 11.5 pounds. This is a big difference, but it wasn't the only difference. The scientists used imaging to detect changes in internal abdominal (visceral) fat. The trans-fat fed monkeys had 30 percent more visceral fat. In these monkeys, ingestion of trans-fats, even in the absence of caloric excess, caused disproportionately large gains in weight and belly fat. The scientists in this case believed that they weren't feeding these primates enough calories for them to gain weight, never mind get fat. They were wrong. It wasn't a matter of how many calories the primates were fed; it was a matter of which calories they were fed. Trans fats were fattening even when caloric intake was strictly controlled.

The Path of Complexity

The types of fat we eat impact the shape we defend. Shape suffers if we don't eat the right types of fat calories, but it also suffers if we eat the wrong types of fats. As in many other areas of life, *quality* is a more important issue than *quantity*. Improving fat quality can be as easy as following a few rules of thumb: If fat occurs naturally in a real food (a nut, seed, avocado, coconut, yogurt, fish, etc.) it's fine to eat that food, and hence the fat it contains. If fat is added to a food, no matter what type of fat it might be, avoid the food, or at the very least, eat less of it. If you are going to eat an added fat or use a fat or oil to cook with, choose "old" fats—butter, lard, olive oil, coconut oil, etc—rather than the newer man-made fats and oils like margarine, vegetable shortening, or colorless/odorless vegetable oils. Oils should have a smell, a taste, and a color. They should smell like, taste like, and be the color of the real food they are from. If they aren't, don't eat them.

Are All Calories the Same? Cases of Sweet Calories

America has a sweet tooth. We consume large amounts of sweet calories, mostly as sugar and corn-derived sweeteners. The U.S.

Department of Agriculture (USDA) estimated that per person in 1980, we consumed an average of about 85 pounds of sweet calories. In 1990, it increased to 94 pounds. In 2000, it was 106 pounds. By 2007, it was about 107 pounds. Between the years 1980 and 2000, a time period that paralleled the expanding American waistline, we have, on average, each increased our annual consumption of caloric sweeteners by about 21 pounds. Put another way, every day in 1980 the average American consumed about 280 sweet calories; by 2000 this number had increased to about 350 daily calories.

There's a big difference in the quantity of caloric sweeteners consumed today compared with a few decades ago. There's also been a shift in the source of sweet calories. This is apparent when consumption data on sweeteners is investigated. Sugar refers specifically to the sweet calories refined from sugar cane and sugar beets. In 1970, an average American ate 72.5 pounds of sugar. By 1980, this had dropped to 59.5 pounds. By 1984, it was down to 47.5 pounds. Our sugar consumption has remained relatively stable since. As a society, we weren't getting fatter because we were eating more sugar; we have been getting fatter despite eating less. But sugar is not the only source of sweet calories. The average American eats less than a pound of honey a year, slightly less than we ate in 1970. So, honey isn't responsible for the overall increase in sweet calories or for replacing sugar in the diet. The same conclusion is reached when the data for edible syrups like maple, agave, or fruit syrups are investigated; the average American eats less than a pound per year of syrups from these sources and our overall consumption of edible syrups has not increased. With sugar, honey, and other edible syrups eliminated, we are left with only one category of sweet calories—corn-derived sweeteners—that can account for (1) the large overall increase in sweet calories and (2) the sweet calories that have replaced sugar. There are four corn-derived sweeteners, (1) high fructose corn syrup, (2) glucose, (3) dextrose, and (4) crystalline and liquid fructose. Consumption of glucose and dextrose has been relatively stable since 1970: They are

HSI CLUE

Don't be fooled by the source of a caloric sweetener. If it's sweet, used in processed foods and sounds too good to be true, it probably is. There are only a few foods that "naturally" contain significant amounts of sweet molecules—sugar cane, sugar beets, honey, or maple syrup. If our great-great grandparents did not use something as a sweetener, the only reason we can is because modern chemical processing allows food scientists to cheaply convert complex foods like corn, agave, grapes, chicory root, etc into simple sugars.

not responsible for the increase in sweet calories or for replacing sugar in foods and beverages. No consumption data exists for crystalline and liquid fructose consumption because the USDA has considered intake to be too low to warrant tracking. While more of it is consumed today than in 1970, its overall use in foods and beverages pales in contrast with high fructose corn syrup.

High fructose corn syrup was first mass-produced in 1967. Prior to that year it contributed zero calories to our diets. In 1970, the average American ate less than a pound of it. Consumption increased to over 13 pounds by 1980. It was a bit more than 26 pounds in 1984. By 1990, it had increased to about 35 pounds. In 2000, it was about 44 pounds. The reason for this big increase in high fructose corn syrup is in large part economic. The price of corn in the United States is kept low by government subsidies. The price of sugar is kept high by tariffs and quotas on imported sugar. This price differential made high fructose corn syrup a more appealing option to the United States soft drink industry, which in the early 1980s, replaced sugar with high fructose corn syrup in soft drinks. This change was a tipping point for high fructose corn syrup consumption. The epidemic of overweight started about the same time and has progressed in tandem with the increase in this new caloric sweetener. This is circumstantial evidence. Correlation does not prove cause. With that in mind, let's explore sweet calories in more detail in an effort to discover (1) whether they cause shape changes, and (2) if, when it comes to our shapes, a calorie of one sweetener is the same as a calorie of another sweetener.

Humans have consumed honey for thousands of years. Refined sugar is a newer introduction to the human diet. High fructose corn syrup is an even newer introduction. If the only important variable were the amount of sweet calories, we should observe similar responses to an equal amount of calories from any source whether it is an old or new sweetener. The same amount of sugar, whether it is in a dry or liquid form, should produce the same effect on shape. Sweet calories, whether from sugar, high fructose corn syrup or honey, should have equivalent effects. And simple sugars, like fructose and glucose should produce the same responses. Is this what we actually observe?

Let's begin our investigation with the *Case of Liquid Sugar*. Sugar has been used as a means to fatten lab animals for many decades. Several interesting observations arise from these experiments. Adding granulated sugar into dry rat chow can increase body weight and body fatness, but it does not *always* produce these responses. Even when it does increase the amount of weight and body fat being defended, dry sugar plus rat chow won't increase weight and body fatness much. In other words, dry sugar's effects are modest and inconsistent. On its own, it can be fattening, but not particularly fattening. A far more effective method of producing an obese rat is mixing sugar into a solution—liquid sugar—and giving rats an option of drinking this solution whenever they like. When this is done, rats will consistently become obese. Dry sugar added to food has a modest effect on how much body fat a rat defends; sugar-sweetened liquids have a big effect.

Soft drinks are the biggest source of liquid sweeteners in our diet. According to the National Soft Drink Association, consumption of soft drinks has doubled for females and tripled for males since the late 1970s. Circumstantial evidence links soft drinks with increased fatness: In one observational study, risk of obesity increased 1.6 times for each additional soft drink consumed daily. There is also evidence that drinking fewer soft drinks improves shape: Among the 810 adults in the PREMIER study, an 18 month randomized, controlled, intervention, a reduction of just one serving a day of sweetened beverages was associated with about 1.5 pounds of weight loss. A similar observation was reported at the fall of 2006 annual meeting of the Obesity Society: Dieters who replaced virtually all drinks containing caloric sweeteners with water lost an extra five pounds a year compared to those who did not. And there is direct evidence that increasing soft drink consumption leads to detectable and quick increases in weight. Normal weight volunteers, who habitually consumed an average of one to two bottles of soft drinks daily, were tasked with drinking four bottles of high fructose corn syrup sweetened soft drinks daily. Three weeks later the male volunteers had gained an average of a bit over one pound and the female volunteers a bit more than two pounds. The evidence, viewed as a whole, suggests that removing sweetened beverages from the diet improves natural weight; increasing them worsens it, quickly.

Let's continue our investigation of sweet calories with the sweet molecule called fructose. Fructose naturally occurs in fruit and honey as part of a complex food. Estimates suggest that the average American gets over 10 percent of daily calories from fructose.

Among teens this percentage is 12 percent of calories, with one out of four teens getting more than 15 percent of daily calories from fructose. This is a lot of fructose; the vast majority of it isn't squeezed out of fruit or coming from honey. The two main dietary sources of fructose are sugar (50 percent fructose) and high fructose corn syrup—HFCS-42, -55, or -90; with the numbers representing the percent of fructose found in that particular version of high fructose corn syrup, 42 percent, 55 percent, or 90 percent fructose, respectively. Other sources include crystalline fructose (about 98 percent fructose), agave syrup (ranges from 58 to 90 percent fructose), fruit juice concentrates and other fruit sweeteners (generally at least 50 percent fructose), and inulin, oligofructose or chicory root sweeteners (when used as sweeteners these generally contain a minimum of 40 percent fructose and can be made to be above 90 percent fructose). In all of these cases, significant processing is done to a complex food to concentrate, or in some instances create, the fructose. In the case of sugar this is refining of sugar cane or beets to strip away everything but a crystalline sugar molecule (glucose bonded chemically to fructose). Getting fructose from corn is a bit more complicated. If you eat an ear of corn you will eat zero calories of fructose. Corn is processed into cornstarch, further processed into corn syrup, and then further processed into pure glucose, which is chemically rearranged into fructose. The fructose can be used in a pure form (crystalline fructose) or added to corn syrup to create the high fructose corn syrup-55 used in many soft drinks. The relevant shape questions are:

- Is fructose fattening?
- Is it more fattening than other simple sugar molecules like glucose?
- Is processed fructose, whether from sugar or corn, more fattening than the fructose found in complex foods like fruit or honey?

The first of these questions is easy to answer: The answer is yes. Evidence indicates fructose is fattening. A relationship between higher fructose intake and obesity has consistently been observed in human studies. This is circumstantial evidence, but direct evidence also exists. This should come as no surprise since, as we have already discussed, sugar, which is 50 percent fructose, can be fattening especially when it's in a liquid form. A more important question is whether fructose is more fattening than other simple sugars. The answer to this question also appears to be yes. In both animal and human experiments conducted to date, fructose appears to contribute disproportionately to metabolic obesity—fatty liver, high blood fats, insulin resistance, etc. Compared with other simple sugars, it also appears to cause far greater gains in overall body fatness, as well as a greater central accumulation of body fat. This can be inferred from several cases

The first case is the *Case of Sugar-Sweetened and Fructose-Sweetened Beverages.* Scientists at the University of Cincinnati allowed mice to freely consume dry chow and either plain water, sugar-sweetened soft drinks (50 percent fructose and 50 percent glucose), or fructose-sweetened water (100 percent fructose). Ten weeks later the mice allowed to drink fructose-sweetened water were the fattest: Compared with the group that drank water, they were 90 percent fatter. The big increase in fatness did not result from consuming far more calories than the mice that were drinking water; they occurred despite similar calorie intake. In this study, sugar was more fattening than water but pure fructose was even more fattening. A recent study in humans— the *Case of Glucose-Sweetened and Fructose-Sweetened beverages*—also provides evidence that fructose is a more fattening sweet molecule than glucose.

HSI CLUE

Sugar, sucrose, cane sugar, evaporated cane juice, beet sugar, high fructose corn syrup, corn syrup, fructose, invert sugar, glucose, glucose-fructose, dextrose, dextrin, agave syrup, concentrated fruit juice, hydrolyzed starch, maltose, maltodextrin, malitol, manitol, sorbitol and xylitol. These are some of the many names found under the ingredients area of a food label that alert you to the presence of refined or processed caloric sweeteners.

Fructose and glucose are simple sugars; they're the building blocks for more complex sweet-tasting molecules like the sucrose found in table sugar. Fructose and glucose have equal amounts of calories. Do they produce equivalent shape effects? To test this question, overweight and obese volunteers consumed enough sweetened beverages daily to account for $1/4^{th}$ of their calories. One group of volunteers consumed glucose-sweetened beverages; the other group consumed fructose-sweetened beverages. Ten weeks later both groups had gained similar amounts of weight. From a weight perspective, it made no difference whether 25 percent of calories were consumed as fructose- or glucose-sweetened liquids: Detectable amounts of weight were gained quickly. But, as is often the case, weight doesn't tell the entire shape story. The scientists used imaging to measure visceral fat. It only increased in the persons drinking fructose-sweetened beverages. Fructose-sweetened and glucose-sweetened beverages might have caused similar weight gain, but only fructose-sweetened beverages increased belly fat.

This leaves us with our final question: Is processed fructose more fattening than fructose found in a complex food like honey? Two pairs of rat and human experiments help answer this question. In one experiment rats were fed a powdered diet that was either sugar-free, or contained an equal amount of fructose and glucose as (1) sugar, (2) a mixture of fructose and glucose as simple sugars intended to mimic the amounts of these sweet molecules found in honey, or (3) honey. The rats were allowed to eat as much food as desired. Six weeks later, gains in weight in the sugar-free and honey-fed groups were similar *despite* the honey-fed rats consuming significantly more calories. Weight gain was significantly lower in honey-fed rats than those fed sugar or the mixture of fructose and glucose as simple sugars despite a similar food intake in all three of these groups. In the second experiment, rats were fed a diet that contained no added caloric sweeteners or diets that contained about eight percent of their calories as either sugar or honey. At the end of the year the rats fed a sugar-enriched diet weighed more and were fatter than the other rats. Rats that were fed a diet with added honey weighed the same and had similar amounts of body fat as rats fed a sweet-free diet. In these experiments the same amounts of sweet calories didn't produce the same shape responses: The source of the sweet calories mattered. The same is true in the pair of human studies.

In the first study, participants were fed identical diets for 15 days with 300 calories of sweeteners added as either (1) a mixture of glucose and fructose as simple sugars intended to mimic the amounts of these molecules found in honey (artificial honey), or (2) honey. In patients who already had high blood fats, the "artificial honey" further increased them, while "real" honey decreased them. In persons with high cholesterol levels, the "artificial honey" further worsened cholesterol levels; "real" honey improved cholesterol. In the second study, 55 overweight or obese volunteers were divided into two groups. Over the next 30 days one group received 280 of their daily calories as sugar and the other group received an equal amount of honey. Eating honey slightly decreased weight, body fat, cholesterol levels, and blood fats. Consuming sugar had none of these benefits.

From the evidence in the **Cases of Sweet Calories** we can make a few inferences. First, the number of calories a sweetener contains doesn't accurately predict shape responses to it. Second, when it comes to shape responses to sweeteners, all calories, and hence all caloric sweeteners, are not the same. The quality of these calories makes a difference. Sweet calories in a liquid form—beverages— might be more fattening than the same amount of sweet calories in a dry form. Fructose might be a particularly fattening source of sweet calories. But this is only true when it is from refined or processed sources (like sugar or corn-derived sweeteners). The existing evidence is that the same amount of fructose, when it is part of a complex *unprocessed* food like honey, is at worst shape neutral and might even contribute to marginal improvements in shape under some circumstances and in some people.

In our experience, all too often reductionist science perspectives dominate the investigations into caloric sweeteners (and other food issues). Calories and the amounts of glucose and fructose become the topic of discussion and theorizing. This misses an important point. Real foods are more than blends of their isolated ingredients. Honey is more than a collection of fructose and glucose molecules. Complexity science informs us that any complex food will be more than the sum of its parts and that we can't fully understand the response to it by studying isolated ingredients found in it. Science backs this up. Animals and humans don't respond equally to honey or something intended to duplicate the calories and amounts of simple sweet molecules that would be in honey: Food science has been slow to learn lessons from complexity science. In fruits and honey fructose is part of a complex food. The big increase in fructose intake hasn't been because we are consuming complex foods that happen to contain fructose. It has come from eating refined sugar and a highly processed product from a food—corn— that in its complex form has no fructose.

Choose the Path of Complexity

If we want to prevent our shape from worsening, or better yet improve it, we can take the following steps with sweet calories. First and foremost, we can choose to consume less of them. For most people this can be accomplished by choosing to drink water instead of soft drinks, fruit drinks or other beverages sweetened with sugar, high fructose corn syrup, fruit juice concentrates, etc. If you are going to indulge in sweet treats, use the most complex—least refined or processed—forms. Unseparated sugar (brand name Rapadura) would be a better choice than "raw" or brown sugars, which would be better choices than white sugar. Grade B maple syrup would be a better choice than grade A maple syrup; both of which would be better choices than imitation maple syrups. Molasses is a better choice than corn, fruit, or agave sweetened syrups. Honey is a better choice than refined or processed sweeteners but there are different qualities of honey—from the more complex to the more purified. Choose the more complex such as an unfiltered rather than a filtered honey. We have lots of *qualitative* choices available to us when it comes to caloric sweeteners. It's our job to choose the most complex ones.

Are All Calories the Same? The Case of Palatability

If you investigate the items listed under the *Ingredients* area of a food label, sugar and high fructose corn syrup turn up in expected places (sweetened cereals, candy, desserts, etc) and in unexpected places (peanut butter, ketchup, etc). Why are they found in these unexpected places? A primary reason has to do with *palatability*—the sweet taste, even in small amounts, makes things "taste" better, increasing how much is eaten. The food science concept of palatability refers to a food's capacity to get us to eat more of it. A food that we'll eat a lot of before feeling like we don't want another bite is more palatable than one that leaves us feeling satisfied after just a few bites. A food that increases appetite is more palatable than one that doesn't. A food that can convince us to continue eating even after we are full, overriding our appetite mechanisms, is more palatable than one which, when full, we would be disinclined to eat.

There is a tendency to naively blame obesity on overeating; we assume people are consciously choosing to eat more and can consciously choose to eat less. But this misses an important point. Obesity can't be reliably produced in either animals or humans by simply making more calories available. To produce obesity the calories must be eaten; appetite must be influenced. David Kessler, M.D., in his book *The End of Overeating*, asks. "Is it possible that eating certain foods can stimulate us to keep eating—and eating and eating?" The answer is yes. Foods can be crafted in ways that cause us to (1) increase how much of them we eat before feeling satisfied, (2) increase appetite, and (3) increase natural weight. As a society, we have been slow to appreciate that eating certain types, forms, or combinations of calories makes us want to eat more of them. The food industry has been way ahead of us. A lot of work goes into getting the sensory attributes of a food or beverage product just right, with the goal being to create something irresistible to consumers. The selection of ingredients, taste and texture, aroma, visual aspects, and more are laboriously honed to produce foods that we will want to eat, and that once eaten, we'll want to eat more of.

Palatability is influenced by the degree to which a food interacts with our senses, including our sense of taste. Science recognizes four basic tastes—sweet, salty, sour, and bitter. Neuroscientists have proposed that at least two, and possibly three, other tastes—fatty, savory (also called umami), and starchy—also exist. Ingredients in processed foods that contribute to these tastes essentially match the category. Caloric and non-caloric (artificial) sweeteners stimulate the sweet taste. Salty taste would be stimulated by salt. Acids (acetic acid, citric acid, lactic acid, malic acid, or tartaric acid) produce a sour (tart) taste. Fatty taste would be stimulated by fats or by ingredients that are intended to simulate the *mouth feel* of fats. Monosodium glutamate (MSG), or other sources of free glutamate, is used to produce the savory taste. As Kessler points out, combining three of these tastes—sweet, salty, and fatty—greatly increases the palatability of a food.

> **HSI CLUE**
>
> Giving a cow twice as much pasture won't make it fatter. To get a cow to be considerably fatter we must change the source of calories. Most livestock are fed *finishing* diets—diets designed to produce the greatest amount of fattening in the least amount of time—prior to slaughter. This is an important lesson: It's the source of calories available that is fattening, not the amount of them.

Sweet taste tends to weakly increase palatability. The same is true for fatty taste. Combining both in the same product produces a far greater increase in palatability. When salt is added to the mix, palatability increases even more. As Kessler states in his book, "Eating foods high in sugar, fat, and salt makes us eat more foods high in sugar, fat, and salt. We see this clearly in both animal and human research." If a food company can find a just right combination of these three ingredients it will succeed in creating a highly palatable food. If we eat this food, we might find ourselves wanting to eat more of it. The same is true for flavor enhancers and the savory taste. Eating foods with added flavor enhancers added to them causes us to want to eat more of these foods.

HSI CLUE

Food makers want their foods to be savory. They also prefer *clean labels*, free of ingredients some consumers wish to avoid. MSG is one of these ingredients: Some consumer won't buy products with MSG. To add MSG-like flavor enhancement without having to put MSG on a label, other free glutamate flavor enhancers are used: Glutamic acid, hydrolyzed vegetable protein, autolyzed protein, textured protein, yeast extract, autolyzed yeast extract, sodium caseinate, protein isolate, modified food starch, and modified corn starch.

Flavor enhancers use the amino acid glutamate (free glutamate) to stimulate the savory taste buds. They're used in many fast foods and processed foods; found in products from soups to salad dressings, processed meats to canned tuna, frozen entrees to ice creams, and bread to crackers; and added to many low-fat and no-fat foods as a way to make up for some of the taste that is lost when fats are removed. MSG is the best-known free glutamate flavor enhancer. Originally introduced in 1947 as a product called Ac'cent, MSG was marketed as something similar to salt that we sprinkle on food to enhance its flavor. The increase in palatability caused by MSG is observed in several ways. Consumers rate foods with MSG as tasting better. Volunteers eat more food and eat it faster when trace amounts of MSG are added: MSG makes us behave as if we are hungrier than we would have been without it. And hunger returns sooner than it would have if MSG had not been added to a food or a meal. Evidence also indicates that when MSG is added to a food, we like the food more initially and we *learn* to like it more and more each time we eat it again. This is even true for novel foods. If we were to eat an unfamiliar food, we *learn* to like it more if MSG is present. Based on our responses to it, the inferences are, in the words of Holmes, elementary: MSG, precisely as its label informs us, is very effective as a flavor enhancer; it does a great job increasing the palatability of a food. Does it also affect shape?

In animal experiments, MSG, in amounts similar to what we might consume in our diets, increases the amount of food consumed, just as it does in human studies. It also increases body fat, liver fat, and blood fats. Despite having no calories, MSG is fattening in mice and rats. What about with humans? While no controlled dietary studies have been done in humans, circumstantial evidence suggests that MSG might be affecting shape self-regulation. This evidence comes from the INTERMAP Study—an international study designed to search for relationships between what is eaten and worldwide patterns of blood pressure. In 752 Chinese men and women from three rural Chinese villages who were followed in this study, there was a strong relationship between how much MSG was consumed and weight. Villagers, who added the most MSG to their food, were three times more likely to be overweight compared to persons who did not add any MSG. This is not proof that MSG caused them to be fatter, but it is evidence of a relationship that merits serious investigation.

MSG and other free glutamate flavor enhancers are being added to many foods for us. We know they increase palatability. We deserve to definitely know whether this increased palatability comes with shape consequences. We don't. Instead what we get are assurances from the companies that profit by making MSG (and other forms of free glutamate) that these flavor enhancers are perfectly safe because they occur naturally in food. Just as was the case with sweet calories, this bait and switch misses an important point. Real foods are more than blends of their isolated ingredients. Humans don't respond identically to honey and a man-made artificial honey even if both contain equal amounts of fructose. From the perspective of complexity science, it is, simply put, unscientific to use the "it's natural" argument. The only way to understand whether adding MSG and other free-glutamate flavor enhancer ingredients to foods is or isn't fattening is to investigate this issue.

The ingredients added to processed foods all have purposes. Preservatives extend shelf life. Texture enhancers add moistness. Taste ingredients are intentionally added to increase palatability. This can be seen in the *Case of Peanut Butter*. Peanuts are the only absolutely essential ingredients for peanut butter, but many brands of peanut butter have more than just peanuts. They have sugar, extra oil (often a trans-fat containing partially hydrogenated

HSI CLUE

Because of the impact palatability can have on our waistlines, it is important that we don't make one of the common dieting mistakes. This mistake is thinking that something that might be low in calories, fat or both, but which tastes like a milk shake or dessert is better for our long-term shape than real food. Highly palatable foods increase natural weight independent of their calories. If something tastes like a milkshake, it's highly palatable.

vegetable oil), salt or all of these ingredients. These are added because they make the peanut butter more palatable than if it was solely made from ground peanuts. This principle can also be seen in the *Case of Low-Fat Foods*. Fat adds palatability to a food; removing it results in a less palatable product. To offset this loss of palatability, many low-fat versions of foods add more sweet taste, as well as other taste ingredients like MSG. In processed foods the combinations of sweet, salty, fatty, and savory tastes are not accidental mistakes; they are intentional additions that are often so skillfully masked by other tastes and flavors that we might not even know they are there.

Palatability influences how much we eat. It also influences shape. This is seen in the *Case of the Cafeteria Diet*. Sugar can make an average lab rat fatter. The same is true for a high fat diet. In both of these instances, the gains in fatness are not particularly dramatic or fast, nor do they occur in all mice or rats. A more reliable method to fatten lab animals was discovered by Anthony Sclafani and Deleri Springer. In the mid-1970s, they purchased foods that can be found in any supermarket— sweetened condensed milk, chocolate-chip cookies, salami, cheese, bananas, marshmallows, milk chocolate, and peanut butter. When allowed to eat as much as they desired of these supermarket foods, the rats did indeed get fatter, and consistently. In less than two weeks a noticeable weight gain was observed. After eight weeks most rats had become obese. This experiment formed the basis of using the so-called *cafeteria diet*— a variety of palatable foods—as a means to promote fattening in lab animals. The foods used in cafeteria diets are generally identical to processed foods that would be found in a supermarket. In most strains of rats a cafeteria diet will increase food intake (between 50 to 90 percent) and produce large increases in weight and fatness. It is a far more reliable dietary method for producing obesity than is adding high amounts of fats and sugars to standard rat chow. Removal of this diet usually results in rapid and spontaneous weight loss. Reintroduction causes rats to once again self-regulate their weight at a higher level. The evidence from the many experiments with cafeteria diets suggests that, at least in rats, the cafeteria diet increases natural weight.

Animal experiments have repeatedly demonstrated that animals will spontaneously eat more when palatable foods are available. They will also do more work to get to these foods. An animal will work hard for foods that are high in sweet and fat calories. It will work hard for salty calories. It will work hard for liquid combinations of these calories especially when they are flavorful. And it will do this even in the absence of overt hunger. Not surprisingly, it will also gain weight and get much fatter. In animals, a more palatable diet causes quick and spontaneous increases in calories consumed, a greater commitment to acquire these calories, and ultimately greater degrees of fatness. Palatability appears to exert the same influence in many humans. Palatable foods increase how much we eat and weigh, and it does this quickly. This was detected in the *Case of the Vending Machine Experiment.* What would occur if volunteers were allowed to freely select whatever foods they wanted, in any quantity desired, with the one constraint being that all of the food had to be chosen from a vending machine? In an experiment designed to answer this question, 34 male volunteers entered a metabolic ward where the amount of calories needed to maintain their weight were fed to them for four days. After these four days they were told to eat as much food as they desired from two free vending machines for the next five days. The vending machines offered a variety of familiar, palatable foods; a variety the researchers described as a mixed cafeteria diet. What happened? They ate about 50 percent more food and they gained an average of about two pounds in just five days.

Choose the Path of Low Palatability

Highly palatable calories affect shape self-regulation—increasing appetite and fatness—far more so than do less palatable calories. The goal is to eat a diet that is lower in palatability. How do you do this without sacrificing all the foods you enjoy? One solution is to be on the alert for *combinations* of ingredients, specifically looking out for the combination of sweet, fatty, and salty taste ingredients. You're better off choosing a food that only has one or two of these tastes than all three. Another solution is to look out for flavor enhancers, like MSG or MSG-like ingredients, and choose similar foods made without these ingredients. In a practical sense this means that if you want to treat yourself to potato chips or tortilla chips, choose a brand with a bare minimum of ingredients. If you are going to eat peanut butter, select a brand with just peanuts, without added sugar and salt.

Adventures in Chewing

How could we make one group of animals or humans fatter than another if we wanted to feed both groups identical foods? One answer to this question is that we would feed one group the food in a rough mixture that requires more chewing and feed the other group the same foods in a form that requires less chewing. We refer to this as the **Chewing Effect**. One experimental example of the **Chewing Effect** is the *Case of Softer Food*. Two groups of rats were fed identical diets in terms of nutritional composition and calories. This was a standard rat chow diet with just one difference between the two groups: One group ate rat chow as hard pellets and the other ate the same rat chow made into softer pellets. Both groups ate diets consisting of identical ingredients. They also ate equal amounts of food. The only difference was the amount of chewing required. Twenty-six weeks later the rats fed the softer pellets were fatter. In this experiment, the rats that ate the softer food did not get fatter because they ate more chow; they got fatter despite the fact that they did not. The texture of the food, not its calories, was the tipping point.

Another example of this effect was observed in the *Case of Puréeing*. Rats were fed a diet comprised of meat, beans, cream, starch, and water. These foods, and only these foods, were given to all of the rats in the study. One group of rats was given them as a rough mixture and another group received them in the form of a purée—a soft paste. All of the rats were allowed to eat as much food as their appetites dictated. Three weeks later the rats given puréed food were eating more calories, and had gained more weight.

Scientific studies of animals have demonstrated that if a food is made easier to swallow—made into a form that requires less chewing—it is more fattening. All else being equal, the same food in a rough mixture is less fattening than in a purée. This effect is put to use in several medical situations, including low birth weight children and institutionalized elderly, where increasing food intake and boosting weight gain are desirable outcomes. Feeding of softer food causes more food to be eaten and more weight to be gained.

The fact that softer texture increases palatability doesn't appear to be lost on the food industry. Kessler, in *The End of Overeating*, informs us that one of the goals of food processing is to turn foods into textures that melt in the mouth. More and more of our calories are made into forms that are easier to swallow. Gristle, fiber, and other aspects of complex foods that require more chewing are removed. Ingredients that hold moisture and soften food are added in their place. The result is that it takes less chewing to eat a processed food diet than it would a diet made up of the more traditional versions of these foods. Cold cuts serve as an example.

Cold cuts, including turkey, chicken, ham, bologna, and other sandwich meats, are an example of an inconsistency in the diet. In the not too distant past, turkey or chicken would have been sliced off, well, a turkey or chicken. The same goes for ham; it would have been sliced off a hambone. European cold cuts like bresaola and prosciutto were made with whole slices of pork cured using traditional old world methods. Sausage-makers put to use meat and animal parts that were edible and nutritious, but not particularly appealing, such as scraps, organ meats, blood, and fat, and then preserved this meat by using natural fermentation. Most modern cold cuts are not made in these manners. They are highly processed foods. Cold cuts might start from a whole cooked chicken, turkey, or ham; most of them don't stop at this point. Gristle, fats, and other harder to chew elements will be removed. The remaining meat will be chopped and made into a texture that is more akin to a meat loaf than a steak. Ingredients like autolyzed yeast extract, sodium phosphate, and soy protein concentrate are added to further soften the texture and to retain moisture and bind the loaf together. Caloric sweeteners, salt, and flavor enhances are often added to increase palatability. Nitrates, nitrites, or sulfites are added as preservatives. The end result is palatable, easy to chew, processed meat products, which have been implicated as contributing factors in metabolic obesity, diabetes, heart disease, and some cancers.

> **HSI CLUE**
>
> Studies on food texture ask, when it comes to shape, is the form of food (or beverages) an important consideration? The answer is an unambiguous yes. The texture of the foods (or beverages) we consume influences appetite, metabolism, hormones, and how much or how little body fat we will defend.

Cold cuts are just a single example of an overall theme: Processed foods require less chewing. Fiber is removed from grains, resulting in easier to chew cereals, breads, and baked goods. Peanuts are ground into crunchy peanut butters, or even easier to swallow smooth and creamy peanut butters. Apples are made into applesauce—a softer apple product—or into apple juice—liquid apple calories. It takes less chewing to eat today than it would have a century ago. This might seem trivial, but available evidence indicates that it is anything but: Softer, easier to chew calories, are more fattening.

A Study in Variety

A cafeteria diet is more fattening than a standard rat chow diet. It's even more fattening than a standard rat chow diet supplemented with high fat and high sugar ingredients. Why? The short answer is that it's more fattening because it's more palatable—rats spontaneously eat more of it. But what exactly causes them to eat more of it? We have already identified two causes: (1) It contains individual foods, some of which, because of the inclusion of sweet calories, fat, salt, flavor enhancers, or a mix of several to all of these, are highly palatable; and (2) it requires less chewing than standard rat chow. A third reason is variety. The cafeteria diet not only contains highly palatable foods; it contains a wide variety of them.

Compared to a less varied diet, a more varied diet consisting of processed, palatable food is more fattening. Scientific experiments have demonstrated this in animals. In humans, much of the evidence for the fattening effects of a varied, palatable foods diet has been obtained from studies designed to detect the presence of a relationship, not necessarily whether the relationship is causative. In these investigations, eating a greater variety of palatable foods— snacks, desserts, sweets, condiments, or processed food entrees—is associated with increased body fatness. Eating a variety of fruits, vegetables, whole grains, and unprocessed meats—foods that are far less palatable—is associated with being leaner. These types of studies suggest that variety is not the issue per se. The issue is variety in the context of palatability and processing. But these types of studies only provide circumstantial evidence. Fortunately, there is direct evidence that variety influences shape self-regulation in humans. One of these cases is the *Case of Monotonous Food*.

In the mid-1970s Dr. Michel Cabanac and Dr. E.F. Rabe decided to intentionally restrict the palatability of the diet. They did this in a way that also reduced the variety of the diet. Volunteers were allowed to consume as many calories as desired with one caveat—all calories were from the same nutritionally complete liquid food. For the next two weeks the volunteers drank as many calories as they desired, and lost about 6.5 pounds. This weight loss occurred without the telltale signs of a person being below natural weight: An increase in hunger, recurring thoughts about food, and increased desire for sweet taste were not observed. This experiment suggested that, at least over a few weeks, a diet that was bland and had no variety changed the shape that was being defended, decreasing natural weight.

Cases of Adding or Omitting Snacks provide another example of variety affecting shape. Volunteers were asked to add a snack to what they were already eating. Adding a snack is a way to increase the variety of palatable foods (especially for people who don't normally snack). On average, the volunteers consumed more calories than they did prior to adding this snack and gained a slight amount of weight. This effect was particularly strong among the volunteers that did not habitually consume snacks and far weaker in those who did. Presumably this difference occurred, in part, because adding a snack food to a diet that contains none is a bigger increase in variety than adding it to a diet that already contains snack foods, where it might substitute for or replace another snack food. A different experiment was the flip side of adding a snack food: Snacking was reduced. Overweight volunteers were divided into two groups. One group was asked to avoid all snack foods on most days. Another group was asked to choose one snack food and to only eat this item when they snacked. Eight weeks later volunteers in both groups had reduced their weight by an average of just less than 7.5 pounds. Whether snack foods were avoided completely, or limited to only one chosen snack food, weight was lost.

A third case is the *Case of More or Less Variety*. It's simple to imagine that it would be easy to consume more calories when there are a

HSI CLUE

Rather than buying processed meat cold cuts, carve your own meat off a chicken, turkey or ham and use this for sandwiches. If you do buy cold cuts, read the ingredients. Choose cold cut options that contain the fewest ingredients. More ingredients are a clue to more processing, higher palatability, and easier swallowing. The same principle applies to a can of tuna fish. Rather than choosing a can of tuna containing tuna, autolyzed yeast, salt, and water, choose a can that contains tuna and water. Applying this fewer ingredients rule of thumb can lead to making less fattening food choices.

wide variety of palatable foods available, some high in fat, some high in sugars, and some high in both. And it is. In this instance, much of the variety comes from the differences in nutritional composition between foods. What would happen if variety were limited to a more narrow range of attributes? In an experiment designed to answer this question, foods were created to be equal in nutritional composition—protein, fat, and carbohydrate—but different in attributes like flavor and texture. Six lean and six overweight volunteers were allowed to eat as much or little of these nutritionally identical foods as they desired for seven days. During this week they were, in random order, allowed to eat 5, 10, or 15 versions of these foods. This experiment eliminated nutritional variety, but not variety that appealed to our senses. More food was eaten on days when there were 10 foods to select from than when there were 5, and more food was eaten when there were 15 foods to choose from than 10. The lean men lost weight when they only had 5 or 10 choices of nutritionally identical foods that varied in flavor and texture to choose from, but gained about one pound in the couple of days when they were offered 15. Overweight men lost weight in all three conditions, but lost more weight when they could only choose from 5 or 10 foods than when they could choose from 15. In this case, flavor and texture variety influenced both how much was eaten and changes in weight. And it did it in a matter of days.

HSI CLUE

Overweight women were asked to eat either an apple or pear 3 times a day. After 12 weeks, the women adding the fruit to their diet had lost an average of about 2.7 pounds. Obese men and women were asked to eat half of a grapefruit before meals. Twelve weeks later they had lost an average of 3.6 pounds. In these experiments, adding several servings a day of real foods—fruits in these cases— improved shape.

These cases suggest that eating a greater variety of *processed* foods is fattening. This doesn't mean that eating a greater variety of *unprocessed* foods produces the same effect. Adding, not subtracting, unprocessed foods, like fruits and vegetables, is the goal. This can be inferred from the *Case of Increased Fruits and Vegetables*. Obese women either (1) reduced fat intake, or (2) reduced fat intake and increased intake of fresh fruits and vegetables. One year later, restricting fat had led to an average weight loss of about 14 pounds. Restricting fats and eating more fruits and vegetables worked even better, resulting in an average weight loss of almost 17.5 pounds. The persons who ate more fruits and vegetables, despite reducing their weight by a greater amount, were less hungry than the other group.

Eating a varied food diet when the foods are naturally high in nutrients and require more chewing is a different thing than eating a varied food diet where the foods have been engineered to be palatable and easy to swallow.

Flavor Variety

Humans crave sensory variety. We might eat more of a highly palatable food, and much less of an unpalatable food, but we'll only voluntarily eat so much of any food before tiring of it. If at this point, a different tasty food were made available, we will usually take at least a few bites of it. Scientists refer to this as *sensory-specific satiety*. We can eat our fill of a food with one set of sensory characteristics, and yet still have room for a food with different sensory characteristics. The brain's satiety mechanisms are affected by flavor, texture, color, and other sensory characteristics of food. When a greater variety of sensory distinct foods are available, we tend to eat more. This was observed in the *Case of More or Less Variety*. Nutritional composition of foods was kept constant. Adding flavors and modifying texture created sensory variety; which led to more food being eaten.

A nutritional bias towards sensory variety makes evolutionary sense. Nutrients are distributed unevenly in whole foods and each food has its own unique sensory characteristics. An apple has more vitamin C than a walnut, but the walnut provides nutrients the apple doesn't—fat-soluble vitamins and essential fatty acids (omega-3 and -6 fats). Both also have unique sensory attributes: There is no mistaking an apple for a walnut. They have different flavors, textures, and colors. Eating a variety of whole foods with distinct sensory characteristics would lead to eating a bigger diversity of nutrients: This would confer a survival advantage; giving a person a greater likelihood of having all of their nutritional needs met. When foods can be engineered to have a variety of flavors, textures, and colors, yet have little to no discernible nutrient differences, the innate sensory variety bias is no longer as advantageous.

HSI CLUE

The diet food industry is massive. As a society, we put a lot of faith in these foods. Most diet foods have not been proven to improve shape or to lower natural weight. Some have ingredients or textures that would, at a minimum, be suspected of doing the opposite. Diet foods are theorized to improve our shape, but in most instances this theorizing is in advance of evidence.

A processed food diet, similar to the foods in the *Case of More or Less Variety*, doesn't get its variety from a cornucopia of different real foods. Variety is produced by combining ingredients from a few foods in many different ways. The diet of the average American is comprised of an inordinately high percent of calories from a few commodity crops. Corn and sugar cane provide most of the sweet calories. Corn and wheat account for most of the starch, soy for the majority of the protein calories, and corn, soy, canola and cottonseed for large amounts of the fat calories in processed foods. By adding specific taste and scent ingredients to the ingredients made from this handful of commodity crops the modern food industry can create thousands of processed foods with distinct sensorial characteristics. These "different" foods appeal to the brain bias towards sensory variety, because they contain a diversity of flavors and textures.

One of the primary ways the brain assesses food variety is through flavor. Every whole food has its own characteristic flavor. If our ancestors ate a variety of flavors, by default they consumed a diversity of nutrients. In our world, flavor is no longer a reliable guide to nutrient diversity. Anything can be flavored to "taste" like a strawberry, as an example, no matter what its nutrient content, by adding natural or artificial strawberry flavorings. To understand these flavoring agents it is important to understand how they work. Flavorings, whether natural or artificial, are fragrance chemicals. They stimulate the sense of smell. Much of what we think of as the "taste" of a food does not come from how it interacts with our taste buds; it comes from its aroma. This is apparent when something like a cold affects our sense of smell and foods no longer "taste" the same to us. Without the sense of smell, foods have little flavor. Fundamental taste attributes (including sweet, salty, bitter, and sour, as well as perhaps savory, fatty, and starchy) are a small part of a food's flavor. Compounds in food that stimulate our sense of smell can be responsible for as much as 90 percent of the flavor experience. Infinitesimal quantities of natural or artificial fragrance chemicals can add fruit, spice, coffee, chocolate, vanilla, or any other desired flavor to a food or beverage.

Fragrance chemicals are essential for the modern food industry. They're used to make things "taste" like something other than what they really are—fooling our brains into thinking we are eating one thing when we aren't. They're also used to add flavors to foods that need them, and to hide flavors we would otherwise find unpalatable. Canning, freezing, and other food processing methods reduce or destroy flavors. Flavor must be added back to replace what was lost. Processing and storage can also create rancidity, freezer burn, and other off-notes or unpalatable flavors. Flavor ingredients are added to cover-up these tastes and scents that, if detected, many consumers would find objectionable. Many ingredients used in processed foods, simply put, add awful flavors to foods: Without using flavoring additives foods with these ingredients would "taste" terrible. If not for the wizardry of the industry that has built up around flavoring foods and beverages, many processed foods would be unpalatable. We wouldn't want to eat a little of them, never mind a lot. The growth in the processed food industry—foods that are estimated to account for about 90 cents out of every dollar spent on food in the United States—has been mirrored by growth in the flavor industry. Without the latter, there couldn't be the former.

Adding natural and artificial flavors to foods increases palatability, and just might make the food more fattening. This occurs despite the fact that these fragrance chemicals, in the amounts used, are essentially free of calories. One piece of evidence for the above inference is the *Case of Flavored Chow*. Female baboons were served diets identical in every way but flavor. Compared to an unflavored diet, a diet flavored with lemon, orange, apple, sugar, fruit punch, or chocolate flavor resulted in increased food intake. It also caused body weight to increase significantly. The only variable that changed in this case was flavor. This one change, flavored verse unflavored chow, increased the palatability of the diet—they ate more food—and contributed to the development of obesity. Flavor was fattening.

The *Case of Natural Food Flavors* indicates that flavor affects palatability in us as well. In this case, six natural flavors were added to the lunch and dinner meals of hospitalized elderly patients for three days. These patients consumed more calories when the foods were flavored than on days when they weren't. This is not the only case in humans where flavor is used to drive palatability. Many elderly individuals lose some of their ability to detect tastes and smells. Certain clinical conditions—most notably cancer and HIV infection—are associated with diminished taste and smell. Use of some medications and exposure to chemical pollutants can also cause a loss of taste and smell. Improving the flavor of food, directly, indirectly, or both, has been proposed as a therapy in these situations. Adding natural and artificial flavors, flavor enhances (like MSG), or strong tastes are direct ways to increase a food's flavor. Improving a person's sense of taste and smell would be an indirect method for improving the flavor of food. Scientific studies where one, or both, of these areas are improved have shown appetite increases and weight gain. In these instances, amplification of the diet's flavor improves food palatability and affects shape.

Flavor is a powerful appetite stimulus. By adding fragrance chemicals that appeal to the sense of smell, processed foods can be made more flavorful and more palatable: We like them more and eat more of them. Eating a variety of flavors is an even stronger stimulus. Advances in the understanding of flavor impact on shape have formed the basis of two diet books—*The Flavor Point Diet* by David Katz, M.D. and *The Shangri-La Diet* by Seth Roberts. The specific recommendations made differ, but both authors share a premise that flavor affects shape and that the flavor variety in processed foods is fattening. They also both suggest steps that, when followed, reduce flavor variety.

Katz's program is aimed at limiting flavor variety (each day has a flavor theme), while we learn to enjoy and appreciate the flavors that occur naturally in whole, unprocessed foods (and avoid the natural and artificial flavors added to processed foods). He reported that weight was reduced by between 10 to 31 pounds in 12 weeks in 16 of his patients by following his flavor reeducation program. He also reported improvements in

HSI CLUE

Many consumers prefer to see natural flavors on a label. This is because of the "it's natural" fallacy. We fall victim to this fallacy when we adopt a belief that, because something is "natural" it is good or healthy. Almost all information on natural flavors is proprietary. It isn't divulged. Not only is there no evidence of how we respond to most natural flavors, we don't even know what's in most of them. The distinction between natural and artificial fragrance chemicals is one of source and how the fragrance is made; not one of health attributes.

shape—waist circumference decreased by an average about 3.5 inches—and body composition—body fat percentage dropped by almost 4.5 percent. This evidence is anecdotal. His program hasn't undergone independent scientific testing.

Roberts is a scientific detective of sorts. One of his strongest interests has been in lowering his natural weight. This interest, along with his self-experimentation, caused him to notice that removing the scent component of some of the calories he consumed reduced the amount of weight he defended. As he ate more low-flavor calories his natural weight got lower and lower. According to Roberts, two foods with an equal amount of calories, one with strong flavor and another with weak flavor, don't have the same effect on natural weight: The food with the stronger flavor might raise natural weight, while the one with weak flavor might lower it. This observation forms the basis for *The Shangri-La Diet*. He recommends consuming two to four tablespoons once daily of extra light olive oil, or some other lightly flavored or unscented oil, at least one hour away from all other things with flavors, including beverages and non-food items like mouthwash, toothpaste, etc. He maintains that as long as we consume enough low flavor calories each day, natural weight will be, in a manner similar to Peck's rats fed quinine, lower. More information about his observations and theories, as well as how real people just like you are using and responding to them, can be found at the online forums he maintains (http://boards.sethroberts.net/).

There is still a great deal to learn about the role flavor variety, in general, and added fragrance chemicals—natural and artificial flavors—impact shape self-regulation. What is clear is that the widespread use of fragrance chemicals in processed food has created a bit of a dilemma for Shape Intelligence. It was once relatively easy for Shape Intelligence to learn which flavors went with which foods, remember the calorie and nutrient benefits and consequences of these foods, and use this stored information to guide future eating decisions and metabolic responses to foods (a process called *flavor learning* discussed in Chapter 20). Today this job is anything but easy.

Isolated Characteristics or Food Complexity?

Humans have always been faced with the question of what to eat. Traditional cultures in every part of the world, based in large part on what was available locally, came up with their unique answers to this question. For generation after generation they ate the same foods. Then, in a span of less than a century, we changed our minds. Our notions about what to eat—food paradigm—shifted: We swapped complexity for simplicity.

HSI CLUE

Obese volunteers who took 1 to 2 tbsp of vinegar diluted in a glass of water for 12 weeks reduced body weight, visceral fat, and waist circumference more than participants who didn't. People who took 2 tbsp of vinegar prior to 2 meals daily for 4 weeks lost several pounds. Perhaps part of the reason for these results is that, while vinegar has a strong taste, it has weak flavor. You can self-experiment by adding 1 to 2 tbsp of vinegar to a glass of water, with or without a tbsp of honey, and drinking this before one or more meals daily.

The modern approach to deciding what to eat, presupposes that, when it comes to food, the really important things are the individual nutritional constituents. Calories, amount of fat, type of fat (saturated, trans-fats, etc), cholesterol, carbohydrates, sugars, fibers, salt, vitamins, antioxidants, and more; these are what really matters when it comes to deciding what to eat. We don't look at food as a whole thing; we look at it as a collection of ingredients. Sometimes we even reduce a complex food down to being essentially one ingredient. An orange becomes known for having vitamin C, milk for calcium, honey for sweet calories, butter for saturated fat, and eggs for cholesterol. It's the job of food science to decide which ingredients are good and which aren't. The modern food industry then engineers foods with more of the good and less of the bad. With this reduction of a complex thing down to a simple thing, it's a small step to convincing consumers that they don't need to eat whole foods. The "good" ingredients can be added to other foods. We no longer need to eat an orange or drink a glass of milk; we can eat something that has been fortified with vitamin C or calcium. Substitute foods—artificial sweeteners, margarine, vegetable shortening, and egg substitutes—are engineered to have the desired benefits of honey, butter or eggs, while having none of the perceived downsides. We are led to believe that if we eat these substitute foods, we'll be healthy and shapely. In the real world things aren't this simple. Despite promises—claims like "heart smart", "low-calorie", "fat-free", "sugar-free", and more—and despite the fact that most adults regularly eat one or more foods engineered to be "better" for us, as a society we are not healthier or leaner; we are chronically ill and fat.

Food is more than a collection of isolated ingredients; it's a complex thing. Trying to understand how an individual will respond to something as complex as food, by trying to understand and apply knowledge about isolated ingredients, is like trying to understand avalanches by studying snowflakes or a rainstorm from drops of water. Complexity science informs us that complex things, like food, are *irreducible*. They are more than the sum of their parts. A whole food is not a car that can be taken apart and reassembled. It is more like Herbie the Love Bug. Whole foods are complex collections of interacting things. While the individual compounds in food are important, the interactions between and relationships among these compounds are also important. Science has, at best, a partial and incomplete understanding about the ingredients in food. It has virtually no understanding about how these ingredients interact. And the complexity doesn't end with food. Foods have complex interactions with us when we eat them.

HSI CLUE

We have more bacteria in our gut, by a wide margin, than we have fat cells in our whole body. Recent research indicates that when mice are fed the equivalent of a Western processed food diet it causes almost instantaneous changes in gut bacteria. This change in gut bacteria results in obesity. Human studies also provide compelling evidence that gut bacteria affect shape. One of the single most powerful ways to improve our gut bacteria is by eating fermented foods.

When isolated ingredients are used as the basis for making food decisions, we replace real foods with things that food scientists create. We are assured this swap is for the best. But evidence indicates the swap is seldom for the better and it's often for the worse. In practical terms, the shift to an ingredient dominated food paradigm means that many of us no longer select butter or eggs because we are told that they are high in saturated fats and cholesterol, respectively. But these foods are more than these single compounds. And the presence of a single compound in a real food doesn't always accurately predict how we respond to eating the *whole* food. In fact, using a single ingredient as the basis for predicting the response to complex foods leads to wrong inferences as often as it leads to correct ones. New information on trans-fats, and the evidence from the *Case of the African Green Monkeys,* provide evidence for this point when it comes to margarine. We were led to believe that margarine was a "better" butter. These cases inform us we weren't better off eating margarine, and the trans-fats it contained; we would have been better off continuing to eat butter. Whole foods are complicated.

Eating margarine or egg substitutes makes sense when food is viewed through an ingredient paradigm. It makes no sense when complexity is used to make food decisions. Using complexity would not lead to engineering substitutes for butter or eggs. It would lead to producing a better butter by feeding a cow better quality food and placing it in a healthier environment—green pastures. Complexity predicts, and science supports that a cow will then, on its own, produce a better butter. The same is true for eggs: Better eggs come from hens living in healthier environments and allowed to eat better food. If we really want the "Real Thing; Only Better", we need to understand what real means and what truly makes one thing better than another. We need to focus on *qualitative* issues around food.

HSI CLUE

Traditionally made sauerkraut, miso, soy sauce, kim chee, cheese, and many other foods are fermented. This does not mean that all sauerkraut or soy sauce in a supermarket is fermented. Most of it won't be. Natural fermentation takes time and time comes with a cost. A clue to fermentation is higher price. Other clues include listing the starter culture under ingredients or finding evidence on the product that indicates it was naturally fermented.

Quality is not a subject that can be judged within an ingredient-centric food paradigm; it is a complexity issue. It has to do with the whole food, not just individual ingredients or isolated attributes. Everything that affects the food—how it was grown, raised, stored, processed and more— impacts its quality. As a society, we have been asking the wrong questions about food. We tend to focus on isolated *quantitative* aspects of food. How many calories does it have? How much fat? How much sugar? Answers to these quantitative questions have been guiding our behaviors. But these are the wrong types of questions. Better questions are; what's in the food? How (and where) was it grown or raised? What's been done to it since?

When it comes to food, improving shape usually entails shifting away from an ingredient-based mindset and into a complexity mindset; a mindset with food that is best described as holism. Holism comes from a Greek word that roughly translates as "all, entire, or total". It means that the properties of a something, in this instance food, can't be determined or explained by its component parts alone. As Aristotle explained in one of his principle works, *Metaphysics*, "The whole is more than the sum of its parts". The individual parts don't explain how a whole system behaves. It is the whole that determines in important ways how the parts behave. This means that it won't be the individual ingredients within an unprocessed or processed food that dictate how we respond to it. It will be the entirety of this food that will determine how we respond to the individual ingredients. Adding ingredients found in an orange, carrot, or some other food into our diet is not the same as eating the orange or carrot. The former might or might not be healthful; the latter most assuredly is.

Eating collections of ingredients formulated into highly processed foods isn't the path to better health or sustainable improvements in shape. Real food is the path. It is our job to learn what is and isn't real food. It's also our job to eat more of the former and less, or none, of the latter. Lastly, it's our responsibility to understand that even when it comes to a whole food—an egg, a glass of milk, butter, fish, meat, produce, etc—there can be big qualitative differences between products that share the same name. No one can do any of these things for us. It is up to each of us.

Investigating Your Diet

Of far more importance than how much we eat is what we eat. All calories are not equal. Some calories increase our appetite far more than others. Some are more fattening than others. What we eat will influence how much we eat, and ultimately, our shape. The starting point for improving what you eat is figuring out precisely what you are currently eating. This entails taking inventory of what you eat at every meal. It requires paying attention to the ingredients on a food label. It means educating yourself on what any unfamiliar ingredient is and does. And it entails learning more and more about qualitative differences between foods. This is a learning process. It takes time. Food is a *very* big topic. The goal is to get started on what we hope becomes a lifelong process of discovery for you.

You can bring yourself a long way on the path to better shape by learning to detect and avoid certain ingredients. These ingredients are used over and over again as the basis for creating highly palatable processed foods: Their presence on a food label serves as a visible clue. Avoiding these ingredients tends to move your diet strongly in a less palatable, and hence less fattening, direction. If one or more of these ingredients appears on a food, a good general rule of thumb is to either avoid this food entirely or shift it into a *treat* category (something you enjoy once in a while but don't eat regularly).

These ingredients include:

- *Trans-fat containing oils*: Look for hydrogenated oils, partially hydrogenated oils, and vegetable shortenings.
- *Highly refined fats and oils*: Look for commodity oils like corn, canola, cottonseed, and soy. Also look for the listing "may contain one or more of the following" followed by several different types of oils. This phrasing means that the food maker switches which oil is used depending on pricing and availability. The reason the oils listed can be swapped without changing the recipe is because they have undergone so much refining and processing that they are indistinguishable.
- *Caloric sweeteners*: By a wide margin, the two most commonly added caloric sweeteners are sugar and high fructose corn syrup. Sugar can be made to sound healthier using a variety of terms including cane sugar, organic cane juice, or turbinado sugar. Substituting a slightly less refined sugar for a more refined sugar is a baby step in a better direction, but let's not fool ourselves; it is a small baby step. Agave syrup (a high fructose syrup) and fruit juice concentrates are increasingly being used as substitutes for high fructose corn syrup, especially in the natural foods marketplace. Agave and fruit juice concentrate (or fruit juice sweetened) might sound more "natural", but they are, nevertheless, highly processed fructose syrups.
- *Flavor ingredients*: Look out for flavorings, natural and artificial, MSG, the word "hydrolyzed", and artificial sugars.
- *Food colorings*: Colorings are added to food to confuse our visual detection system. Look for words like annatto, caramel coloring, & any color (such as red, usually listed with a number like "red 40").
- *Salt*: Increasing the salty taste improves palatability. Choose versions of food with no added salt when possible.
- *Any ingredient you don't completely understand*: If you don't understand the purpose(s) and ramification(s) of an ingredient, write it down, and find out more about it before you eat a product with it.

Brand is another clue. Nationally advertised brands of foods and beverages are, in many cases, engineered to be palatable. If the foods weren't highly palatable, they would be hard pressed to carve out large enough market shares to merit their advertising budgets;

budgets that are often much larger than all the money spent annually on promoting fruits and vegetables. As a general rule, if your diet consists largely of nationally advertised foods and beverages, you will be eating a highly palatable diet. The same goes for foods sold at fast food restaurants and restaurant chains; they are often, though not always, highly palatable.

The better something tastes, and the more it seems to melt in the mouth, the more palatable it is. In addition to doing a better job in avoiding things that "taste" great, we want to use our powers of detection to monitor texture. Weight loss experts sometimes tell people to chew their food more. This advice misses the mark. When it comes to shape, the problem is not chewing food too few times. It is eating foods that require less chewing. The solution to this isn't chewing what you eat more; it is eating foods that require more chewing. To investigate this aspect of your diet, it is your job to begin to take notice of the texture of what you eat. Does it require a little chewing or a lot? Is it easy to swallow or does it still have gristle, fiber, or other things that make the swallowing process a bit more complicated? Is the texture soft? We want to shift our food choices towards foods, or versions of a food, that require more chewing. Gristle, fiber, skins and other constituents that make the chewing processes more complex aren't things to be avoided; we want to eat things that are hardier. When it comes to shape, the most important things to avoid are foods that have been made to be fattening. This does not mean avoiding natural foods—unprocessed foods—which happen to have high amounts of fat like an avocado, almonds, butter, coconut, olives, etc. It's a mistake to mix up dietary fat with fattening. The former does not always lead to the latter. A food, which naturally has high amounts of fat, is not the same thing as a food with added fat. The former generally improve shape; the latter tends to be fattening. Our investigations in this chapter have identified ingredients and characteristics that make food fattening.

H S I   C L U E

Yogurt, from a texture perspective, is easier to swallow than cheese, but more viscous than milk. But yogurt, because it is a *fermented food*—made with a starter culture—has shape effects that are not entirely predicted by its calories and texture. In experiments, eating yogurt is far healthier and makes a more positive impact on shape, than its calories or texture would predict. The starter culture used to ferment milk into yogurt changes this food and has its own complex effect on our body. The net result is that yogurt, like many fermented foods, has an effect that is more than the sum of its parts.

Investigating for these things, not things we might have previously thought were the problem, is the goal.

The *Heuristics* Solution

Most of us use one to a few simple rules of thumb to guide food decisions. A synonym for rules of thumb is *heuristic*—a loose strategy that helps us come up with a rapid solution to a dilemma. Our brain uses heuristics for all manner of complicated decisions. In some instances, we will be consciously aware that we used a heuristic. In most instances, we won't: They will be running in the background. We are born with some heuristics. The preference for sweet and aversion to bitter tastes is an example. The rule of thumb is, if it is sweet, eat it; if it is bitter, don't. We can watch an infant's food behaviors and see this heuristic in action. An infant is not consciously aware of using this loose strategy to make food choices; nor did they learn it. Similar to an infant, adults will rarely be consciously aware of using food heuristics. Unlike with a newborn infant, the ones we use are often acquired; they have been learned.

Heuristics are used to simplify decision-making, taking what would otherwise be a difficult problem and chopping it down to a more manageable size. This is often done by focusing on a single attribute of the problem, rather than on the entirety of the dilemma. This simplification process can be observed with *diet heuristics*— commonly used rules of thumb for selecting what to eat when the goal is weight loss. With the state of current nutritional science it is impossible to know everything about even a single food, much less *all* possible foods. There is also no way to perfectly predict how your shape will respond to eating anything until after it is eaten. And after eating a food, it would require measuring and tracking small or subtle changes to learn what the food actually did. Because of these and many other hurdles, the decision about what to eat for weight loss is complicated. Most people don't spend even a moment trying to compute the answers to all of the questions that would need answering. They take a shortcut, simplifying the problem, by focusing on a few readily available attributes of a food. They might use the *low-fat or fat-free heuristic*. This rule of thumb goes something like; when in doubt choose the item lowest in fat. They might use its close cousin, the *low-calorie heuristic*. Choose the food lowest in calories. Whether we use one, both, or some other simple decision making rules of thumb, we are usually using some heuristic(s) to solve the *what to eat* problem.

Heuristics are not intended to be perfect; they are intended to help us make a good enough decision quickly. Sometimes they do this; other times they don't. Many of the most widely used food heuristics in our society fall into the latter camp. They don't improve shape. At best they are neutral, and at worst, they worsen shape. They are akin to Holmes's obvious facts, being, in a phrase, common sense. But Holmes did not use the term obvious facts in a flattering way. He used it to describe educated guesses, intuitive judgments, and popularly held notions that sounded right, but actually interfered with solving a problem. The food heuristics many of us use act in much the same way. They seem like they should work but they don't. To impact our shape positively through food usually requires abandoning the heuristics we have been using and learning some new, better ones.

Our world has *lots* of information. This poses several dilemmas. When there is a lot to learn, it takes a lot, in terms of time, effort, or both to learn it. Having access to lots of information, can also lead to a tendency towards using much, or all of it, to make decisions. We complicate the decision-making process. It seems obvious that using a complicated decision-making strategy that takes advantage of large amounts of information would lead to better decisions. It can; it often doesn't. When behavioral scientists have compared the actual results of complicated decision strategies to ones that rely on simpler aspects of a problem, heuristics often win: Simple loose strategies can outperform more complicated ones, leading to better decisions. Decision-making can suffer as much from too much information as it would from too little. The goal is to strike the correct balance, focusing on only the most *pertinent* information. This is what a useful heuristic will do.

Before we list a few heuristics you might want to practice, let's discuss a few you might consider *unlearning*. We have already mentioned two—the *low-fat or fat-free heuristic* and the *low-calorie*

HSI CLUE

Michael Pollan, author of *The Botany of Desire*, *The Omnivore's Dilemma* and *In Defense of Food*, has been writing about food for more than a decade. This left him wiser, but how could he pass this wisdom to his readers? As he writes in the *New York Times* article 'Unhappy Meals', "[he opted for a] few (flagrantly unscientific) rules of thumb, collected in the course of my nutritional odyssey... [to]at least point us in the right direction." He chose to give his readers heuristic solutions.

heuristic. Making a food choice based on how much fat or calories something has is a naïve rule of thumb. It will cause us to avoid many foods that are great for our shape and get us to replace these real foods with ones that aren't. These rules of thumb also focus on *quantitative* attributes of food. The goal, when it comes to food, is to move away from focusing on quantitative clues while shifting our focus to *qualitative* attributes.

The next heuristic to be aware of is called the *recognition heuristic.* This heuristic would lead to a decision-making strategy of: If you recognize one object but not another, choose the recognized one. Our instincts are to go with what we already know or have heard of. We are prone to believe that something we recognize is in some way better, safer, or of higher quality. In many areas, there is significant correlation between recognition and quality. Unfortunately, food is not one of them. Many of the most recognizable food items in North America are highly palatable foods, not high quality foods. Brand-name recognition and a familiar label, not the quality of the item, cause us to prefer it. Blindly following the *recognition heuristic* generally leads to two behaviors that can hinder shape outcomes:

1. We choose nationally recognized brands of foods and beverages; which are often engineered to be highly palatable and contain several, often many, ingredients that have been identified as being shape negative in this chapter.
2. We choose to eat things we have already eaten—familiar foods—which, if our shape is not what we desire, are often part of the problem.

The next loose strategy we can be done, or undone by is the *follow the herd heuristic.* This heuristic boils down to: Watch what others are doing and do the same thing. We learn from and copy other people, both consciously and unconsciously. We have a tendency towards conformity. Other peoples' actions can have big influences on ours. This can be good; it can also be bad. With foods, since the items consumed by many North Americans contribute to shape challenges, following the herd gets us into trouble. We can use this tendency to our advantage if we surround ourselves with one or more persons, preferably a community of people, who are committed to eating higher quality foods and making more informed food decisions. We don't want to blindly follow the crowd; we do want to surround ourselves with a crowd that, with our eyes wide open, we would want to follow.

Now that we have discussed a few loose decision-making strategies to avoid, or at least to be aware of, it's time to discuss some that are worth consciously implementing. The goal of these heuristics is to make it easier to select foods that are less palatable, and hence, less fattening. The heuristics listed are broadly divided into two categories: Rules of thumb intended to get us to change our overall approaches to eating, and rules of thumb designed to get us to focus on more pertinent information about a food. The goal of the former is to use these loose strategies to change our *behaviors* around food and eating in ways that will better support our desired shape. The goal of the latter is to use this information as the basis of making individual food choices.

Eat calories; don't drink them. We want you to eat food, not drink calories. The easiest way to move in a positive direction is to make water your primary beverage, using it to replace servings of soft drinks, fruit juices, fruit drinks, energy drinks, and shakes, as examples. Have one to two large glasses of water immediately after waking, and another one to two with each meal. This rule of thumb does not mean you should avoid soups.

> **HSI CLUE**
>
> One of Pollan's rules of thumb rephrased is: If your great-great-grandmother would have recognized something as food, eat it. If she wouldn't, don't. Pollan offers many other rules of thumb in his writing. We encourage you to read his book *Food Rules: An Eater's Manual* to discover some of his other favorite rules of thumb.

Choose foods that require more chewing; avoid easy-to-swallow calories: Unprocessed foods require more chewing before they can be swallowed, so the easiest way to improve in this area is to eat whole foods. As you eat familiar foods, try new foods, eat at home or out at restaurants, pay attention to whether things seem to melt in your mouth. If they do, choose something else. Do your best to find versions of food that require more chewing. Using peanuts as an example, this would mean eating peanuts rather than peanut butter. If you do choose peanut butter, it would mean choosing a crunchy peanut butter instead of smooth peanut butter.

Consume foods; avoid collections of ingredients: Food is what we want to eat, collections of ingredients, well, not so much. Many foods are easily identified. A fruit, a vegetable, brown rice, a piece of fish, a cup of plain yogurt would be items a person from several hundred years ago would have recognized as food. They are still food.

Some things in supermarkets are entirely made from collections of processed ingredients. Pollan describes these as edible food-like substances. They might not list a single thing under the ingredients section of a food label that someone from several hundred years ago would recognize as food. Many items fall between these extremes. The goal is to eat fewer and fewer ingredients and more and more actual food.

Eat meals, minimize grazing and snacking: Meals are what we want to eat more of (many of us don't eat enough). Snacks are what we want to eat less of (many of us snack too much). In the 25-year period between 1977 and 2002, the percentage of Americans eating three or more snacks daily increased from 11 percent to 42 percent. The percentage of us eating three or more meals daily plummeted. The goal is to, as an individual, reverse this trend. If you do snack, good choices include soup, fruits, vegetables, nuts, cheese, yogurt, or other items that are real foods and would be at home as part of a complete meal.

Consume at least one flavor-lite serving of calories a day, away from all other food:. A flavor-lite food is something with little to no scent. Many real foods will qualify as long as they don't have any added flavor ingredients. A cup of plain yogurt would qualify. The same is true for a baked potato eaten on its own or a serving of brown rice. Eat at least one serving, preferably large enough to be meal-like, of a low flavor real food by itself away from other foods daily. Seth Roberts' extra light olive oil protocol would also qualify (described earlier in the chapter).

Increase the variety of foods eaten in a month; decrease the variety of foods eaten in a meal or a day: Many of us eat a variety of highly palatable foods (including meals, snacks, and beverages), if not at every meal, at least every day. We also eat a relatively narrow range of foods overall: We eat the same familiar, often highly palatable, foods over and over again. This approach to variety is a recipe for poor shape. To improve our shape, we want to turn variety on its head, so to speak. The goal is to eat a narrower range of foods, especially palatable foods, in a meal or during a single day, while increasing the variety of whole foods we eat in a week or a month. This can be accomplished by eating simpler meals (fewer different foods each eating episode) each day, but more complex menus over a week or month (see the next heuristic). We also do this by eating a greater diversity of fruits, vegetables, nuts, cheeses, meats, whole grains, and other whole unprocessed foods over the course of several weeks to a month.

Keep individual meals as simple as possible: Jon Franklin said, "Simplicity, carried to an extreme, becomes elegance." The most elegant diet is one made up of a variety of simple whole foods, combined a few at a time during each meal, with different meals relying on different simple foods. The result of this approach is simplicity of nutrients, flavors, and foods at a single meal, and complexity of nutrients, flavors, and foods in our overall menu. When thinking in terms of meal simplicity, it can be helpful to place things on a continuum. A meal consisting entirely of hard-boiled eggs, or any other single whole food, would be as simple as it gets. A *Cafeteria Diet* situation—all-you-can-eat buffets, cafeterias with many food choices, etc—if indulged in, represents the other end of this continuum. Each single food item we add to a meal increases its complexity by a factor of one. Hardboiled eggs, plain yogurt, and a piece of fruit would be 3 simple items—a simplicity rating of 3. A yogurt with many ingredients, sweetened and flavored, even though it is a single thing in terms of coming in one container, might be far more complicated. Multi-ingredient items—foods with many ingredients, a condiment like ketchup or steak sauce, a pre-made salad dressing, etc—can complicate the meal exponentially. They don't count as adding a single thing; they add all of the separate ingredients they contain to the meal. At a single meal, eating a few single ingredient foods, results in a relatively simple meal. Adding a single complicated condiment to even a single food might result in a far more complicated meal. With the above in mind, the goal is to, without being neurotic, simplify at each meal—move the eating episode a bit towards the simpler end of the continuum. The goal isn't to make eating devoid of pleasure. Do your best to, when it comes to a meal, apply the Albert Einstein quote, "Make everything as simple as possible, but not simpler". This might mean using fewer condiments. It might mean putting one fewer thing on your plate. It might include skipping desert or having water instead of a soft drink. Start small and progressively simplify.

Keep only one "treat" in the home at a time: It's fine to enjoy a dessert, favorite snack, or other items that fall into the "treat" category occasionally. An occasional treat won't make or break most shape efforts. If you are going to be having treats consistently, since you won't be significantly decreasing the quantity, it is important to significantly decrease the variety. One way to accomplish this is to pick one treat to keep around your home, and for a few weeks at a time, make this item your staple treat. If you want a different treat during this time, it's fine to enjoy it, if you are willing to make a special trip to buy it.

HSI CLUE

Spices including black pepper, Chile pepper, cinnamon, ginger, licorice, and turmeric have shape benefits. This does not mean you should add these flavors to your diet. It means you should consider adding the actual spices—the root, bark, herb, etc—to your diet. Cinnamon flavor and cinnamon are not the same. The candy called licorice is not the same as the spice called licorice. The candy might or might not have any actual licorice in it, and it most certainly has other ingredients, some of which might be better avoided.

Trust foods that humans have been eating for centuries and be suspicious of "new" food innovations: If your great-great grandmother would have recognized something as food, eat it. If she wouldn't, don't. Application of this rule of thumb would lead to being suspicious of margarine, egg substitutes, and other foods that are engineered as substitutes for real foods. It's not only fine, but recommended to eat oily parts of fish, high fat foods like avocados, coconut, or olives, and nuts and seeds. Fat is not the enemy; new fangled fats are.

Eat foods that have been processed using traditional methods; be suspicious of modern shortcuts: Since the most universal traditional form of food processing is fermentation, let's use fermentation to illustrate this point. Examples of fermented foods include yogurt, buttermilk, sourdough bread, soy sauce, miso, and traditionally made sauerkraut. To ferment a food, a starter culture is needed. Starter cultures for dairy are usually lactobacillus or other probiotic bacteria. Fermented soy products, including soy sauce, often use koji as a starter culture. The clue to whether a food has been fermented is the listing of a starter culture under ingredients. Words such as "cultured" or "fermented" are also clues. Fermented soy sauces are available, but most soy sauce in supermarkets isn't fermented: They are made by modern methods, usually protein hydrolysis. The result is two different products, which both share the soy sauce name, one of which— fermented soy sauce—has anti-cancer compounds; the other— hydrolyzed soy sauce—contains carcinogens. The way soy sauce, and other products, is made makes a qualitative difference in the product. Traditional food processing has generally stood the test of time. New methods haven't.

Flavor foods yourself; minimize or avoid pre-flavored items. Flavor includes the taste and the scent. Highly palatable foods add taste ingredients—sweeteners, fats, salt, MSG (or similar free glutamate ingredients)—and scent ingredients—natural or artificial flavors. One of the strongest steps we can take to make our diet less palatable, but still very enjoyable, is to take over the role of flavoring our foods ourselves. Rather than buying something with an added sweetener—usually sugar or high fructose corn syrup—buy an unsweetened version of the food, and if the item is not sweet enough for you, add your own sweetener (preferably honey, a less refined sugar (such as rapadura sugar), or real maple syrup). The same goes for salt; buy versions of foods that are unsalted and add a salty taste by salting it yourself with an unrefined salt, or sprinkling it with traditionally brewed (fermented) soy sauce. Fermented soy sauce, miso, and wine are great ways to add the savory taste to foods. Lemons, limes, lemon grass, or apple cider vinegar add a sour taste. Use butter, extra virgin olive oil, or other natural fats for a fatty taste. Scent chemicals—natural and artificial flavors—are ubiquitous in processed foods. Anything can be made to taste like anything. But the goal isn't to have anything taste like a blueberry or strawberry, as examples. The goal is to have only one thing in your diet with a blueberry flavor, a blueberry. The same goes for the strawberry flavor. Get it from strawberries. The best way to overhaul the flavor component of the diet is to scale way back on foods that have natural or artificial flavors as ingredients. Replace them with "plain" versions of foods and add the flavors yourself by adding whole foods, the blueberry or strawberry. As a single example, this would mean buying plain yogurt, instead of a flavored yogurt, and adding fruit to it.

Make food decisions based on quality, not quantity: One of the better methods for decreasing the quantity of what we eat is to improve the quality of what we eat. We accomplish this by ceasing to be overly concerned about the number of calories or grams of fat and instead learning (1) whether the calories come from food, or, in the words of Michael Pollan, edible food-like substances, (2) what processing has been done to the calories, and (3) what ingredients make up the calories. A serving of margarine and a serving of olive oil might have an identical amount of calories and fat, yet be qualitatively extremely different. All olive oil is not the same. Some is better than others. The same goes for all real foods, products made from them and even items closer to the edible food-like substances end of the continuum. The goal is to choose the highest quality version of food available to us on as many eating occasions as possible.

There are two ways to approach food quality. We can learn more and more about individual foods; using the information we acquire to guide eating decisions. There are very few areas that merit the time and effort food merits, so this area is a tremendously worthwhile investment. One of the better resources for improving our knowledge in this area is Marion Nestle's book *What To Eat*. Another option is our free online ebook resource on Food Quality (the *Food Quality Traffic Light Guide*) available at our website. A third option would to be to enroll in our online Food Investigation course (this course has a fee). The message boards (forums) at our website, as well as at culinary websites, can also be valuable resources for improving our food IQ. Improving our knowledge on what does and doesn't constitute quality choices is one approach. But, even if we are committed to this approach, we will still need to be eating while we are acquiring new information. Having good rules of thumb can be an indispensable interim crutch, as well as a time saving shortcut even when we have lots of information. Placing a series of rules of thumb into a fast and frugal *decision tree* can be even better.

A decision tree is a series of sequential questions. Ideally, each question in the tree forces us to consider one piece of pertinent information—one reason. We start with the first question: If it allows us to make a decision, we make it. If it doesn't, we move to the next question, considering the next piece of information, and whether or not it allows us to make a decision. At each level of the tree the goal is take the best available option. If there is clear winner, we stop. If there isn't, we continue down the tree. Decision trees aren't intended to make a perfect choice every time. They are intended to help simplify the decision making process and to help us make a sound choice most of the time.

The rules of the game for the food quality decision tree below are as follows:

- This decision tree asks only yes-no questions.
- The questions are in descending order of importance. The first question is a better clue to high quality food than the second, which is a better clue than the third, etc.
- When using the decision tree the goal is to identify a food product and then use the tree to consider it as well as *similar* competing products.
- If at any point the answer to a question is a clear yes, stop and choose the food option that allows for the yes answer.
- If the answer is no, or if you are unsure of how to answer the question for the particular food item, go to the next question down in the sequence.
- The more levels you descend, the more likely that the food item you are considering is lower in quality and higher in palatability, hence more likely to be fattening.
- Questions will point you toward what is, and by extension isn't, pertinent information. It's up to you to actually obtain the information about a food item.
- If you find yourself unable to answer a question about food, be inquisitive. Ask questions, look things up, and by all means learn more.

The Fast and Frugal Food Quality Decision Tree
1. Did you grow it, raise it, catch it, or make it from whole real foods yourself?
2. Could you visit, within a reasonable drive, the place where the food was grown (for produce), raised (for meat, eggs, dairy, etc), or caught?
3. For meat or dairy products, is the food labeled as "grass-fed"? For seafood is it "wild caught" (as opposed to farmed)?
4. Is the food visibly the same as it would be in nature—unmodified in any way by processing? [Note: If it is, select the most colorful version of the food available.]
5. Is this a plain—unsweetened, unsalted, and unflavored—version of the food?
6. Would your great-great grandmother recognize every ingredient in the item?
7. Are all of the ingredients organic?

8. Is the food product free of high fructose corn syrup, sugar, artificial sweeteners, hydrogenated/partially hydrogenated oils, commodity oils (canola, corn, cottonseed, palm, peanut, soy, or sunflower), mono- and/or diglycerides, natural or artificial flavors, and MSG-like flavor enhancers?
9. Does this product have fewest ingredients than other similar products?
10. Will this product require more chewing than other similar products?
11. Is it packaged in glass rather than plastic or a can?

Let's give a few examples of how this decision tree might work using peanuts and peanut products as examples.

Example 1: Should I choose peanuts in the shell or canned or bottled peanuts?
Since few of us grow our own peanuts, and most of us won't live in areas where peanuts are grown, the first two questions in this example would be answered with no. In nature, peanuts come in a shell, not in a can. When we ask ourselves question #4, peanuts in the shell become the clear winner so we choose and eat them.

Example 2: Which bottled, canned or packaged peanuts should I buy?
For this example, imagine that our choices are between (1) a leading brand of canned peanuts made with peanuts, peanut and/or cottonseed oil and salt as ingredients; (2) a leading brand of bottled dry roasted peanuts made with peanuts, sea salt, sugar, cornstarch, monosodium glutamate, gelatin, torula yeast, corn syrup solids, paprika, onion and garlic powders, spices, and natural flavor; and (3) a less well known brand of dry roasted peanuts that only contains peanuts (no added salt, sugars, oils, etc.). The best choice in this case would be option (3). We would not be able to get to a clear answer until question #5, but at that point the winner would be crystal clear.

Example 3: What if I wanted to decide between the leading brand of canned peanuts and bottled dry roasted peanuts described in example 2?
Great-great grandmother would not have recognized cottonseed oil as food so the canned peanuts receive a no to question #6. The same goes for several of the ingredients in the bottled dry roasted peanuts. Both also get a no answer for question #7 because all of the ingredients aren't organic and a no answer for question #8 because of one or more ingredients. This brings us to question # 9,

which leads to picking the canned peanuts because they have fewer ingredients.

Example 4: Should I buy a crunchy or smooth (creamy) version of a leading brand of peanut butter?
Let's assume that everything about the two types of peanut butters is the same. The ingredients are identical: Both have added sugar, salt, mono and diglycerides, and hydrogenated oils. No matter which we choose we will be eating a highly palatable food. The first question that separates the two is question #10. Our best choice of two relatively low quality choices, in this case, would be crunchy peanut butter since it will require a bit more chewing.

Example 5: Should I buy a leading brand of crunchy peanut butter or an organic crunchy peanut butter?
For this example, the organic crunchy peanut butter contains organic dry roasted peanuts, organic palm oil, organic cane juice, and sea salt. The leading brand in this instance contains roasted peanuts, sugar, hydrogenated vegetable oils, and salt. Both products contain sugar and salt. The organic brand in this instance dresses these ingredients up a bit by calling the sugar "organic cane juice". It is open to debate whether your great-great grandmother would recognize "organic cane juice" as an ingredient. She might but she probably wouldn't. It is a new way of describing sugar. This leaves us with question #7. Since all of the ingredients are organic, select the organic crunchy peanut butter. While the organic peanut butter will be a better choice, let's not fool ourselves into thinking it is a great choice in this case. Even though it's organic, it's still engineered to be highly palatable; containing the taste triad described by Kessler—sweet (organic cane juice), salty, and fatty (because of the peanuts). It has also been processed into a more palatable texture/consistency—peanut butter rather than peanuts. Less palatable organic peanut butter options exist. Example 6 illustrates.

H S I C L U E

Food and beverage cans are coated on the inside with epoxy resin to prevent corrosion and contamination. These resins often contain bisphenol A, which can migrate into foods. In November 2009, Consumer Reports tested for the presence of bisphenol A in leading brands, including organic versions of canned soups, juice, tuna, and green beans. Bisphenol A was found in most of the tested products. If you desire to minimize your chemical exposure, cutting back on canned foods is a smart choice.

Example 6: Which brand of organic crunchy peanut butter should I buy?
In this instance the choices are the peanut butter in example 5 (organic dry roasted peanuts, organic palm oil, organic cane juice, and sea salt) and an organic crunchy peanut butter with only 1 ingredient—organic roasted peanuts. Question #5 picks a clear winner, the latter peanut butter, which has no added sugars or salt.

The above examples are intended to provide guidance in how to apply the decision tree. In areas where there's lots of information—food for example—some of which is helpful and much of which is distracting, learning to pay attention to the most pertinent information can improve decision-making. The decision tree is intended to help get you to the most pertinent information and help with decision-making. It isn't intended to replace the need for learning more about food and what makes one item higher quality than another.

When it comes to answering the what to eat question, many of us use either familiarity (brand recognition, past behaviors, etc), a few pieces of information—total calories or grams of fat; buzzwords (like "natural", "diet", "organic", "low-fat", etc), or label claims (like "heart healthy")—or some combination of all of these to guide decisions. There is nothing inherently wrong with familiarity or using a few pieces of information as the basis for decisions. The problem is when we confuse familiarity with better quality, or when the few pieces of information we use as the basis for our decision aren't the most pertinent bits of information. The most visible aspects on food products—branding, product names, images, buzzwords, and health claims—is information, but it often isn't the information that allows for making the best predictions about actual product quality. Familiar brand names, images that give the impression of farms or fresh produce, buzzwords, and other aspects on the front of a food label are skillfully designed to play to our emotions; to comfort our brain into believing we have made sound choices. With few exceptions, the front of the label won't contain either sufficient information or the most pertinent pieces of information. Our investigation into this area has revealed that there is a big gap between what a consumer believes the words and images on the front of a food label mean and what they actually do mean. It has revealed instances of misrepresentation—errors of omission and errors of commission. Rarely will the front of a label reveal all of the information needed to legitimately measure quality. Quality begins with how something is raised and grown. It doesn't end there. It is a big topic. Please don't allow yourself to be distracted by what amounts to *obvious facts*. Investigate.

Conclusion

Diets with the same exact amount of calories can have very different effects on shape, body fat, muscle mass, metabolism, and voluntary food intake (appetite). It is not so much how much we are eating, but what we are eating that is the core issue when it comes to food and shape. We could feed two genetically identical people an equal amount of calories, but if one ate highly palatable calories and the other didn't, we would expect them to defend very different natural weights. Calories are an incidental clue; the source of the calories is vital. If we eat certain foods, we will be fatter, weaker, and crave foods that do not support our shape and health goals even if these foods are produced to be low in calories. Yet if we eat different foods, even foods that might be higher in calories, we could end up leaner, stronger, and find it easier to eat healthy foods. When it comes to our shape all calories are not created equal. There are certain ingredients/foods that, when included in our diet, keep us leaner and healthier. When these foods are dropped from the diet, we tend to crave fattening foods, get lazy, gain weight and experience diminished health. There are other foods that, as long as they are included in the diet, contribute to making us fatter and less healthy than we would be without them. If we want to improve our shape in a sustainable manner we need to discover which ingredients in foods and beverages lower natural weight and eat (drink) more of them. And we need to discover which ingredients in foods and beverages increase natural weight and eat (and drink) much less (or none) of these items. We also need to discover whether other aspects of food make a difference when it comes to natural weight. Texture is one of these "other aspects". The most important question, when it comes to food and beverages will never be how many calories, grams of fat, or carbohydrate the food or beverage might have. It is how and where it was grown or raised, what ingredients it has, its texture, the types and extent of processing it has undergone, its flavor, its bite-to-bite consistency, and other factors that are far from obvious. These aren't quantitative clues; they are qualitative clues.

What our body really needs is high quality real food. We need its texture, its tastes, and its nutrition. Real food sends powerful messages to our body that can't be duplicated in a lab with designer ingredients. When we alter the textures, tastes, and compositions of what we eat, when we add concentrated ingredients that enhance taste, extend shelf-life, increase palatability, and cater to some scientist's sense of nutrition, we rapidly head in the wrong direction with our shapes. It is up to each of us to make a course correction.

Closing Dialogue

Health Scene Investigator: Now that we have reviewed the evidence for food and shape, what are your thoughts?

Apprentice: My first thought is that most of us, me included prior to our investigation, focus on the wrong things when it comes to food. I have made many of my food decisions because an item is lower in fat or calories and never paid attention to what made it lower.

Health Scene Investigator: You are not alone. Many of us have been deceived by obvious facts when it comes to what we eat. But the question is not only what you have done; it is also what you will do moving forward. Where we are is important. The direction we are heading can be even more important.

Apprentice: Moving forward I am going to learn far more about food. I will become more informed on what constitutes food quality. And I will act on this information.

Health Scene Investigator: A commendable goal. Food merits thoughtful investigation. It is up to each of us to be participants in this investigation because the food industry has their own, not our interests in mind. And their interests and ours are not always aligned.

Apprentice: Is this your way of hinting that I should expect to uncover some inconsistencies and deceptions as I educate myself and become more informed?

Health Scene Investigator: I think that would be a fair expectation. I also want to encourage you to think of your education with food in terms of a statement Holmes made in *The Red Circle*; "Education never ends. It is a series of lessons with the greatest for last." With this quote in mind, let's go to lunch.

Chapter 20

The Mystery of Food Instincts

All my instincts are one way, and all the facts are the other, and I much fear that British juries have not yet attained that pitch of intelligence when they will give the preference to my theories over Lestrade's facts

Sherlock Holmes

Opening Dialogue

Health Scene Investigator: Our last lesson will be the selection of lunch. I have had a variety of appetizers, entrees, and desserts prepared. They are laid out on the table before you. The question for you is two-fold. The first question is, "What are you going to eat?" Please show me by putting the items you intend on eating on a plate.

Apprentice: (Fills a plate with food).

Health Scene Investigator: How did you choose what you took to eat?

Apprentice: Well, I looked at all the foods, divided some into healthy choices and others as unhealthy, and then did my best to choose mostly healthy items.

Health Scene Investigator: Ah. You took an intellectual approach. Can you think of some other way you could have gone about selecting what to eat for lunch?

Apprentice: I am not sure what you mean.

Health Scene Investigator: We can use intellectual intelligence to select foods. We can also use instinctual intelligence. Let me explain.

About Instincts

In the opening quote (from *The Norwood Builder*) Holmes wasn't calling the jury stupid, but he feared that, when it came to detection, they had not developed similar instinctive faculties to his *yet*. And because they hadn't, they would instead opt for something that more closely matched their less developed instincts, *obvious facts* that, in this instance, would be wrong.

HSI CLUE

Appetite, food cravings, metabolism, and other aspects of the biobehavioral defense of shape are not under volitional control. We can't control any of these things and can't even consciously monitor most of them. If we can't monitor our energy deposits and withdrawals accurately, never mind adjusting finer details of metabolism, what makes us think we can keep track of something like calories with anywhere near the precision needed to regulate shape?

In a strict sense, an instinct is an *unlearned* inborn complex behavior. Holmes wasn't using instinct in this way; he was describing something more akin to educated guesses, hunches, intuitions, or gut feelings. We'll also use instinct in this looser sense. These types of instincts are complicated processes, relying on aspects of the conscious and unconscious. They are often dependent on past experiences, education, and training. This can be seen in the *Case of Temperature*. People raised in the United States have an instinctual grasp of what 75°F means. They might not feel as sure how hot or cold it is if we told them the temperature was 24°C. The instincts are reversed in a person raised in a country using metric units. While 75°F and 24°C are two different ways to describe what is essentially the same temperature, our instinctual grasp of what these numbers mean is going to be influenced by the temperature education we have received in the *past*. This principle applies to other areas where instincts play a big role. One of these areas is food. Humans have the capacity for food instincts, but our *expertise* in this area will be strongly influenced by how our palate has been educated.

Complex adaptive intelligence learns and draws inferences about our world, using past experience to make best guesses. These best guesses can sometimes be felt as intuitions or instincts. They are automatic and represent an instinctual intelligence. This is a very different form of intelligence than reflective, thinking about things or figuring it out, intelligence. Instinctual and reflective intelligence are different approaches each have strengths and weaknesses. As a generality, instinctual intelligence is better when it comes to solving complex problems where (1) computation would be extensive, (2) there are lots of variables to consider, (3) access to the information needed to make the computation is imprecise or unavailable, and (4) feedback on our decisions is remote. Food and shape is an area where all of these issues apply.

William Bennett, M.D., and Joel Gurin make this point in their book *Dieter's Dilemma*, arguing that trying to manage weight by taking a reflective approach—counting calories—isn't as easy as it sounds. They write: "Consider what it would take, theoretically, to gain ten pounds in one year—the fastest rate at which most normal adults ever gain weight, except those coming off a diet. This gain requires no more than 100 "extra" calories a day. The excess amounts to one tablespoon of butter *or* a plain muffin without butter *or* a pear *or* a cup of minestrone *or* a biscuit of shredded wheat. And the caloric mistake is not being made at a single meal. It is spread out over an entire day in which 2,000 to 3,000 calories are being consumed and burned away. A few extra flakes of cereal at breakfast, three more bites of cheese at lunch, a couple of Life Savers in the afternoon, a chicken breast instead of a drumstick at dinner—and the jig is up. Indeed, this error is so subtle that a trained nutritionist, shadowing someone all day long, could not guess to within 300 to 400 calories how much the subject had eaten."

If a trained nutritionist can't accurately figure out how many calories are being consumed, what hope does an average person really have? As Bennett and Gurin point out, accurately figuring out how many calories we eat is where computation issues begin. Figuring out how many calories one uses in a day is even more complicated. We need to know precisely how much energy is used for every daily task and activity. We would need to keep track of how long we did each thing. We would have to have some way of knowing how much energy our body is using for all of our internal processes. We would have to invest the mental energy into making these calculations every day and balancing the amount we use against how many calories we consumed. This would be an immense amount of computational work. Even if we could access all of this information and were willing to do all of the needed calculations, things would still breakdown because of complex adaptation. Many of the variables we would need to gather for our computations aren't constant; they are constantly changing. As Bennett and Gurin so aptly conclude: "It strains belief to think that people—even those who lead very well regulated lives—can supervise their own weight with anything like the precision commonly achieved by non-dieters". Consciously making the necessary fine adjustments in food intake simply cannot be done…"

Bennett and Gurin believe that an internal automatic system of some sort must exist that can do all of this for us. This is akin to what we refer to as Shape Intelligence; a system designed to precisely supervise shape *automatically*. We don't need to make all the necessary fine adjustments in food intake and activity levels to precisely self-regulate shape because we have an intelligence that makes these adjustments for us. Shape Intelligence can strongly influence what and how much is eaten. Evidence for this inference has been discussed in previously described cases. The question is not whether it can do this; it is how expertly it *is* doing this important job.

Expertise is acquired. Holmes developed a high level of it when it came to detection. Lestrade had not acquired the same "pitch of intelligence": The jury even less so. As a result, Holmes' instincts and the jury's were likely to take them in different directions. The same principle applies to food instincts. Aside from the few innate taste biases an infant is born with, our palate starts out as a blank slate. Each time we eat, especially in early life, we educate it. The food instincts we have by late childhood are acquired by this education process. We have the capacity for intelligent food instincts, but it must be acquired.

Cases of Food Instincts

In the 1920s and 1930s, Dr. Clara M. Davis performed an experiment intended to test whether young children had food instincts. Fifteen children, ranging in age from newly weaned infants to about four years old, were placed in a specially designed orphanage where the amount of every single thing eaten or spilled at all meals was recorded. Health and medical data were tracked for each child. All of the children were followed for at least six months, many of them for several years, and two for more than four years. During this observation period, each child, even while in infancy, was allowed to entirely *self-select* what they ate at all meals from 33 different whole foods. Foods included fresh vegetables (both raw and cooked), fruits, whole grains, meats, chicken, fish, organ meats, milk, and fermented (soured) milk. The preparation of each food was kept as simple as possible. At each meal, foods were placed where children could easily access whatever foods they desired. Adults weren't allowed to so much as hint at what should be selected or give any overt or covert feedback that the choices made were good or bad. What happened when children were allowed to entirely self-select what they ate from these whole foods?

Initially, these infants and young children didn't have any observable instincts when a variety of foods, each in a separate dish, were placed before them. Many of them didn't even appear to instinctually know what was and wasn't food; chewing on whatever was in reach including spoons, dishes, trays, or paper. They were, in a sense, blank slates. While they started out with no food instincts, they didn't remain this way for long. In what appeared to be an entirely random process, they smelled and tasted the foods that were offered. Almost every child chose to sample all 33 foods, in most cases several times, during the first few weeks. This random sampling led to strong individual food preferences, many emerging in just days, which guided food choices.

> **HSI CLUE**
>
> None of the self-selected diets were identical. The 15 infants chose what amounted to 15 different diets based on extremely different taste preferences. After observing this Dr. Davis concluded that "Such successful juggling and balancing of the more than 30 nutritional essentials that exist in mixed and different proportions in the foods from which they must be derived suggests at once the existence of some innate, automatic mechanism for its accomplishment."

While the foods offered were not nutritionally foolish, it is easy to imagine that a child could have eaten themselves sick by choosing some of the offered foods to the exclusion of others. This never occurred. The children thrived despite what were extremely varied choices child-to-child, selection of unorthodox combinations of foods (such as a meal consisting entirely of orange juice and liver), and other idiosyncratic food behaviors. While each separate meal wasn't well-balanced, and even for several meals in a row an infant or child might feed largely on one or two items, left to completely self-select a diet, these very young children somehow managed to chose foods over weeks, months, and years that kept them healthy. The medical check-ups provided objective evidence for this inference. That a healthy infant could remain healthy by entirely self-selecting what to eat from a variety of whole foods is noteworthy. There was something that was at least, if not more noteworthy. All of the orphans did not start out healthy. Five had vitamin D deficiency. After using their sensory system—smell and taste—to sample the available foods, these children self-selected a diet that corrected the deficiency. Not only could food instincts keep a healthy infant healthy, they could be used to get an unhealthy child to become healthy.

Dr. Davis's experiment provides evidence for the *emergence* of food instincts. This food wisdom wasn't something the children were born with; they acquired it through sensory experience and a trial and error process of food sampling. This learning took some, but not much time. It was complete for the foods offered within a few weeks. Once sensory experience had been acquired for each item, an internal automatic system appeared to guide food choices flawlessly. It's also important to point out what Dr. Davis's experiment did and didn't show. It showed that when *whole foods* were the sole options available, a healthy diet could be self-selected by infants and young children. It didn't investigate what would occur if *processed foods* were available. Dr. Davis intended to investigate this question, but because of the Great Depression, was unable to. Her writings indicate that she felt processed foods might corrupt food instincts; making them less reliable. We concur with her assumption here.

Dr. Davis isn't the only person to conduct food instinct experiments with children. Leann Birch, Ph.D., Jennifer Fisher, Ph.D., and Susan Johnson, Ph.D. have done a series of experiments to test whether children have the ability to self-regulate food intake. Their findings indicate that children have the potential to accurately compensate for calories. Calorie compensation means (1) if we are given food that is higher in calories, we eat less of it, and (2) if we eat some calories now, we eat fewer later. But just because children *can* compensate for calories, doesn't me they *will* do it, or will do it accurately. Birch, Fisher, and Johnson found that the best predictor of a child's calorie compensation expertise was the parent's approach to feeding. Children, whose parents strictly controlled the child's food intake, showed less expert calorie compensation. A child with parents who allowed a high degree of food autonomy showed greater expertise. The implication is that parents who do not allow children to have some degree of self-determination with regard to food choices and amounts may inadvertently create a situation that results in less expert food instincts.

If a parent is controlling all food-related behaviors, the child presumably doesn't learn to listen to, or trust, their own body: How can they when they are busy listening to their parents? As a result, they don't develop a functional internal food guidance system. And, eventually, they come to rely on the one thing they did learn. External control is the way to select food, only now, they are the ones who must apply this control. And they do. This is the bad news. The good news is that Birch, Fisher, and Johnson have found that children can be taught to focus on internal cues of hunger and satiety, and acquire the expertise to more accurately self-regulate calories.

Birch, Fisher, and Johnson feel that early experiences might be the most critical for the development of food instincts. Dr. Davis's work supports this inference. Research published in the August 2006 issue of the medical journal *Pediatrics* also lends credence to this contention. This study, conducted by doctors from the United Kingdom, suggested that babies whose mothers gave them more autonomy in their early attempts at eating solid food might do a better job of self-regulating their weight. It should not be a surprise that early childhood is such a pivotal period for the development of food instincts. A massive amount of learning occurs during infancy in many areas including language and movement skills. An enormous amount of information must also be acquired about food in what amounts to a very short period of time. Infants are born with a few "unlearned" preferences. They are biased to like sweet or salty tastes and dislike bitter tastes. Everything else, when it comes to food, must be learned.

> **HSI CLUE**
>
> Children and adults can compensate for calories. But Kessler points out, in his book *The End of Overeating,* that "...in the 1980s, children ages two to four were compensating for about 90 percent of any extra calories added to their diet. By the 1990s, they were compensating for only about 45 percent of those added calories." What is causing this change in the ability to compensate accurately? Could it also be contributing to shape problems?

Humans can learn whether foods are higher or lower in calories, and compensate by lowering or increasing their intake accordingly. They can learn the benefits and consequences of foods. Benefits were once mostly, if not entirely nutritional—nutrients and calories. Now, because of engineered palatability and variety, a common benefit is pleasure—the food stimulates reward centers. When a food has a benefit, whether nutritional, reward, or both, it's a lot easier to learn to like it. But this learning doesn't come about by studying food charts, labels, or notes about the benefits of foods. This learning takes place outside of our conscious mind's awareness. The same is true for the application of this learning. We can quickly learn if food offers more or fewer calories per serving and we can automatically adjust the portions we eat accordingly. Studies that touch on this learning capacity offer some useful insights into how this automatic system works. One of these lessons is that we can only learn about things we experience. If we have never eaten a certain food, we won't have any information stored away to draw on when we do encounter it.

HSI CLUE

Birch, Fisher, and Johnson have also found that ingredients like artificial sugars, fat substitutes, flavor additives—things that make it difficult for the body to learn how many calories a food might have—result in poorer compensation. The automatic system appears to have trouble making sense of modern taste and flavor ingredients.

A study highlighting this point was conducted at the University of Bristol in the United Kingdom. Dr. Jeff Brunstrom presented results of the study in a talk he gave entitled *The Role of Learning in Expectations About Satiation and Satiety* at the British Nutrition Foundation's conference held during June 2009. He reported that children, whose parents restricted their consumption of high-calorie snack foods, were more likely to underestimate how many calories snack foods contained, and to eat much larger portions, when they were given these snack foods. Children who had not had an opportunity to *learn* about snack foods did poorly in *predicting* the caloric consequences. Children who had consumed them many times in the past, made far more accurate predictions. Our food instincts will only be as expert as the education our palate has received. But as **Cases of Specific Appetites** indicate, properly educated food instincts are capable of amazing feats.

Cases of Specific Appetites

Scientists refer to the drive to eat things with a specific flavor, or other characteristics, as *specific appetite* (or *specific hunger*). Specific appetite can be highly intelligent. This was apparent in Dr. Davis's experiment. Five of the orphans started the experiment with an existing vitamin D deficiency. Vitamin D had been a missing ingredient, in a quantitative sense, from their previous diets. In two of the infants its level had been so low prior to coming to the orphanage that severe rickets, the vitamin D deficiency disease, had developed. Allowed to completely self-select foods, all five infants, including the two with severe rickets, corrected the deficiency. They did this by, after sampling the variety of foods offered, having a strong preference for the specific foods that were high in vitamin D. One of these foods was cod liver oil. Dr. Davis wrote, "The first infant received for the study was one of the two with severe rickets, and, bound by a promise to do nothing or leave nothing undone to his detriment, we put a small glass of cod liver oil on his tray for him to take if he chose. This he did irregularly and in varying amounts until his blood calcium and phosphorus became normal and x-ray films showed his rickets to be healed, after which he did not take it again." Anyone who has tasted cod liver oil can attest that it isn't the most palatable food. It tastes, in a word, fishy. Any parent who has tried to get their child to take cod liver oil can also attest that it is easier said than done. Yet, in this instance, a specific appetite for cod liver oil—a rich source of vitamin D—emerged when the previous diet was missing this nutrient, and it remained until the nutritional need was fully corrected, after which, it vanished.

Similar to what was observed with vitamin D in Dr. Davis's experiment, when the diet has had a missing substance, animals show a strong appetite preference for the specific foods that contain this substance. This was detected in the *Case of the Thiamin Deficient Rat*. There is a strong bias towards the familiar, and against novelty, when it comes to food. Humans show this bias. So do animals. While this bias is normally evident, there are times of the life cycle and specific circumstances where it disappears, and, in fact, is reversed. One of these circumstances is when the diet is deficient in a needed nutrient. A thiamin (vitamin B1) deficient rat does not show the typical drive towards familiar, and aversion to novel foods. It eagerly tries new foods. If we were to give it free access to a new food that was still low in thiamin, it would show an immediate and marked, but short-lived preference for this food. It seemingly learns quickly that the new food doesn't contain what it needs and loses interest. If a new food is made available and it does contain thiamin, the animal will eat enough of the

HSI CLUE

Allowed to self-select its own food, a thiamin-deficient rat will eat more thiamin-rich foods. It will continue to eat more of these foods until the thiamin deficiency is corrected. Not only does it self-select a wise diet when it comes to getting the substance that was missing, it will often continue to eat higher amounts of thiamin-rich foods even after the deficiency is corrected. It becomes more Scrooge-like with thiamin-rich foods, building in a cushion for thiamin, just in case, which under the circumstances seems intelligent.

food to correct the deficiency and it will develop a lasting preference for the food. It learns to like it. This willingness to reverse course when it comes to exploratory behaviors with food, shunning the familiar and trying new things, allows a rat to potentially find and exploit new sources of the missing nutrient. If it does find a food with the missing substance, it eats more of it. Under the circumstances, these behaviors appear to be intelligent.

Specific appetites for other B vitamins, vitamin C, salt, calcium, magnesium, phosphorous, selenium, zinc, essential omega fats, and amino acids have been demonstrated. Most of the experiments on the specific appetite for missing nutrients have been conducted in animals (rats, mice, domestic livestock like fowl, lambs and pigs, and monkeys). The few human studies indicate that we too have the capability for intelligent specific appetites. Deficiencies in the body, at least when it comes to some nutritionally important substances, produce a specific appetite for foods which can correct the deficiency. With the exception of salt, these specific appetites are not inborn. They arise through a trial and error process that requires sampling of foods.

Could Some Food Cravings Be Intelligent?

It isn't a big stretch to imagine that having a specific appetite for a food that provides a missing vitamin might be the smart thing under the circumstances. It also isn't difficult to imagine that having a craving for watermelon, after being out in the sun all afternoon, might be sensible. The same goes for cravings for other foods that would generally be considered as being healthy. If we crave a healthy food like a fruit, vegetable, or salad, most people have no issues indulging in this craving without viewing it as foolish. The same can't be said for all cravings. Carbohydrate cravings are an example. Many people experience them at one time or another. Some people experience them frequently. Conventional wisdom holds them as being undesirable. This is understandable when what is actually craved is stated more specifically.

When a person has a carbohydrate craving, generally speaking, they don't crave a baked potato or bowl of brown rice. They want refined starches, deserts, sweets, snack foods, or junk foods. It's a lot easier to imagine a craving for a food with a missing nutrient or for watermelon after a hot day in the sun as being intelligent: It's not quite as easy to imagine a specific appetite for carbohydrate-rich, and usually high-fat foods as being intelligent. But what if there was some circumstance that was akin to vitamin deficiency or hot sun, except in this instance, the need it creates isn't satisfied by a food with the missing vitamin or watermelon, respectively, but by fattening foods? If there were this type of circumstance, perhaps carbohydrate cravings might not look so insensible.

A circumstance that appears to fit the bill is sleep deprivation. In investigations conducted on human volunteers, sleep deprivation increases overall appetite but this increase is especially pronounced for foods that (1) are high in carbohydrates, and (2) pack lots of calories in a small serving size. Is what amounts to a craving for high fat, carbohydrate-rich foods actually intelligent under these circumstances? The *Case of the Sleep-Deprived Rats* suggests that it just might be. Total sleep deprivation is stressful. If rats are continuously deprived of all sleep it is fatal without exception. Before dying, the rats will exhibit a variety of symptoms, some of which are suggestive of protein malnutrition. In one experiment, scientists decided to feed sleep-deprived rats a "normal" amount of chow augmented with protein to test whether this could help attenuate the negative consequences of sleep deprivation. They also allowed other sleep-deprived rats to freely eat a diet augmented with calories. If a rat appears to be suffering from protein malnutrition, feeding it a diet higher in protein seems like a sensible thing to do. Was it? Or, was allowing the rats to eat according to their appetite—an appetite that resulted in eating about two and one half times more calories than normal by the end of the experiment—smarter under the circumstances?

> **HSI CLUE**
>
> Water-deprived rats crave carbohydrates. Why? One possible explanation is that water is a by-product of carbohydrate metabolism. If we aren't getting sufficient water to drink, making water from carbohydrates in the body sounds like a pretty intelligent thing to do. Craving carbohydrates might not look like a smart thing, but sometimes appearances are deceiving.

In the *Case of Sleep-Deprived Rats* one group of rats lived much longer than the other. Which group do you think it was? Was it the group that did the "sensible" thing when it came to diet? Or was it the group that "overate"? It turned out that being allowed to eat a "normal" amount of food augmented with extra protein wasn't such a great strategy when it came to survival; eating far more calories was. Rats allowed to indulge their appetite, for what amounted to absurdly large amounts of fattening food, outlived the other rats by

40 percent. Inner intelligence appeared to have had a better sense of what it really needed than outer intelligence (the scientists). Food instincts, even when they led to a behavior that it might be tempting to judge as "bad"—eating lots of high calorie food—helped these animals survive in the face of a stress (sleep deprivation) that would have otherwise killed them much more rapidly.

HSI CLUE

An animal habitually fed a high protein diet will often, if allowed to self-select its food, avoid high protein foods. It will have had its fill of protein and want something else. This is an example of *specific satiation*. If a person gets sick after eating a certain food, even if they liked the food before, they might now want no part of eating it. This is an example of a learned *specific aversion*. When it comes to what we eat, we are always learning.

In *The Boscombe Valley Mystery* Holmes said; "Circumstantial evidence is a very tricky thing. It may seem to point very straight to one thing, but if you shift your own point of view a little, you may find it pointing in an equally uncompromising manner to something entirely different." When rats, and as it turns out humans, are deprived of sleep, there tends to be a large increase in hunger and specific cravings for high-fat, carbohydrate-rich foods. The knee-jerk reaction to carbohydrate cravings is usually to assume it points towards a behavior that needs to be resisted or corrected. Yet, in the *Case of Sleep-Deprived Rats*, when our point of view is changed to include the bigger picture—survival—the same observation, of eating large amounts of fattening foods, seems to point in an entirely different direction. Instead of appearing to be foolish, it now seems to have been the smart thing to do.

Context is a powerful influence on behavior. We can crave a food, even if it is a food we might judge as a "bad" choice, because eating it is the intelligent thing to do under the circumstances. Carbohydrate cravings often emerge when a person does not get enough sleep. In animal experiments, water deprivation causes carbohydrate cravings. In persons with seasonal mood disorders— SAD—short days can lead to carbohydrate cravings. Carbohydrates can be craved at other times when we are feeling blue. And, in many of these circumstances, indulging the craving might be the sensible thing to do, tantamount to self-medication. While it might not be the optimal strategy for correcting things, it might be a better strategy than doing nothing. A carbohydrate craving is probably best interpreted as making the best of a bad situation. It might be intelligent under circumstances such as sleep or water deprivation, but a far more intelligent thing would be for us to meet the actual need—get more sleep or drink more water, respectively.

Cravings can be intelligent. This doesn't mean they're always intelligent. Given free access to delicious milk shakes, many animals will drink themselves obese for no apparent reason other than the beverage is highly palatable. We shouldn't blindly trust cravings, nor should we cavalierly assume the craving has no merit. A better course is healthy skepticism. There is often a reason for food cravings. When the entire health scene is investigated, the reason becomes evident, and what appears on the surface to be foolish might end up looking wiser. Rather than assuming that cravings for unhealthy or fattening foods are bad, perhaps we should at least approach them with a blank mind. If we broaden our perspective, we might find that they are more intelligent than they appear at first blush. But even in these instances, we would be better served finding the underlying cause, and correcting it.

Specific appetites, including cravings, are learned. They will only be as expert as the education our palate has received. If our palate hasn't been educated in ways that allow for easy identification of which foods have which substances, or if it has never experienced a food with a certain nutrient, it will be hard pressed to find what it needs. It might still behave intelligently, and yet fail to find what it is missing. Let's conduct a thought experiment to highlight this point. Assume for a moment that inner intelligence knows it needs something but has no idea where to get it. What might an intelligent food instinct look like? One intelligent response would be to crave a variety of different foods. This response works great when we eat whole foods. In nature, nutrients occur unevenly. If a wider variety of foods are sampled, the odds of finding what's missing go up. This response doesn't work as well when processed foods are the backbone of the diet. The variety in processed foods is based on a variety of ingredients, flavors, and textures, but not on nutrient variety. A food instinct and craving for variety is smart, but it still might not solve the problem if most of our diet is made up of processed foods. Another intelligent thing to do might be to increase appetite tremendously in the hope that by eating more, somehow it will get what it needs. Now let's imagine that in this desperate search it finds what it needs: The substance is in potato chips. If the food instinct system needs something, and the only thing it is aware of that has the something are potato chips, it would be expected to crave the potato chips even if there are far healthier sources of the needed substance. If it hasn't sampled and learned about these healthier sources, it won't crave them because it has no way of knowing they exist. Food instincts, in this thought experiment, are acting as intelligently as they can, given what they know and don't know. If we want them to behave more intelligently, we will need to provide them with a better education.

Flavor Learning

Flavor plays a large role when it comes to gathering and applying information about food. Our brain is constantly engaged in trying to learn what flavors go with what foods. It does this because it helps it remember what to eat and what to avoid, what is safe and what isn't. It does this because it is part of its global strategy for determining which foods are higher in calories and which are lower. And it does this as part of its mechanisms for identifying and remembering which nutrients are found in which foods. Complex adaptive intelligence is designed to learn, remember, and make predictions. It gathers and applies information, trying to make sense of things. In this instance, the intelligence is trying to make sense of what we put in our mouths. One way it does this is by learning to associate certain flavors (and possibly other attributes like color and texture) with the calorie, as well as the nutrient content, of a food. Scientists refer to this as *flavor learning*. Flavor learning is the food equivalent of odor-associative learning (discussed in Chapter 15). Odor-associative learning causes us to have strong preferences for some scents, weaker preferences for others, and aversions to others. Detection and evaluation of flavors is also an exercise in associative learning and recall. It is a learning process in which Shape Intelligence learns to associate certain flavors with certain foods. Flavor learning goes by different names—flavor-flavor conditioning, flavor-calorie association, flavor-nutrient learning, and flavor-preference learning—depending upon what is being associated with what. Flavor-flavor learning implies that we can learn to

HSI CLUE

Rats were placed on a diet that resulted in a deficiency in brain levels of omega-3 essential fats. They were then allowed to self-select from chow sources including one enriched with the missing essential fats. A gradual preference for the omega-3 enriched chow emerged. But this behavior only emerged through trial and error. They did not have any inborn instinct that led them to prefer the chow with the needed nutrient; they only preferred it as they somehow learned that it could correct the deficiency and they only learned this *after* trying it.

like a new or even disliked flavor, if it is presented repeatedly in combination with a second flavor that is already liked. A young child might learn to like broccoli, a food with a bitter taste, if it is dipped in diluted honey. By pairing broccoli with the sweet taste that most children are biased to strongly like, they learn to like a vegetable they otherwise wouldn't. Flavor-calorie learning implies that we associate certain flavors with the calorie content of a food. It means, among other things, that if we always use non-caloric sweeteners to add a sweet taste to foods and drinks, we might learn that there are less caloric consequences to sweetness. Flavor-nutrient learning means that it's not just calories, we also learn to associate a flavor with the nutrients—vitamins, minerals, etc.—found in foods. Flavor-preference learning means that we learn to prefer certain flavors. As a general rule of thumb, we learn to prefer flavors that do something useful, providing some type of benefit. In all of these instances, flavor is used as a sort of learning and memory aid.

Humans can learn if a food offers more or fewer calories, or whether it contains certain nutrients. They can use this acquired knowledge to automatically adjust what and how much they eat. If we have experienced a food with high amounts of certain nutrients or calories, we'll tend to gravitate to this food in times when the nutrient or calories are needed in higher amounts. We observe this with calories in the participants in *Survivor*; they crave fattening (calorie-rich) foods. We detect this with nutrients in cases of specific appetites. If we have had an experience with a certain food, and need something it provides, our appetite for the food goes up. This food seeking behavior is typically not a conscious process. We don't think to ourselves, "I'm a bit low in iron, I'll have a steak" or "I'm a bit low in calories, I think I'll eat something fattening". All we know is that we feel like having a steak or have a craving for a high calorie food. But what exactly are we remembering and craving in these instances? Most nutrients (salt being an exception) don't have discernible tastes or scents. They can't be directly detected by our senses. What we can detect is flavor and it is the flavor of the food with the substance, not the substance, that is remembered and for which there is a strong preference. When an iron-deficient woman craves a piece of red meat, it is because their complex adaptive intelligence remembers that eating that food will give them the specific nutrient they need. But it is not the nutrient (iron) that they are remembering or craving; it is the flavor of the food that was high in that nutrient. In other words, food instincts (including specific appetites and cravings) tend to be for a remembered flavor.

In nature there is only one food with the flavor of an orange…an orange. In a 21st century supermarket there might be dozens of different foods with orange flavor. It's relatively easy for complex adaptive intelligence to learn how many calories and which nutrients oranges have, to store this information, and to use it to make future predictions about a food. It is far more difficult to do these things when anything can be made orange flavored. With the ubiquity of chemical flavorings in our food supply a monkey wrench has been thrown in the smooth functioning of flavor learning. When the only thing that has an orange flavor—an orange—always has high amounts of vitamin C, it is relatively straightforward for our brain to learn and remember that eating an orange is a good idea when we need some extra vitamin C. When anything can be orange flavored, whether it has high amounts of vitamin C, low amounts of vitamin C, or no vitamin C, there is no recognizable pattern. Our brain has no idea where to turn to when it needs extra vitamin C. Our food instincts malfunction. They no longer reliably attract us to the foods that support good health and might even steer us towards foods that don't. When the only thing that tasted like an orange was an orange, and the same was true of other foods, Shape Intelligence's job was easier. When anything can be flavored to "taste" like anything, things get confusing. We see this confusion with things that stimulate the sweet taste.

Neuroscientists believe that the brain is biased to use the presence of a sweet taste as a way to predict that a food is going to be a good source of calories. We don't need to acquire this information. It is evident in infants' innate preference for sweet tastes. This makes sense since in nature there are only a few foods, including honey, sugar cane, sugar beet, sweet potato, maple syrup, and fruits, that have a strong sweet taste. These foods are a good source of calories, nutrition, or both. Non-caloric sweeteners—artificial sweeteners—

create a strong sweet taste without adding any calories or having any nutrients. Shape Intelligence must be able to understand the benefits *and* consequences of eating a food with a certain taste in order to accurately self-regulate shape. A sweet taste in nature comes with calories and nutrition. A sweet taste from artificial sweeteners doesn't. Are there consequences for this conflicting information? Scientists attempted to answer this question in the *Case of Sweet Taste and Calorie Prediction*.

One group of adult rats were fed yogurt sweetened with sugar and another group the same yogurt sweetened with saccharin (an artificial sweetener). Rats that were fed the saccharin-sweetened yogurt ate more calories, gained more weight, and got fatter. Presumably, they had learned, at least in part, that there was no caloric consequence to a sweet taste, so they didn't learn to compensate for these calories. The scientists also detected one other important clue: Rats that had learned to associate a sweet taste with no added sweet calories, when eventually fed sugar-sweetened foods, failed to respond metabolically to the same degree *in advance* of eating the sweet food compared to sugar-fed rats. Aspects of metabolism begin to ramp up before we eat, to deal with the calories we will be eating. This can't be based on how many calories we have eaten; we haven't eaten any yet. Notionally it is based on how many calories Shape Intelligence is *anticipating* eating. The scientists in this case theorized that the reason metabolism didn't ramp up to the same degree in the rats that had been fed saccharin-sweetened yogurt was that these rats had learned that the sweet taste had no caloric consequences, so there was no need to prepare metabolism to deal with them. They were now at a metabolic disadvantage when a sweet taste did come with caloric consequence, because their prediction about sweet taste and calories was wrong. Since they couldn't predict accurately, they couldn't compensate accurately. And, as a result, they gained weight. Shape intelligence appears to predict how it should align its metabolic capabilities in advance of eating something based upon *past* experiences with a food. When a calorie-free sweetener consistently produces the sweet taste, past experience is no longer a reliable guide for future encounters with sweet taste produced by a sweetener that has calories.

The *Case of Sweet Taste and Calorie Prediction* is not the only evidence suggesting that certain modern flavor ingredients can weaken Shape Intelligence's ability to accurately learn from flavor. The *Case of*

Confusing the Tastes of Rat Pups provides further evidence. Scientists at the University of Alberta in Canada designed an experiment intended to test flavor learning in rat pups. Higher calorie and lower calorie (diet) versions of the same food were flavored with artificial sweeteners or salt. Rats were fed the food long enough to learn what flavor was associated with a certain amount of calories. Once this learning stage had been completed, the experiment moved into the next stage—testing compensation. Animals and humans fed some food slightly before an actual meal will automatically compensate by eating fewer calories during the subsequent meal. We will also adjust intake up or down if we are fed foods that have been made more or less calorie dense. The accuracy of these compensations is influenced by a number of variables. One of the variables is past flavor learning. In this case, after rat pups had learned that certain flavors meant a low calorie food, they failed to compensate when fed unfamiliar higher calorie foods with these same flavors. Put another way, once young rats had learned that a certain flavor meant a diet food, they tended to overeat when given a similarly flavored non-diet version of the food. The scientists theorized that the reason for the failure to accurately compensate was because of flavor learning. Rat pups had learned that foods with certain flavor were low in calories. They then applied this information when exposed to novel foods with the same flavor(s). But, in this case, because the flavors were now added to higher calorie foods, past experience was not predictive. And, as a result, the rats ate more food.

One more case—the *Case of Consistency or Inconsistency*—shows a similar tendency towards there being a cost to flavor confusion. Scientists at Purdue University gave rats free access to rat chow supplemented with potato chips. One group (Consistency) was fed potato chips that always had the same flavor, amount of calories, and amount of fat. Another group (Inconsistency) was fed regular potato chips on some eating occasions and "diet" potato chips on others. The diet potato chips used a fat substitute to replace the fat in the potato chips and resulted in potato chips that were lower in fat and calories. The rats in the "Consistency" group were given a clear lesson: A certain flavor accurately predicted a high calorie food. Rats in the "Inconsistency" group were given mixed and contradictory information. A potato chip with a certain flavor might be high in fat and calories, but then again it might not be. When the relationship between flavor and calories was consistent, rats ate less food on a routine basis and less food when a new high-fat, high-calorie snack chip was offered. The opposite tendencies occurred in the rats fed regular and diet versions of potato chips—they ate more routinely and failed to compensate as accurately when an unfamiliar chip was offered.

Flavor learning has gotten much more difficult because of chemical ingredients that can change the taste and scent of processed foods. In a modern supermarket there might be thousands of foods that stimulate sweet taste buds and dozens that are orange flavored, as examples. It is easy to be exposed to many flavor inconsistencies today. How does instinctual food intelligence make sense of all of the conflicting information? Could there be shape consequences to confusion? This latter question has not been investigated in humans, but in the *Case of Uncoupling the Flavor-Calorie Relationship*, the answer in rats was yes. Scientists attempted to determine what, if any, influence consistency of the sensory properties of the diet, or the lack of it, had on food intake and weight. Chow with different calorie densities—high calorie, medium calorie, and low calorie—were paired with different flavors and fed to rats. Some rats received chow with a medium amount of calories per gram of food and it was always the same flavor. Other rats received chow of a medium calorie density flavored with one of three different flavors. They were rotated through the three flavors every three days. Other rats rotated daily between high, medium, and low-density chows. Some of these rats always had the density of chow matched with a certain flavor—high density chow was one flavor, medium another flavor, and low a third flavor. The rest of the rats were rotated through the chows with differing calorie densities, but the flavors were not consistently paired with calorie density. In other words, these rats were fed chow where it was impossible to make any sense out of the relationship between flavor and calories. Based on our investigations to this point, which group would you speculate might have had the worst weight outcomes? It was the last group. In this experiment, when chow was always equally calorie dense, no matter how it was flavored, it was not fattening. Varying the calorie density of the diet when it was clear which flavors signaled high, medium, or

---

HSI CLUE

Elizabeth D. Capaldi, Ph.D., author of *Why We Eat What We Eat: The Psychology of Eating,* has used the capacity for flavor-flavor learning to teach children to like cauliflower, broccoli, grapefruit and other foods. By pairing a taste that is already enjoyed—sweet—with a food that isn't, grapefruit or broccoli, the un-liked food becomes liked. At this point, the sweet taste can be gradually decreased and eventually eliminated

low calorie foods was not fattening either. The flavors sent a clear and unambiguous message about the calorie content. The animals could use flavor to predict calories and compensate. Weight gain occurred when there was no ability to make sense out of what was being eaten. Flavor-calorie confusion was fattening.

Like animals, humans are capable of flavor learning. Shape Intelligence will be using its education in this area to determine the benefits and consequences of foods. If it has a Ph.D. in flavor learning, it might nudge us in one direction when it comes to choosing specific foods. If its education was cut off at the kindergarten level, we might be nudged towards very different foods. If we have a Ph.D. we might respond to a high-calorie, high-fat food by spontaneously choosing to eat a smaller portion (appetite compensation), increasing our metabolism (metabolic compensation), or both. If we have never eaten this food, Shape Intelligence will have no idea how to respond to it. If we have eaten it but had a confusing education in the past, our response might not be particularly "smart". We won't compensate accurately. The *pitch of intelligence* we have with food will be dependent on the flavor learning education we have received.

Key Point

Scientists fail to agree on the effect of artificial sweeteners on humans: Some research shows weight loss, some shows weight gain, and some shows no effect. In other words, we have a lack of consistency, and as Holmes advises us, we must expect deception. Some of this deception might arise from funding bias, since much of the artificial sweetener research has been industry funded. Part of the inconsistency might also arise from the failure to account for flavor learning. Flavor learning predicts that a person who has routinely consumed artificially sweetened foods and beverages would not respond to them in the same way, as would a person with no experience with them. If a person routinely uses artificial sweeteners as the source of a sweet taste, they would, notionally, learn that a sweet taste doesn't have any additional calorie consequences. If they do eat a sugar-sweetened food or beverage, they would not compensate, either with appetite or metabolism for the added calories. They would be *under-compensating*. If switched to foods that were sweetened with caloric sweeteners, they would be expected to gain weight; at least until they can learn that a sweet taste has caloric implications. Conversely, a person who has learned that a sweet taste has caloric consequences, who is now switched to artificially sweetened items, would respond as if these items contained more calories than they do. They would be *over-compensating* to these food and beverages and likely to lose weight, until their body learns that sweet taste comes with no calorie penalties. If a person was inconsistent in what has been producing the sweet taste in their diet—eating some items sweetened with caloric sweeteners and others with artificial sweeteners—they will be leaving Shape Intelligence confused.

[Note: Funding bias means that if a study is industry-funded, it is more likely to report a positive finding or bigger benefits than if it the study had been paid for by some uninterested party (like the government).]

The Solution:
Educating Our Palate and Using Food Instincts

The goal is to build *expert* food instincts and to allow them to guide more and more of our eating behaviors. The expertise of our food instincts, the automatic system's ability to recognize the benefits and consequences of a food and compensate accordingly, will depend on the education our palate has received. So, ultimately, the goal is to better educate our palate. We do this by taking *baby steps*. In many areas, and with most skills, starting small is an advantage. This is the case with infants when it comes to movement and language skills. Children learn to crawl before walking, and to walk before running. They learn to make simple sounds before simple words, proceed to more complicated sounds and words, and eventually mix and match these together to make phrases. Parents intuitively grasp the importance of starting small and use baby talk and encourage baby steps. Building food instincts is a lot like moving and language skills; we want to start small, focusing on the most basic elements, and build from here. Because of this, we are wise to model how infants, such as those in Dr. Davis's food orphanage, developed food instincts. Let's summarize a few important inferences from her experiment.

- We acquire food instincts through trial and error.
- Sensory experience (smelling and tasting) is needed for this trial and error process.
- We only have food instincts for things we have previously sampled.

- There is a strong willingness to sample when everything is unfamiliar, but this willingness goes away as familiarity is gained.
- If food instincts are adequately educated, and sufficient healthful options are available, they can get a sick child healthy, and keep an already healthy child healthy. They might also support shape efforts (No child got too fat or too thin).
- When using food instincts a healthful diet can be selected over the course of weeks or longer, but won't necessarily be selected in any single meal or day.
- Food instincts work well when educated on whole foods; it is unknown how well they would work if educated on modern processed foods.

In our experience it's possible to improve food instincts by focusing on some of these *lessons learned* and taking advantage of the capacity for flavor learning. This requires using sensory experience and works best when we build a large food vocabulary, so to speak, with whole foods.

My Flavor Learning Education

Sensory experience with a wide variety of different foods is the foundation of a well-rounded flavor education. We can only be intelligent about things we have previously smelled and tasted. The goal is to expand our flavor learning education; primarily in the realm of whole, unprocessed foods. We do this by sampling unfamiliar foods, on their own, with no distractions from other foods, flavors, or background distractions, like TV. This type of sampling creates an opportunity to unconsciously learn about the food and to acquire information about its calorie and nutrient benefits and consequences, knowledge which Shape Intelligence can use in the future. We recommend educating your palate on *at least* one simple food each week using the below approach.

1. A simple food is a single ingredient item like a piece of fruit, a vegetable, a nut, plain yogurt, unprocessed meat, baked potato, etc.
2. Choose the food and buy enough of it to have several samples.
3. Sample it, preferably by itself away from other foods, three to six times during the next week.

4. Sampling means smelling, tasting, chewing and concentrating on the sensory characteristics of the food.
5. The best time to sample is when we are slightly hungry but before we are starving.

    EXTRA CREDIT: After sampling the food, check-in and ask your body questions. How did that make you feel? Is it something you want to experience again? When?

Simple foods form the foundation for food instincts. Each exposure, every sample, will increase our knowledge. With sufficient repetition we become an expert. After you have gained experience with a simple food, feel free to combine it with other foods or integrate it into more complicated menus. As you are improving your single food education, concentrate on the sensory experiences of the other things you are eating as well. Smell them before eating them and then ask yourself whether or not you really want to eat the food *right now*. When you do eat something, concentrate on fully experiencing its flavors and textures (this is often easier to do with our eyes closed). Focus on keeping meals simpler, but having a greater variety of whole foods over weeks or longer. Continue to broaden your food instinct education by sampling a variety of meals when you go to restaurants, as opposed to always ordering the same items. Keep in mind that the human brain is biased against food novelty; which by default causes us to go with what is familiar. This

> **HSI CLUE**
>
> If one has never acquired sensory experience with a food, there will be no "knowledge" of it within the automatic food guidance system. We can't know whether we like it or dislike it. We won't know if it has benefits for us. And we won't ever be guided to it. We can only be guided to choose or eat more of things we have already sampled and are knowledgeable about.

hinders efforts to expand our food education and it can contribute to getting stuck in a flavor rut, so to speak; eating the same foods over and over again. We break out of this rut by consciously choosing to sample novel foods. In addition to focusing on improving our exposure to novel foods, it's also important to get a better education with any mixed foods (even processed foods like snacks) we eat, whether regularly or periodically, so that we will have better food instincts when it comes to these foods. Approach these foods in a manner similar to the above. Sample them on their own away from other foods, as if you were eating them for the first time.

As you educate your food instincts, start to pay attention for what your body seems to be wanting. During at least one eating episode daily, check in with your body, asking what exactly it is that would best satisfy its current need for food. Look in the refrigerator and see if anything seems to jump out to you in some way. If you are at a restaurant, and you look at the menu with a blank mind, does any item seem really appealing? Is there something that, if you knew nothing intellectually about the things on the list, you would want to eat much more than everything else? As we broaden our flavor learning education, and check in with the body more frequently as part of the eating decision process, in our experience, food instincts become more intelligent.

While we want to produce food novelty, we want to do our best to avoid creating confusion. Confusion, especially because of conflicting information, does not improve education; it hinders it. If we sat in a classroom where one day we were taught that $2 + 2 = 4$, the next day we were taught it equaled 5, and on another day we were taught it equaled 3, we wouldn't develop very good math skills. The same principle applies to flavor learning. Much of the confusion in flavor learning arises from modern food ingredients, some of which are intentionally designed as substitutes for tastes, and others, flavoring agents especially, that are designed to confuse our flavor detection abilities. A 1 gram serving of artificial sugar will have 0 calories, while 1 gram of sugar has 4 calories. The fatty taste in an avocado, nut, butter, or other unprocessed foods come with a cost of 9 calories per gram. Ingredients that give the mouth feel of fat—fat substitutes or diet versions of food—have fewer calories per gram. In nature the only thing flavored like a strawberry is a strawberry. In a supermarket dozens of things might be strawberry flavored, many of which will not only have different calorie and nutrient profiles than a strawberry, but also widely different calorie and nutrient profiles from each other. When we eat these modern processed food ingredients, or the foods made from them, we are providing Shape Intelligence a confusing education. As a result, food instincts can be less reliable, perhaps even unreliable. The body can have a difficult time predicting how much of something it should eat and how it should respond to it metabolically. If a teacher has taught us that $2 + 2 = 9$ sometimes, 0 others, and 4 still other times, we won't be very good at math. It is no different when it comes to Shape Intelligence's efforts to do math with food. This can be inferred from some of the cases we have already investigated. It can also be inferred from the *Case of Watered-Down Fat*.

Rats were given access to a source of fats, a source of protein, and a source of carbohydrates, and allowed to self-select their own diets. After a period of time eating from these sources, the fat source was diluted. Dilution of the fat source promoted intake of fat that was not simply compensatory in nature. The rats didn't just eat sufficiently more of the diluted fat source to make up for what amounted to watered down calories. They ate more fat calories overall when fat was diluted. Diluting the fat seemed to throw a wrench in the ability for the automatic system to accurately regulate how much was eaten. When fat was in essence watered down, food instincts were as well.

In the *Case of Watered-Down Fat*, confusion originated from tampering with fat by diluting it. In a modern diet there are many sources of tampering and potential confusion. The best way to avoid confusion is consistency. Our body can learn to associate fatty foods with having more calories when the only foods we eat with a fatty taste contain fat. Once it learns this lesson, it can apply it to future meals and we can compensate with both appetite and metabolism. But it can't do an accurate job in this area when it is fed confusing information. If we are eating low-fat versions of foods which are made to be low in fat by what amounts to in essence watering down the fatty taste, Shape Intelligence won't know whether $2 + 2 = 4$ or whether it equals something else. If Shape Intelligence can't accurately predict how it should respond, it won't respond accurately. The same principle applies with sweet taste and artificial sweeteners. It also applies with flavoring agents (MSG, natural and artificial flavors, etc.); they create inconsistent, and hence, confusing information. We create improved consistency by avoiding ingredients and foods that substitute for, or in any way water down actual foods. We eliminate flavor inconsistency by doing our best to make sure that we only eat one thing with a specific flavor, preferably the whole food that naturally has this flavor. If the only thing in our diet that tastes like butter is butter, our body can figure out how to adapt, with appetite and aspects of metabolism, to this concentrated source of calories. If multiple things have a buttery flavor, prediction is more difficult and less likely to be reliable. The same principle applies to other food flavors.

Learning to Listen For Feedback

No matter what the skill, we perform poorer in areas where we don't get prompt feedback. This is a bit of an issue with food. Take drinking soft drinks as an example. The enjoyment we experience from drinking them is immediate, but some of the downsides (weight gain, increased risk of chronic disease, etc.) might not occur until weeks, months or even years later. This presents a feedback problem: In an ideal setting we receive immediate feedback on both the benefits and consequences. We can overcome this problem to some degree by being more attentive to the signals the body gives us. This requires being mindful, which leads to an important point. Food instincts are an automatic system; this is not the same as eating on autopilot. When we are eating mindlessly, we aren't checking in with the feedback the body is giving. It is impossible in this state to fully develop food instincts, never mind use them. Learning to listen for and pay attention to the body's feedback is a big part of using food instincts. We can improve the way the food feedback system works by, similar to flavor learning, starting small. The baby step, in this instance, is shifting our focus internally and *paying attention* before, during, and after we eat, to how we feel. While we are doing this, especially when we are learning to do it, asking ourselves questions can be immensely helpful. Questions might include:

Before eating ask:
- What am I feeling?
- Is it hunger or is it something else (thirst, sleepiness, stress, an emotion, etc.) I am feeling? (Note: If some other need is identified, take steps to satisfy it.).
- What is it I really feel like having?

As you begin to sample the food ask:
- How does this food smell and taste to me?
- Does it make me want to have more of it?

After taking a few bites ask:
- How does this food smell and taste to me now?
- How have I satisfied my hunger so far?

- Will a few more bites satisfy it even more or will it put me past the good place?
- Is there something else I am still hungry for?

The goal is to develop better abilities to eat when we are feeling a bit hungry (but before we are starving) and to cease eating when we are satisfied (but before we feel stuffed). It's also to make eating an activity that serves primarily as a means to satisfy hunger and nutrient needs, rather than using it as a distraction from boredom, stress, or emotions. The first and most important step in this process is becoming reacquainted with the feelings of hunger and satiety. This requires paying attention and minimizing external distractions while eating. TV is a form of distraction. The same is true for watching a movie, computer use, playing video games, reading, carrying on a conversation, and other activities. If our attention is split, or even worse, mostly elsewhere, it is very difficult to improve our ability to be in tune with hunger and satiety. The cure for this is to do away with multi-tasking when we eat. Make eating episodes about experiencing what is being eaten as often as possible. As we gain experience by paying better attention, it will become more apparent why we are eating and what it is we really need.

> **HSI CLUE**
>
> Large differences exist in how individuals experience hunger. The most common experience is a subjective sensation in the stomach of a hunger pang. This can be painful but typically isn't. Commonly, it is simply a sense that the stomach is, in its way, calling for food. If food isn't provided, the call gets louder. Other sensations that can be clues to hunger include weakness, headaches, dizziness, anxiety, difficulty in concentration, food craving, watering of the mouth, nausea, and thirst.

Using food instincts also requires learning to differentiate between hunger and a craving. Hunger is a generalized sense that food is needed. When we are only hungry, most foods will do. A craving is more exact. It is a desire, often an intense desire, to consume a specific food. Most people experience cravings at some point. They can arise if a food is being intentionally restricted. They can also be a clue that we might need something and that Shape Intelligence believes this need will be met by eating the craved food. In this instance, the craving will be akin to a specific appetite. Eating the food, even if we can't figure out why our body might want it, might be a better strategy than using willpower to resist. Resisting food cravings requires using some of our willpower reserves. Generally speaking, this is a counter-productive strategy.

HSI CLUE

If you crave chocolate, you are not alone. By a wide margin, it is the most craved food. In studies, people who are actively resisting the craving to eat chocolate tend to eat it less frequently than those who aren't *but* end up eating greater quantities when they do yield to the craving. Net, net, they eat the same amount of chocolate. They also tend to experience far more anxiety in the interim, and guilt after. This highlights the futility of fighting cravings.

Willpower is too important a commodity to waste on countering food cravings, many of which are possibly more intelligent than we can see in the moment. And resisting cravings rarely works as intended because humans tend to want what they are denied even more. Food cravings don't just go away when we resist them; they generally persist and often increase. It's not unusual to eventually yield to a craving for what we've been resisting. When we do, not only do we eat the craved food, we often eat large amounts of it, and can feel anxious before and guilty after, emotions that as far as we can tell, are indigestible. In our experience, it is better to trust in the food instinct educational process and indulge in cravings. Paraphrasing Oscar Wilde, satisfy the craving by yielding to it. If you find yourself craving foods that don't appear to be sensible, investigate other areas of your diet, lifestyle, and environment. Are you getting enough sleep? Do you need to relieve stress more effectively? Are you exercising too much, or too little? Food cravings don't occur in a vacuum. They can be a clue that we need more of a specific substance or more calories. They can be a clue that some other area could benefit from attention, and once attention has been given, the craving vanishes on its own. They can also be a clue to past learning. In this case, past learning that we might be better off unlearning.

We can crave something solely because we have become habituated to having it at a certain time. If we consistently have a treat mid-morning, late in the evening, or after supper, as examples, guess what we crave when this time comes around. If past experience has taught our body that treats come at predictable times, it learns to expect them at these times. This is intelligent in the sense that it shows how our body learns from and uses past experience to anticipate the future. It isn't intelligent in the same sense as a specific appetite that arises because our body actually needs something. Yielding to this type of craving isn't generally the best solution. Interrupting the pattern, until our body learns something else, is. We can interrupt the pattern by going for a short walk. We can have a glass of water. We can do many things. The goal in this instance is to do whatever we are going to do consistently enough to give our body a chance to learn to expect something else at this time.

A similar type of craving occurs if we have become habituated to having one item with another. If we routinely have coffee and a donut, our body will learn to pair these things together. When we drink coffee, we will tend to want a donut. When we have a donut, we want coffee. This same principle applies to other food-food or food-beverage pairings. This craving isn't indicative of physiologically needing something; it simply demonstrates how capable the body is when it comes to learning to associate one thing with another. Once again, the solution is interrupting the pattern until our body learns that these things don't always go together.

> **HSI CLUE**
>
> What is a food or beverage with artificial or natural flavors preventing us from smelling and tasting? In many instances, it is one too many aversive flavors; rancid oils, bitter chemicals, chemical burns from preservatives, warmed-over flavors, and metallic notes. Most of us find these tastes objectionable for a good reason. Our brain knows that items with these tastes aren't good for us. If we could taste these compounds, we would avoid these food products, but we can't, so we don't.

We can also learn to crave specific foods, or types of foods, because of repeated experience of eating the craved food when we have been hungry in the past. If we routinely wait to eat until we are already very hungry, the body will learn that the best way to satisfy a strong hunger signal is to eat the things we habitually eat in this state. It will crave these things when it is hungry because it has learned that they satisfy hunger. Eating before we get too hungry is one way to counter these cravings. Consciously choosing a food other than what the body is craving until it learns to associate this new food with satisfying hunger is another way. A similar theme can occur when we are sleepy. If we routinely eat something when we are feeling sleepy, our body will learn to associate eating this food with being sleepy. It will then tend to express a craving for the food when it needs sleep. By investigating our past behaviors and tendencies, we can often figure out whether a craving is occurring because of past repeated behaviors. Since complex adaptive intelligence is always learning, if we give it new opportunities to learn something else, over time, it will.

It is perfectly fine to indulge in cravings but the goal is to learn from them as we indulge them. Rather than resisting them, or blindly yielding to them, use them to further educate your palate. Before taking a few bites of the craved food, or sips of a craved beverage, smell it, and ask yourself if it is really what you feel like having. After having a few bites or sips, smell it once again. Now ask yourself, if you have had enough? Do I want more now or am I satisfied with what I have eaten? After finishing eating, check in with your body. How did the food make you feel immediately after eating it? How about 30 minutes later? Pay attention to the process and over time, in our experience, it improves the outcomes.

When your body craves something, eat it, but eat the highest quality version of it you can find. If you are craving chocolate, have chocolate but have a *great* chocolate, with the best ingredients. The same goes for butter, ice cream or any other food. When you satisfy a craving do it with the highest quality version of the items you can find (Refer to chapter 19 for guidance on what higher quality looks like.) We want you to satisfy your cravings, but we also want you to do it in a way that gives the body what it is most likely to actually need. If we are used to satisfying our need for basic tastes—sweet, salty, fatty, savory, etc.—from substitutes or poor quality ingredients, we'll crave food items that contain these ingredients. How can you satisfy, or yield to this craving, while still practicing eating habits that improve overall food quality? The solution to this dilemma is getting these tastes satisfied from eating the real foods that contain them.

If you feel like you are craving something sweet, try a teaspoon of honey or real maple syrup. If you are craving something fatty, have something with real fat, like avocado or nuts. If you are craving something with lots of flavor or a snack food that has MSG, have a teaspoon of fermented soy sauce, a cup of miso soup, or a bit of aged cheese. These are rich sources of savory taste. The goal is to indulge in real foods that naturally have strong flavors, the types of foods that our ancestors would have used to satisfy their flavor cravings.

As we are learning to identify and respond to food cravings, as well as hunger and satiety signals, we also want to learn to decipher other feedback clues the body provides. We aren't all the same. A food might agree with one person and disagree with another. As the saying goes, one person's food can be another's poison. Foods, even "healthy" foods, can sometimes cause allergic or other intolerance reactions. Food can have an immediate impact. We might eat something and almost immediately notice that it doesn't agree with us. It can also have a delayed effect. Something might make us feel better in the moment but worse an hour or even several days later. It is up to each of us to discover what, if any, immediate and delayed effects foods have on us when we eat them. It's also important to recognize that complex adaptive systems aren't fixed and rigid. They change. A food that makes us feel better today might make us feel worse if we eat it every day, or at some future time. Food and eating is a lifelong process of self-experimentation.

The feedback clues to pay attention to include:
- Allergy and Congestion Clues: Sniffling, runny nose, post-nasal drip, sneezing, scratchy throat, itchy eyes or nose
- Digestion Clues: Gas, bloating, heartburn loose stools, or constipation
- Energy Level Clues: Fatigue, sleepiness, brain fog or irritability

Ideally, we want to stop while eating foods and check-in to determine if we detect any of these clues. We also want to check-in again after we have eaten them (1 to 2 hours later), because something can seem to agree with us in the moment but leave us feeling worse an hour or two later.

Conclusion

What we choose to eat at any given meal is a complex decision that is guided by the Shape Intelligence we each possess, attempting to match our unique genetics to our individual diet/lifestyle/environment. Our appetite and food cravings at our next meal will be largely determined well in advance of when we sit down to eat. Stress, sleep debt, body clock function, activity levels, recent dieting behaviors, what we ate at our last meal and when we ate it, past flavor learning, and much more will interact to influence the pressure we feel to make better or worse choices and whether we eat a little or a lot. Appetite is complex and it is an effect of many causes. One approach to appetite, a common one in a weight-obsessed culture, is the control approach. Another approach—the opposite one in this case—is a trust approach. Rather than trying to figure it all out, to eat only what we consciously think would benefit our shape, and avoid everything else; we place our faith in Shape Intelligence and its ability for intelligent food instincts. We trust that these food instincts will outperform control over time. We prefer this trust approach.

Food instincts can be intelligent, but keep in mind that they aren't infallible; especially if the child (or adult) has no reference for healthy foods or if much of its education has been based upon modern food ingredients and foods engineered to be highly palatable. Shape Intelligence might need to learn, and in a sense unlearn, a great deal before it demonstrates a "pitch of intelligence." Also, keep in mind that if our instincts are guiding us repeatedly towards "fattening" foods, and we have an excellent base for food instincts—lots of sensory experience with a variety of whole foods—it can mean that something else needs to be corrected. This might be sleep. It might be high stress. It might be that we have just quit smoking or are taking a medication that causes fat gain. There are many smart reasons why Shape Intelligence would decide to defend more body fat and then choose the foods that make attaining the higher weight easier. If your food instincts are leading you to consistently want, or choose foods that aren't conducive to having the shape you desire, there is probably a reason. Don't be too quick to judge Shape Intelligence. It will be doing the best it can under the circumstances, given what it currently knows. It always is.

Just like with the children in Dr. Davis's experiment we want to remember that exceptional nutrition plays out over weeks and months not over a single meal or day. The goal is more simplicity of foods and different flavors in single meals and days, and more variety over weeks and months. We want to also keep in mind that, not only do we learn from our experiences; we also learn from what other people around us do: people's words, actions, thoughts, and behaviors convey information, and we act in our own self-interest on the salient aspects of this information. In a tangible sense, this means that if we want to improve our food instincts, it is usually going to be easier to do if we are around people who have expertise in this area and who use food instincts to guide eating decisions. If we surround ourselves with people who approach food and eating through a control relationship, this rubs off on us as well. Birch, Fischer, and Johnson observed this in the infants and children they studied. If parents followed diet behaviors, the child learned to as well. They modeled what they observed. We all do. Exposing ourselves to others who already know how to do what we aspire to do can be an incredibly important step when it comes to learning something new. With this in mind, we want to extend to you, your family, and your friends, an invitation. Please join us online. Participate in the community that is developing around the HSI approach to shape. Learn from others in the community and share your experiences. Together, we make a difference. Join us at healthsceneinvestigation.com

Closing Dialogue

Health Scene Investigator: In *A Study in Scarlet*, Holmes said, "It was easier to know it than to explain why I know it. If you were asked to prove that two and two made four, you might find some difficulty, and yet you are quite sure of the fact." Can you see the relevance of this quote when it comes to choosing food?

Apprentice: I believe I can. A person who relies on food instincts to select foods can know what food to eat but might not be able to easily explain why they know what to eat.

Health Scene Investigator: Precisely so. They might have learned very early in life the food equivalents of basic math, and while they are sure that they need what they need, they would have difficulty proving why they know what they know to a person who relies upon external food rules.

Apprentice: And by following these food instincts, by doing what they know rather than what they can explain, they end up making better food choices?

Health Scene Investigator: Yes. This has been my experience. While it might seem obvious that the sensible way to eat would be to consciously choose what and how much to eat, sometimes, the obvious is misleading and something far less obvious is of far more importance.

Apprentice: This has been the case in many of the areas we have investigated.

Health Scene Investigator: Yes, it has. We have investigated many areas. You have learned a great deal. I have one more request of you. Please take ownership of this learning.

Apprentice: How do I go about this?

Health Scene Investigator: You decide what you will be doing and when you will be doing it. You then live this life. A good start is to create a daily schedule that will serve as a blueprint of sorts.

Appendix A - Resources and Tools

We Are Smarter Than Me
Join Us: HealthSceneInvestigation.com

We don't accomplish anything in this world alone...and whatever happens is the result of the whole tapestry of one's life and all the weavings of individual threads from one to another that creates something.

Sandra Day O'Connor

The Online Shape Scene Investigation Community

- Investigate Your Own Shape Scene Using Our Assessment Questionnaire (FREE!)

- Interact with and learn from others in the message boards

- Hear the latest news from Dr. Greg, Dr. Mark, and the HSI Team

- View our Medication and Shape Database

- Diet, Fitness, and Lifestyle Videos

- Get Access to FREE Shape Shift® Resources and Tools

- Find Links to Useful Products, Resources, and Services

- Take Advanced Shape and Health Courses

- Find Out More about Our Shape Shift® America Campaign and What You Can Do To Make a Difference in Your Community

Visit us at HealthSceneInvestigation.com

Coupon code

Get Support in Shifting Your Shape

MY SHAPE AND WEIGHT GOALS

Please reflect on the below and fill in your individual answers and goals then review this goal sheet at least once daily for the next 30 days.

Which is the most important to you?
- How much I weigh ☐
- How I look and feel ☐

Past and Future Actions and Commitments
- Have you done things in the past that only caused temporary changes in your shape and weight? ☐ Yes ☐ No
- List these things
- _____
  _____
  _____
  _____
  _____

- Would you be willing to do other things if they could help you to more permanently improve the way you look and feel? ☐ Yes ☐ No
- How much effort are you willing to put into these things? None ☐ A little bit ☐ A moderate amount ☐ Whatever it takes

My Shape and Weight Goals
- Weight my body naturally gravitates to (My Current 'Natural Weight') _____
- My desired 'Natural Weight' _____
- My desired body shape _____
  _____
- I will need to deplete ~ _____ pounds of body fat to meet this goal
- I will need to add ~ _____ pounds of muscle to meet this goal
- Achieving this weight & shape is a realistic goal? ☐ Yes ☐ No
- Keeping the improvements I make is a realistic goal? ☐ Yes ☐ No
- How many months do you realistically expect it will take to get to this improved shape and weight? ☐ 1-3 ☐ 3-6 ☐ 6-12 ☐ More than 1 year

Note: We recommend you find a picture of a person who has or create a drawing/picture of a body shape that you desire and can realistically aspire to as part of setting your "desired body shape" goal. Having a visual picture of our goals is important to clarify what we really want and to unleash our creative potential.

MY SHAPE SHIFT® SUPPORT COMMUNITY

LIVING THE SHAPE SHIFT® LIFESTYLE is about community. A vibrant online community is part of this; our part. There is something even more powerful when it comes to reshaping our bodies, our lives, and the world our children will inherit. This 'something' is the power of small groups of people (6-7 people). A small group can do things that an individual or a larger group can't. We can help each other understand new concepts. We can pick each other up when we fall down during the process of making changes in our diets and lifestyle habits. And, we can share our solutions to the challenges we encounter on our journey to reshape our bodies and our lives.

This does not mean LIVING THE SHAPE SHIFT® LIFESTYLE can't be used by one person who is committed to shifting their shape. It absolutely can be used in that way. We have just found that it is usually easier to produce long-lasting shape and health changes when we have the support of other people. If you don't have or want to be involved in a small group, please share your goals with the important people in your life. Let them know where you are going and give them the gift of helping you get there.

Below is a box to place your signature and the signatures of people who will be supporting you. Please feel free to print this page out, have each person sign it, and place it in a place where you will see it daily. You are not alone and "We" are more capable than "Me".

MY SHAPE SHIFT® SUPPORT COMMUNITY

My Signature _____

Signature _____

Signature _____

Signature _____

Signature _____

Signature _____

Signature _____

Mark Percival and Gregory Kelly

Appendix B

HSI Health Professional Support

Below you will find the names, addresses and contact information for the health professionals who have engaged our Shape Shift® courses over the past several years. Each is an extraordinary person and should prove very helpful to you, should you desire the input of a properly trained "shape" professional. Most are available for consultation by internet and in-person.

Canada

Katherine Ackland, N.D.
Health and Wellness Vitality Centre
3 Waterloo St
New Hamburg, Ontario
N3A 1S3
519.662.2123

Mark Percival, D.C., N.D.
Kitchener-Waterloo, Ontario
Kelowna, British Columbia
888.888.8565
www.healthsceneinvestigation.com

Timothy Houlton, D.C.
King City Natural Health Centre
1229 King Rd.
King City, Ontario
L7B1K5
905.773.5122
www.kcnh.ca
drtim@kingkom.com

J. Todd Norton, D.C.
Holistic Clinic
2211 Riverside Dr., Suite 200
Ottawa, Ontario
K1H 7X5
613.521.5355
www.holisticclinic.ca
tnorton@holisticclinic.ca

United States – HSI Health Professional Support

Mark de Dubovay, D.C., C.T.N.
Advanced Wellness Center
6423 Pacific Coast Highway
Long Beach, California 90803
562.795.6680
www.advancedwellness.org

Richard Perryman, D.C.
Phoenix, Arizona
San Diego, California
888.888.8565

Richard Powers, D.C.
Holistic Medical Center
969 Central Pkwy
Stuart, Florida 34994
772.283.4046
 www.HealthCoachDoctor.com
HiDrPowers@HealthCoachDoctor.com

Donald Huml, D.C.
Huml Integrative Healthcare
430 – 79th St.
Brooklyn, New York 11209
718.748.6644
www.doctorhuml.com

Russel Sher, D.C.
Asheville Center for Health Excellence
118 Charlotte St.
Asheville, North Carolina 28801
828.253.1727
www.ashevillehealthcoach.com

Debra Martin-Belleville, N.D.
Anti-Aging and Wellness Clinic
911 Country Club Rd., Ste. 270
Eugene, Oregon 97401
541.683.4071
www.drdebra-nd.com
drdebra82@yahoo.com

David H. Haase, M.D.
Maxwell Clinic for
Proactive Medicine
556B Fire Station Rd., Suite B
Clarksville, Tennessee 37043
931.648.9595
www.maxwellclinic.com
info@maxwellclinic.com

Kenneth A. Gilman, D.C.
Clarksville Chiropractic Center
1636 Madison St.
Clarksville, Tennessee 37043
931.647.3692
www.clarksvillechiropractic.com
professorgilman@hotmail.com

Steven Bircher, D.C.
Optima Health and Vitality Center
3321 Golf Rd.
Eau Claire, Wisconsin 54701
715.832.1953
www.optimahvc.com

Notes and References

Chapter 1

- **Thomas Kuhn, author**... *The Structure of Scientific Revolutions* is published by University Of Chicago Press.
- **In December 2001, the U.S. Surgeon General issued a health warning**... Epidemic nature of overweight and obesity issue was pointed out in the *Surgeon General's Call To Action To Prevent and Decrease Overweight and Obesity 2001*. A PDF of this report is available at www.surgeongeneral.gov/topics/obesity/calltoaction/CalltoAction.pdf.
- **Estimates suggest that 65% of adults**... Statistics reported by National Center for Health Statistics. www.cdc.gov/nchs/
- **The latest government statistics indicate that obese Americans outnumber overweight Americans**... This research was mentioned in *Obese Americans now outweigh the merely overweight* (www.reuters.com/article/idUSTRE50863H20090109) and *Severely obese fastest-growing U.S. overweight group* (www.reuters.com/article/idUSN0934626920070410).
- **By the year 2025 40-45% of individuals in the US will be**... Source is Wang Y, Beydoun MA. The obesity epidemic in the United States—gender, age, socioeconomic, racial/ethnic, and geographic characteristics: a systematic review and meta-regression analysis. *Epidemiologic Reviews*. 2007;29:6-28. Newer estimates have suggested we might reach this point by 2015 (See reuters article *Study predicts 75 percent overweight in U.S. by 2015* at www.reuters.com/article/idUSN1841918320070718).
- **In a 2009 Newsweek article**... *Born to be Big: Early exposure to common chemicals may be programming kids to be fat* by Sharon Begley was published in the September 11, 2009 issue of Newsweek

Chapter 2

- **The concept of tipping points**... Political Scientist Morton Grodzins studied integrating American neighborhoods in the early 1960s. He discovered that most of the white families remained in the neighborhood as long as the comparative number of black families remained very small. But, at a certain point, when "one too many" black families arrived, the remaining white families would move out en masse in a process known as white flight. He called that moment the "tipping point". He wrote about his observations in *The Metropolitan Area as a Racial Problem*, 1958. Pittsburgh: University of Pittsburgh Press.
- **Malcolm Gladwell**... *The Tipping Point: How Little Things Can Make a Big Difference* was first published by Little Brown in 2000.
- **The *Case of Neutering a Pet***... Studies used for this case include:
    - Fettman MJ, Stanton CA, Banks LL, et al. Effects of neutering on bodyweight, metabolic rate and glucose tolerance of domestic cats. *Res Vet Sci* 1997 Mar-Apr;62(2):131-6.
    - Flynn MF, Hardie EM, Armstrong PJ. Effect of ovariohysterectomy on maintenance energy requirement in cats. *J Am Vet Med Assoc* 1996 Nov 1;209(9):1572-81.
    - Harper EJ, Stack DM, Watson TD, Moxham G. Effects of feeding regimens on bodyweight, composition and condition score in cats following ovariohysterectomy. J Small Anim Pract. 2001 Sep;42(9):433-8.
    - Kanchuk ML, Backus RC, Calvert CC, et al. Weight gain in gonadectomized normal and lipoprotein lipase-deficient male domestic cats results from increased food intake and not decreased energy expenditure. *J Nutr* 2003 Jun;133(6):1866-74.
- **Fundamental Attribution Error**... In social psychology, the fundamental attribution error is also known as correspondence bias or attribution effect. It is the tendency to over-value dispositional or personality-based explanations for observed behaviors of others while under-valuing situational explanations for those behaviors. Lee Ross coined the term. Wikipedia has a page dedicated to this topic that provides an overview of this concept and references to experiments that form the underpinning of this concept.
- **In 1965 about 10 of these 40 hours**... Statistics on free time and TV viewing from Robinson JP. Changes in American Daily Life: 1965–2005. *Social Indicators Research* 2009:93;47-56.
- **In 1975, the average American slept 7.5 hours**... Data taken from polls conducted by the National Sleep Foundation.
- **Per capita fructose consumption**... Per capita fructose consumption is estimated from information published by the Economic Research Service of the United States Department of Agriculture.

Chapter 3

- **Complexity Science, the science of complex adaptive systems**... Many good books are available on complexity science. Some ones to consider reading include:
  The Genius Within: Discovering the Intelligence of every living thing by Frank T. Vertosick, Jr. (ISBN 0-15-100551-6)
  Complexity: Life at the Edge of Chaos by Roger Lewin (ISBN: 0-02-570485-0)
  Chaos: Making a New Science by James Gleick (ISBN: 0-14-009250-1)

- **Reductionism and Complexity**... A useful starting point to appreciate differences between these two scientific models is Marc H.V. Van Regenmortel's review article titled Reductionism and complexity in molecular biology (published in the journal *European Molecular Biology Organization* (EMBO) 2004 November; 5(11): 1016–1020 and available online at http://www.ncbi.nlm.nih.gov/pmc/articles/PMC1299179/)

- **Collective Intelligence and Decentralized Intelligence**... Our favorite book on these types of intelligence and its ramifications for health is *The Genius Within: Discovering the Intelligence of every living thing* by Frank T. Vertosick, Jr. (ISBN 0-15-100551-6)

- **Superorganisms**... To read more about superorganisms we recommend reading the books:
  The Superorganism: The Beauty, Elegance, and Strangeness of Insect Societies by Bert Hölldobler and E. O. Wilson (ISBN-10: 0393067041)
  The Buzz about Bees: Biology of a Superorganism by Jürgen Tautz and Helga R. Heilmann (ISBN-10: 3540787275)

Chapter 4

- **The *Case of Army Rangers*...** based on information from Friedl KE, Moore RJ, Hoyt RW, et al. Endocrine markers of semistarvation in healthy lean men in a multistressor environment. *J Appl Physiol* 2000; 88:1820–1830.

- **The *Case of the Minnesota Experiment*...** based on information from
  - Dulloo AG, Jacquet J, Girardier L. Autoregulation of body composition during weight recovery in human: the Minnesota Experiment revisited. *Int J Obes Relat Metab Disord* 1996 May;20(5):393-405
  - Dulloo AG, Jacquet J. Adaptive reduction in basal metabolic rate in response to food deprivation in humans: a role for feedback signals from fat stores. *Am J Clin Nutr* 1998 Sep;68(3):599-606
  - Dulloo AG, Jacquet J, Girardier L. Poststarvation hyperphagia and body fat overshooting in humans: a role for feedback signals from lean and fat tissues. *Am J Clin Nutr* 1997 Mar;65(3):717-23.
  - Kalm LM, Semba RD. They starved so that others be better fed: remembering Ancel Keys and the Minnesota experiment. *J Nutr* 2005 Jun;135(6):1347-52.
  - Keys A, Brozek J, Henschel A, Mickelsen O, Taylor HL. *The Biology of Human Starvation, Vols. I-II.* University of Minnesota Press, Minneapolis, MN. p. 837

  To read more about this experiment and the people involved we recommend the book *The Great Starvation Experiment: The Heroic Men Who Starved so That Millions Could Live* by Todd Tucker (ISBN-10: 0743270304)

- **The *Case of and Starving in the Desert*...** based on information from:
  - Silverstone SE. Food production and nutrition for the crew during the first 2-year closure of Biosphere 2. *Life Support Biosph Sci* 1997;4(3-4):167-78
  - Verdery RB, Walford RL. Changes in plasma lipids and lipoproteins in humans during a 2-year period of dietary restriction in Biosphere 2. *Arch Intern Med* 1998 Apr 27;158(8):900-6
  - Walford RL, Mock D, MacCallum T, Laseter JL. Physiologic changes in humans subjected to severe, selective calorie restriction for two years in biosphere 2: health, aging, and toxicological perspectives. *Toxicol Sci* 1999;52:61-5
  - Walford RL, Mock D, Verdery R, MacCallum T. Calorie restriction in biosphere 2: alterations in physiologic, hematologic, hormonal, and biochemical parameters in humans restricted for a 2-year period. *J Gerontol A Biol Sci Med Sci* 2002 Jun;57(6):B211-24
  - Weyer C, Walford RL, Harper IT, et al. Energy metabolism after 2 y of energy restriction: the biosphere 2 experiment. *Am J Clin Nutr* 2000 Oct;72(4):946-53

Chapter 5

- **Data from 7767 patients with previous heart failure**... From Curtis JP, Selter JG, Wang Y, et al. The obesity paradox: body mass index and outcomes in patients with heart failure. *Arch Intern Med* 2005 Jan 10;165(1):55-61.

- **Let's list some of the most consistent observations...** In many areas the apparent consensus is more fragile than it looks. The certainty we are sold is based on data that is anything but certain, and often rife with conflicting facts. This is exactly the case with weight and health. To get a better feel for this uncertainty we recommend reading books such as:
  - *The Diet Myth: Why America's Obsession with Weight is Hazardous to Your Health* by Paul Campos (ISBN-10: 159240135X)
  - *Big Fat Lies: The Truth about Your Weight and Your Health* by Glenn A. Gaesser (ISBN-10: 0936077425)
- **In one study, over a 24-year observation period...** Source is Sørensen TI, Rissanen A, Korkeila M, Kaprio J. Intention to lose weight, weight changes, and 18-y mortality in overweight individuals without co-morbidities. *PLoS Med* 2005 Jun;2(6):e171.
- **The *Case of the News Media*...** The various wire services news releases were reporting on research that was published as Flegal KM, Graubard BI, Williamson DF, Gail MH. Cause-specific excess deaths associated with underweight, overweight, and obesity. *JAMA* 2007 Nov 7;298(17):2028-37.
- **The *Case of Overfeeding Identical Twins*...** based on information from:
  - Bouchard C, Tremblay A, Despres JP, et al. Overfeeding in identical twins: 5-year postoverfeeding results. *Metabolism* 1996 Aug;45(8):1042-50.
  - Bouchard C, Tremblay A, Despres JP, et al. The response to long-term overfeeding in identical twins. *N Engl J Med* 1990 May 24;322(21):1477-82.
  - Bouchard C, Tremblay A. Genetic Influences on the Response of Body Fat and Fat Distribution to Positive and Negative Energy Balances in Human Identical Twins. *J Nutr* 1997;127:943S–947S
  - Pritchard J, et al. Plasma Adrenal, Gonadal, and Conjugated Steroids before and after Long Term Overfeeding in Identical Twins. *J Clin Endocrinol Metab* 1998;83:3277–3284
- **The *Case of the Vermont Overfeeding Study*...** based on information from:
  - Salans LB, Horton ES, Sims EA. Experimental Obesity in Man: Cellular Character of the Adipose Tissue. *J Clin Invest* 1971:50;1005-11
  - Simms EA, et al. Experimental obesity in man. *Transactions of the association of American Physicians* 1968;81;153-70
  - Simms EA. Studies in Human Hyperphagia. In Bray G, Bethune J. *Treatment and Management of Obesity*. New York, Harper and Row 1974;29
- **The *Case of Guru Walla*...** based on information from:
  - Pasquet P, Apfelbaum M. Recovery of initial body weight and composition after long-term massive overfeeding in men. *Am J Clin Nutr* 1994 Dec;60(6):861-3.
  - Pasquet P, Brigant L, Froment A, et al. Massive overfeeding and energy balance in men: the Guru Walla model. *Am J Clin Nutr* 1992 Sep;56(3):483-90.
- **Economist John Kenneth Galbraith coined the term conventional wisdom...** This term originally appeared in Galbraith's 1958 book *Affluent Society*.

Chapter 6

- **The *Case of Conserved Calories*...** based on information from Foster GD, Wadden TA, Kendrick ZV, et al. The energy cost of walking before and after significant weight loss. *Med Sci Sports Exerc* 1995 Jun;27(6):888-94.
- **The *Case of the Damaged Hypothalamus*...** We recommend reading *Fat: Fighting the Obesity Epidemic* (ISBN-10: 0195118537) by Robert Pool for a very readable orientation to the experiments done that led to better understanding of the role of the hypothalamus in shape regulation.
- **Set Point Theory...** Set point theory is not a new idea. Many scientific articles have been written on the subject over the past 4 decades. Out of print books including *Dieter's Dilemma: Eating Less and Weighing More (The Scientific case against dieting as a means of weight control)* by William Bennett, M.D. and Joel Gurin; and *Breaking the Diet Habit: The Natural Weight Alternative* by Janet Polivy & C. Peter Herman, were based on set point theory. *Fat: Fighting the Obesity Epidemic* (ISBN-10: 0195118537) by Robert Pool also touches on set point theory. A newer book, *The Shangri-La Diet: The No Hunger Eat Anything Weight-Loss Plan* by Seth Roberts (ISBN-10: 0399533168), also uses a set point theory premise.
- **Douglas Coleman published research that predicted the existence of a substance he referred to as *satiety factor*...** We recommend reading *Fat: Fighting the Obesity Epidemic* (ISBN-10: 0195118537) by Robert Pool for a more detailed introduction into Coleman and his experiments.
- **A communication molecule that would be named *leptin*...** We recommend reading *Fat: Fighting the Obesity Epidemic* (ISBN-10: 0195118537) by Robert Pool for a more detailed introduction into the people involved in the discovery of leptin.
- **Sweet things taste better longer...** This has to do with a concept called Alliesthesia. Scientific articles on this subject include:
  - Cabanac M, Rabe EF. Influence of a monotonous food on body weight regulation in humans. Physiol Behav. 1976 Oct;17(4):675-8.

- Rodin J. Effects of obesity and set point on taste responsiveness and ingestion in
- humans. J Comp Physiol Psychol 1975 Nov;89(9):1003-9
- **Sleep eating**... This is more accurately called Nocturnal Sleep-Related Eating Disorder (NSRED) in clinical medicine. Wikipedia has a page dedicated to this topic.

Chapter 7

- **Chile peppers adjust the amount of spicy compounds...** Information is from the article *Chiles' live-and-let burn philosophy is good for humans, bad for fungus* by Joe Rojas-Burke Newhouse News Service August 28, 2008
- **Evidence published in the *American Journal of Sports Medicine* calls this assumption into question...** This information is from the article Gwinup G. Weight loss without dietary restriction: Efficacy of different forms of aerobic exercise. *American Journal of Sports Medicine* 1987,15,275-279
- **This is not the first piece of perplexing evidence arising from studies of swimming...** Studies used for the purpose of this paragraph include:
  - Almeras N, Lemieux S, Bouchard C, Tremblay A. Fat gain in female swimmers. *Physiol Behav* 1997 Jun;61(6):811-7.
  - Flynn MG, Costill DL, Kirwan JP, et al. Fat storage in athletes: metabolic and hormonal responses to swimming and running. *Int J Sports Med* 1990 Dec;11(6):433-40.
  - Jang, KT., Flynn, MG., Costill, DL., et al. Energy balance in competitive swimmers and runners. *Journal of Swimming Research* 1987 3, 19-23
  - Tuuri G, Loftin M, Oescher J. Association of swim distance and age with body composition in adult female swimmers. *Med Sci Sports Exerc* 2002 Dec;34(12):2110-4.
- **In one study, a group of 11 men swam for 45 minutes in neutral (86 degrees F) and cold (68 degrees F) water...** Source is White LJ, Dressendorfer RH, Holland E, et al. Increased caloric intake soon after exercise in cold water. *Int J Sport Nutr Exerc Metab*. 2005 Feb;15(1):38-47.
- **Insulative adaptation as an adaptation to cold water exposure...** This concept comes from studies including:
  - Anderson GS. Human morphology and temperature regulation. *Int J Biometeorol* 1999 Nov;43(3):99-109.
  - Bittel J. The different types of general cold adaptation in man. *Int J Sports Med* 1992 Oct;13 Suppl 1:S172-6.
  - Brito NA, Brito MN, Bartness TJ. Differential sympathetic drive to adipose tissues after food deprivation, cold exposure or glucoprivation. *Am J Physiol Regul Integr Comp Physiol* 2008 May;294(5):R1445-52.
  - Dulac S, Quirion A, DeCarufel D, et al. Metabolic and hormonal responses to long-distance swimming in cold water. *Int J Sports Med* 1987 Oct;8(5):352-6.
  - Frisch RE, Hall GM, Aoki TT, et al. Metabolic, endocrine, and reproductive changes of a woman channel swimmer. *Metabolism* 1984 Dec;33(12):1106-11.
  - Harri M, Kuusela P. Is swimming exercise or cold exposure for rats? *Acta Physiol Scand* 1986 Feb;126(2):189-97.
  - Hayward MG, Keatinge WR. Roles Of Subcutaneous Fat and Thermoregulatory Reflexes in Determining Ability To Stabilize Body Temperature in Water. *J. Physiol.* 1981;320:229-251.
  - Karl I, Fischer K. Why get big in the cold? Towards a solution to a life-history puzzle. *Oecologia* 2008 Mar;155(2):215-25.
  - Keatinge WR, Khartchenko M, Lando N, Lioutov V. Hypothermia during sports swimming in water below 11 degrees C. *Br J Sports Med* 2001 Oct;35(5):352-3.
  - Koska J, Ksinantova L, Sebökova E, et al. Endocrine regulation of subcutaneous fat metabolism during cold exposure in humans. *Ann N Y Acad Sci* 2002 Jun;967:500-5.
  - McArdle WD, Magel JR, Spina RJ, et al. Thermal adjustment to cold-water exposure in exercising men and women. *J Appl Physiol* 1984 Jun;56(6):1572-7.
  - McMurray RG, Horvath SM. Thermoregulation in swimmers and runners. *J Appl Physiol* 1979 Jun;46(6):1086-92.
  - Park YS, Rennie DW, Lee IS, et al. Time course of deacclimatization to cold water immersion in Korean women divers. *J Appl Physiol.* 1983 Jun;54(6):1708-16.
  - Rennie DW. Tissue heat transfer in water: lessons from the Korean divers. *Med Sci Sports Exerc* 1988 Oct;20(5 Suppl):S177-84.
  - Veicsteinas A, Rennie DW. Thermal insulation and shivering threshold in Greek sponge divers. *J Appl Physiol* 1982 Apr;52(4):845-50.
  - Vybiral S, Lesna I, Jansky L, Zeman V. Thermoregulation in winter swimmers and physiological significance of human catecholamine thermogenesis. *Exp Physiol* 2000 May;85(3):321-6.

- **The *Case of Brown Fat*...** A good article (*Calorie-Burning Fat? Studies Say You Have It*) on recent brown fat findings was written by Gina Kolata and appeared April 9, 2009 edition of the New York Times. Her articles is based on research including:
    - Cannon B, Nedergaard J. Developmental biology: Neither fat nor flesh. *Nature* 454, 947-948 (21 August 2008)
    - Saito M, Okamatsu-Ogura Y, Matsushita M, et al. High incidence of metabolically active brown adipose tissue in healthy adult humans: effects of cold exposure and adiposity. *Diabetes* 2009 Jul;58(7):1526-31.
    - van Marken Lichtenbelt WD, Vanhommerig JW, et al. Cold-activated brown adipose tissue in healthy men. *N Engl J Med* 2009 Apr 9;360(15):1500-8.
- **Body Fat Fingerprints...** Information in this section is based on evidence from studies including:
    - Arner P. Control of lipolysis and its relevance to development of obesity in man. *Diabetes Metab Rev* 1984;4:507–515.
    - Arner P. Regulation of lipolysis in human fat cells. *Diabetes Rev* 1996;4:1–13.
    - Bjorntorp P. Adipose tissue distribution and function. *Int J Obes* 1991 Sep;15 Suppl 2:67-81.
    - Bjorntorp P. The regulation of adipose tissue distribution in humans. *Int J Obes Relat Metab Disord* 1996 Apr;20(4):291-302.
    - Caspar-Bauguil S, Cousin B, Galinier A, et al. Adipose tissues as an ancestral immune organ: site-specific change in obesity. *FEBS Lett* 2005 Jul 4;579(17):3487-92.
    - Garaulet M, Hernandez-Morante JJ, Lujan J, Tebar FJ, Zamora S. Relationship between fat cell size and number and fatty acid composition in adipose tissue from different fat depots in overweight/obese humans. *Int J Obes (Lond)* 2006 Jun;30(6):899-905.
    - Garaulet M, Pérez-Llamas F, Pérez-Ayala M, et al. Site-specific differences in the fatty acid composition of abdominal adipose tissue in an obese population from a Mediterranean area: relation with dietary fatty acids, plasma lipid profile, serum insulin, and central obesity. *Am J Clin Nutr* 2001 Nov;74(5):585-91.
    - Hudgins LC, Hirsch J. Changes in abdominal and gluteal adipose-tissue fatty acid compositions in obese subjects after weight gain and weight loss. *Am J Clin Nutr* 1991 Jun;53(6):1372-7.
    - Leibel RL, Edens NK, Fried SK. Physiologic basis for the control of body fat distribution in humans. *Annu. Rev. Nutr* 1989;9:417–443.
    - Lin DS, Connor WE, Spenler CW. Are dietary saturated, monounsaturated, and polyunsaturated fatty acids deposited to the same extent in adipose tissue of rabbits? *Am J Clin Nutr* 1993 Aug;58(2):174-9.
    - Malcom GT, Bhattacharyya AK, Velez-Duran M, et al. Fatty acid composition of adipose tissue in humans: differences between subcutaneous sites. *Am J Clin Nutr* 1989 Aug;50(2):288-91.
    - Mattacks CA, Sadler D, Pond CM. Site-specific differences in fatty acid composition of dendritic cells and associated adipose tissue in popliteal depot, mesentery, and omentum and their modulation by chronic inflammation and dietary lipids. *Lymphat Res Biol* 2004;2(3):107-29.
    - Perrini S, Leonardini A, Laviola L, Giorgino F. Biological specificity of visceral adipose tissue and therapeutic intervention. *Arch Physiol Biochem* 2008 Oct;114(4):277-86.
    - Phinney SD, Stern JS, Burke KE, et al. Human subcutaneous adipose tissue shows site-specific differences in fatty acid composition. *Am J Clin Nutr* 1994 Nov;60(5):725-9.
    - Pittet PG, Halliday D, Bateman PE. Site differences in the fatty acid composition of subcutaneous adipose tissue of obese women. *Br J Nutr* 1979 Jul;42(1):57-61.
    - Pond CM. Adipose tissue, the immune system and exercise fatigue: how activated lymphocytes compete for lipids. *Biochem Soc Trans* 2002 Apr;30(2):270-5.
    - Power ML, Schulkin J. Sex differences in fat storage, fat metabolism, and the health risks from obesity: possible evolutionary origins. *Br J Nutr* 2008 May;99(5):931-40.
    - Ren J, Dimitrov I, Sherry AD, Malloy CR. Composition of adipose tissue and marrow fat in humans by 1H NMR at 7 Tesla. *J Lipid Res* 2008 Sep;49(9):2055-62.
    - Sabin MA, Crowne EC, Stewart CE, et al. Depot-specific effects of fatty acids on lipid accumulation in children's adipocytes. *Biochem Biophys Res Commun* 2007 Sep 21;361(2):356-61.
    - Sadick NS, Hudgins LC. Fatty acid analysis of transplanted adipose tissue. *Arch Dermatol* 2001 Jun;137(6):723-7.
    - Schoen RE, Evans RW, Sankey SS, et al. Does visceral adipose tissue differ from subcutaneous adipose tissue in fatty acid content? *Int J Obes Relat Metab Disord* 1996 Apr;20(4):346-52.
    - Summers LK, Barnes SC, Fielding BA, et al. Uptake of individual fatty acids into adipose tissue in relation to their presence in the diet. *Am J Clin Nutr* 2000 Jun;71(6):1470-7.
    - Tan CY, Vidal-Puig A. Adipose tissue expandability: the metabolic problems of obesity may arise from the inability to become more obese. *Biochem Soc Trans* 2008 Oct;36(Pt 5):935-40.

- Tang AB, Nishimura KY, Phinney SD. Preferential reduction in adipose tissue alpha-linolenic acid (18:3 omega 3) during very low calorie dieting despite supplementation with 18:3 omega 3. *Lipids* 1993 Nov;28(11):987-93.
- Tremblay A, Doucet E. Obesity: a disease or a biological adaptation? *Obes Rev* 2000 May;1(1):27-35
- Tiikkainen M, Bergholm R, Vehkavaara S, et al. Effects of identical weight loss on body composition and features of insulin resistance in obese women with high and low liver fat content. *Diabetes* 2003 Mar;52(3):701-7.

- **Complex Adaptive Intelligence...** Many good books are available on complex adaptive intelligence, networks, and decentralized intelligence. Some to consider reading include:
  - *The Genius Within: Discovering the Intelligence of every living thing* by Frank T. Vertosick, Jr. (ISBN 0-15-100551-6)
  - *Complexity: Life at the Edge of Chaos* by Roger Lewin (ISBN: 0-02-570485-0)
  - *Six Degrees: The Science of a Connected Age* by Duncan J. Watts (ISBN-10: 0393325423)
  - *The Superorganism: The Beauty, Elegance, and Strangeness of Insect Societies* by Bert Hölldobler and E. O. Wilson (ISBN-10: 0393067041)
- **Natural Weight...** We began using the term natural weight in our teaching and writing about shape and weight in the year 2002 only to eventually discover that Janet Polivy and C. Peter Herman had used it in the early 1980's in their book *The Natural Weight Alternative*.

Chapter 8

- **The *Case of the Framingham Heart Study* and The *Case of the Tecumseh Community Health Study*...** The source for these cases is Allison DB, Zannolli R, Faith MS, et al. Weight loss increases and fat loss decreases all-cause mortality rate: results from two independent cohort studies. *Int J Obes Relat Metab Disord* 1999 Jun;23(6):603-11.
- **A *Study in Hormone Replacement Therapy*...** The source for this case is Delibasi T, Berker D, Aydin Y, et al. Effects of combined female sex hormone replacement therapy on body fat percentage and distribution. *Adv Ther* 2006 Mar-Apr;23(2):263-73.
- **The *Case of Lipodystrophy*...** Wikipedia has a page dedicated to lipodystrophy and one dedicated to HIV-associated lipodystrophy.
Sources used for this case include:
  - Dinges WL, Chen D, Snell PG, et al. Regional body fat distribution in HIV-infected patients with lipodystrophy. *J Investig Med* 2005 Jan;53(1):15-25.
  - Estrada V, Martinez-Larrad MT, Gonzalez-Sanchez JL, et al. Lipodystrophy and metabolic syndrome in HIV-infected patients treated with antiretroviral therapy. *Metabolism* 2006 Jul;55(7):940-5.
  - Guaraldi G, Murri R, Orlando G, et al. Severity of lipodystrophy is associated with decreased health-related quality of life. *AIDS Patient Care STDS* 2008 Jul;22(7):577-85.
  - Hansen AB, Lindegaard B, Obel N, et al. Pronounced lipoatrophy in HIV-infected men receiving HAART for more than 6 years compared with the background population. *HIV Med* 2006 Jan;7(1):38-45.
  - Herranz P, de Lucas R, Pérez-España L, Mayor M. Lipodystrophy syndromes. *Dermatol Clin* 2008 Oct;26(4):569-78, ix.
  - Huang JS, Becerra K, Fernandez S, et al. The impact of HIV-associated lipodystrophy on healthcare utilization and costs. *AIDS Res Ther* 2008 Jul 1;5:14.
  - Huang JS, Harrity S, Lee D, et al. Body image in women with HIV: a cross-sectional evaluation. *AIDS Res Ther* 2006 Jul 6;3:17.
  - Mulligan K, Parker RA, Komarow L, et al. Mixed patterns of changes in central and peripheral fat following initiation of antiretroviral therapy in a randomized trial. *J Acquir Immune Defic Syndr* 2006 Apr 15;41(5):590-7.
- **The *Case of Normal Weight Big Belly Syndrome*...** The source for this case is Koster A, Leitzmann MF, Schatzkin A, et al. Waist circumference and mortality. *Am J Epidemiol* 2008 Jun 15;167(12):1465-75.
- **In a 2009 study, shape was also a far better predictor of risk for dementia and cognitive decline...** Source is West NA, Haan MN. Body adiposity in late life and risk of dementia or cognitive impairment in a longitudinal community-based study. *J Gerontol A Biol Sci Med Sci* 2009 Jan;64(1):103-9. Epub 2009 Jan 23.

Chapter 9

- **Researchers decided to follow 4107 elderly...** Source is Wannamethee SG, Shaper AG, Lennon L, Whincup PH. Decreased muscle mass and increased central adiposity are independently related to mortality in older men. *Am J Clin Nutr* 2007 Nov;86(5):1339-46.

- **Approximately 19 percent of men and 25 percent of women were classified as obese**... Source Romero-Corral A, Somers VK; Sierra-Johnson J, et al. Accuracy of body mass index in diagnosing obesity in the adult general population. *Int J Obes (Lond)* 2008 Jun;32(6):959-66.
- **The *Case of T⌐ xifen*...** Sources used for this case include:
  - Ali PA, al-Ghorabie FH, Evans CJ, et al. Body composition measurements using DXA and other techniques in tamoxifen-treated patients. *Appl Radiat Isot* 1998 May-Jun;49(5-6):643-5.
  - Bilici A, Ozguroglu M, Mihmanli I, et al. A case-control study of non-alcoholic fatty liver disease in breast cancer. *Med Oncol* 2007;24(4):367-71.
  - Hoskin PJ, Ashley S, Yarnold JR. Weight gain after primary surgery for breast cancer--effect of tamoxifen. *Breast Cancer Res Treat* 1992;22(2):129-32.
  - Nguyen MC, Stewart RB, Banerji MA, et al. Relationships between tamoxifen use, liver fat and body fat distribution in women with breast cancer. *Int J Obes Relat Metab Disord* 2001 Feb;25(2):296-8.
  - Nishino M, Hayakawa K, Nakamura Y, et al. Effects of tamoxifen on hepatic fat content and the development of hepatic steatosis in patients with breast cancer: high frequency of involvement and rapid reversal after completion of tamoxifen therapy. *AJR Am J Roentgenol* 2003 Jan;180(1):129-34.
  - Ozet A, Arpaci F, Yilmaz MI, et al. Effects of tamoxifen on the serum leptin level in patients with breast cancer. *Jpn J Clin Oncol* 2001 Sep;31(9):424-7
  - Rohatgi N, Blau R, Lower EE. Raloxifene is associated with less side effects than tamoxifen in women with early breast cancer: a questionnaire study from one physician's practice. *J Womens Health Gend Based Med* 2002 Apr;11(3):291-301.
  - Wallen WJ, Belanger MP, Wittnich C. Sex hormones and the selective estrogen receptor modulator tamoxifen modulate weekly body weights and food intakes in adolescent and adult rats. *J Nutr* 2001 Sep;131(9):2351-7.
  - Wallen WJ, Belanger MP, Wittnich C. Body weight and food intake profiles are modulated by sex hormones and tamoxifen in chronically hypertensive rats. *J Nutr* 2002 Aug;132(8):2246-50.
- **The *Case of Insulin*...** Sources for this case are:
  - Rigalleau V, Delafaye C, Baillet L, et al. Composition of insulin-induced body weight gain in diabetic patients: a bio-impedance study. *Diabetes Metab* 1999 Sep;25(4):321-8.
  - Sinha A, Formica C, Tsalamandris C, et al. Effects of insulin on body composition in patients with insulin-dependent and non-insulin-dependent diabetes. *Diabet Med* 1996;13:40-6.

Chapter 10

- **During the past few decades, science has uncovered many new details about fat**... For further reading in this area we recommend:
  - Avram MM, Avram AS, James WD. Subcutaneous fat in normal and diseased states: 1. Introduction. *J Am Acad Dermatol* 2005 Oct;53(4):663-70.
  - Bjorntorp P. Adipose tissue distribution and function. *Int J Obes* 1991 Sep;15 Suppl 2:67-81.
  - Cinti S. The adipose organ: morphological perspectives of adipose tissues. *Proc Nutr Soc* 2001 Aug;60(3):319-28
  - Klaus S. Adipose tissue as a regulator of energy balance. *Curr Drug Targets* 2004 Apr;5(3):241-50.
  - Pond CM. Adipose tissue and the immune system. *Prostaglandins Leukot Essent Fatty Acids* 2005 Jul;73(1):17-30.
  - Pond CM. Long-term changes in adipose tissue in human disease. *Proc Nutr Soc* 2001 Aug;60(3):365-74.
  - Power ML, Schulkin J. Sex differences in fat storage, fat metabolism, and the health risks from obesity: possible evolutionary origins. *Br J Nutr* 2008 May;99(5):931-40. Epub 2007 Nov 1.
  - Trayhurn P, Beattie JH. Physiological role of adipose tissue: white adipose tissue as an endocrine and secretory organ. *Proc Nutr Soc* 2001 Aug;60(3):329-39
- **The *Case of Overfeeding Identical Twins*...** based on information from:
  - Bouchard C, Tremblay A, Despres JP, et al. Overfeeding in identical twins: 5-year postoverfeeding results. *Metabolism* 1996 Aug;45(8):1042-50.
  - Bouchard C, Tremblay A, Despres JP, et al. The response to long-term overfeeding in identical twins. *N Engl J Med* 1990 May 24;322(21):1477-82.
  - Bouchard C, Tremblay A. Genetic Influences on the Response of Body Fat and Fat Distribution to Positive and Negative Energy Balances in Human Identical Twins. *J Nutr* 1997;127:943S–947S

- **Where we store fat is an important clue**… A vast amount of evidence on body fat distribution has accumulated over the past decade. For further reading in this area we recommend beginning with some of the following references.
    - den Tonkelaar I, Seidell JC, Collette HJ. Body fat distribution in relation to breast cancer in women participating in the DOM-project. *Breast Cancer Res Treat* 1995 Apr;34(1):55-61.
    - Iemura A, Douchi T, Yamamoto S, et al. Body fat distribution as a risk factor of endometrial cancer. *J Obstet Gynaecol Res* 2000 Dec;26(6):421-5.
    - Koh-Banerjee P, Wang Y, Hu FB, et al. Changes in body weight and body fat distribution as risk factors for clinical diabetes in US men. *Am J Epidemiol* 2004 Jun 15;159(12):1150-9.
    - Kopelman PG. The effects of weight loss treatments on upper and lower body fat. Int J *Obes Relat Metab Disord* 1997 Aug;21(8):619-25.
    - Moreau M, Valente F, Mak R, et al. Obesity, body fat distribution and incidence of sick leave in the Belgian workforce: the Belstress study. *Int J Obes Relat Metab Disord* 2004 Apr;28(4):574-82.
    - Ozbey N, Sencer E, Molvalilar S, Orhan Y. Body fat distribution and cardiovascular disease risk factors in pre- and postmenopausal obese women with similar BMI. *Endocr J* 2002 Aug;49(4):503-9.
    - Rosmond R, Bjorntorp P. Quality of life, overweight, and body fat distribution in middle-aged men. *Behav Med* 2000 Summer;26(2):90-4.
    - Tanne D, Medalie JH, Goldbourt U. Body fat distribution and long-term risk of stroke mortality. *Stroke* 2005 May;36(5):1021-5. Epub 2005 Mar 31.
    - Thalmann S, Meier CA. Local adipose tissue depots as cardiovascular risk factors. *Cardiovasc Res* 2007 Mar 14;
    - Wallner SJ, Luschnigg N, Schnedl WJ, et al. Body fat distribution of overweight females with a history of weight cycling. *Int J Obes Relat Metab Disord* 2004 Sep;28(9):1143-8.
    - Walton C, Lees B, Crook D, et al. Body fat distribution, rather than overall adiposity, influences serum lipids and lipoproteins in healthy men independently of age. *Am J Med* 1995 Nov;99(5):459-64.
- **The *Case of Lipodystrophy*…** Notes and references for this case were provided in chapter 8.
- **The *Case of the Disproportionate Loss of Peripheral Fat*…** Source is Wang J, Laferrere B, Thornton JC, Pierson RN Jr, Pi-Sunyer FX. Regional subcutaneous-fat loss induced by caloric restriction in obese women. *Obes Res* 2002 Sep;10(9):885-90.
- **The *Case of Menopause*…** Source is Franklin RM, Ploutz-Snyder L, Kanaley JA. Longitudinal changes in abdominal fat distribution with menopause. *Metabolism* 2009 Mar;58(3):311-5.
- **During the same three decades population-wide triglyceride levels (blood fats) have increased**… Source is Earl S. Ford, MD, MPH; Chaoyang Li, MD, PhD; Guixiang Zhao, MD, PhD; William S. Pearson, PhD; Ali H. Mokdad, PhD Hypertriglyceridemia and Its Pharmacologic Treatment Among US Adults. Arch Intern Med. 2009;169(6):572-578.
- **Cases of Subcutaneous and Visceral Adipose Tissue**… Wikipedia has pages dedicated to "Adipose tissue". A great deal of research has been done on visceral and subcutaneous adipose tissue. For further reading in this area we recommend beginning with some of the following references.
    - Chaston TB, Dixon JB. Factors associated with percent change in visceral versus subcutaneous abdominal fat during weight loss: findings from a systematic review. *Int J Obes (Lond)* 2008 Apr;32(4):619-28.
    - Ibrahim MM. Subcutaneous and visceral adipose tissue: structural and functional differences. *Obes Rev* 2009 Jul 28.
    - Kuk JL, Saunders TJ, Davidson LE, Ross R. Age-related changes in total and
    - regional fat distribution. *Ageing Res Rev* 2009 Oct;8(4):339-48.
    - Matsuzawa Y. The role of fat topology in the risk of disease. *Int J Obes*
    - *(Lond)* 2008 Dec;32 Suppl 7:S83-92.
    - Ohman MK, Wright AP, Wickenheiser KJ, et al. Visceral adipose tissue and atherosclerosis. *Curr Vasc Pharmacol* 2009 Apr;7(2):169-79.
    - Pi-Sunyer FX. The epidemiology of central fat distribution in relation to disease. *Nutr Rev* 2004 Jul;62(7 Pt 2):S120-6.
    - Santosa S, Jensen MD. Why are we shaped differently, and why does it matter? *Am J Physiol Endocrinol Metab* 2008 Sep;295(3):E531-5.
    - Snijder MB, Visser M, Dekker JM, et al. Low subcutaneous thigh fat is a risk factor for unfavourable glucose and lipid levels, independently of high abdominal fat. The Health ABC Study. *Diabetologia* 2005 Feb;48(2):301-8.Westerbacka J, Corner A, Tiikkainen M, et al. Women and men have similar amounts of liver and intra-abdominal fat, despite more subcutaneous fat in women: implications for sex differences in markers of cardiovascular risk. *Diabetologia* 2004 Aug;47(8):1360-9.

- Wajchenberg BL, Giannella-Neto D, da Silva ME, Santos RF. Depot-specific hormonal characteristics of subcutaneous and visceral adipose tissue and their relation to the metabolic syndrome. *Horm Metab Res* 2002 Nov-Dec;34(11-12):616-21.

- **Rats were fed diets containing lard, corn oil, or fish oil for six months**... Source is Hill JO, Peters JC, Lin D, et al. Lipid accumulation and body fat distribution is influenced by type of dietary fat fed to rats. *Int J Obes Relat Metab Disord* 1993 Apr;17(4):223-36.

- **Chronic stress tends to result in a disproportionate increase of belly fat**... This topic will be discussed in more detail in chapter 14.

- **The *Case of Thin Outside, Fat Inside*...** There are many news articles on the work of Dr. Jimmy Bell that can be found by doing a search for "thin outside, fat inside" or "TOFI". A good starting place to read about his findings is an article written by the guardian (Are you a Tofi? (That's thin on the outside, fat inside)) available online at:
  http://www.guardian.co.uk/science/2006/dec/10/medicineandhealth.health

- **Cases of Marbled Steak and Foie Gras**... A huge amount of information is available on fatty liver and a growing amount of research is available on the fat inside muscle tissues. The information links these sites of fat deposition as being associated with increased risk of disease. We suggest reading the Wikipedia "Marbled Meat" page for information on meat marbling, and the Wikipedia "Foie Gras" for information on this food. For those interested in reading more about human intermuscular fat we recommended beginning with the following references.

  - Gallagher D, Kuznia P, Heshka S, et al. Adipose tissue in muscle: a novel depot similar in size to visceral adipose tissue. *Am J Clin Nutr* 2005 Apr;81(4):903-10.
  - Hilton TN, Tuttle LJ, Bohnert KL, et al. Excessive Adipose Tissue Infiltration in Skeletal Muscle in Individuals With Obesity, Diabetes Mellitus, and Peripheral Neuropathy: Association With Performance and Function. *Phys Ther* 2008 Sep 18.
  - Manini TM, Clark BC, Nalls MA, et al. Reduced physical activity increases intermuscular adipose tissue in healthy young adults. *Am J Clin Nutr* 2007 Feb;85(2):377-84.
  - Miljkovic-Gacic I, Gordon CL, Goodpaster BH, et al. Adipose tissue infiltration in skeletal muscle: age patterns and association with diabetes among men of African ancestry. *Am J Clin Nutr* 2008 Jun;87(6):1590-5.
  - Song MY, Ruts E, Kim J, et al. Sarcopenia and increased adipose tissue infiltration of muscle in elderly African American women. *Am J Clin Nutr* 2004 May;79(5):874-80.
  - Yim JE, Heshka S, Albu JB, et al. Femoral-gluteal subcutaneous and intermuscular adipose tissues have independent and opposing relationships with CVD risk. *J Appl Physiol* 2008 Mar;104(3):700-7.
  - Yim JE, Heshka S, Albu J, et al. Intermuscular adipose tissue rivals visceral adipose tissue in independent associations with cardiovascular risk. *Int J Obes (Lond)* 2007 Sep;31(9):1400-5.

Chapter 11

- **Eleven volunteers were allowed free access to meals and snacks during two 14-day stays in a sleep laboratory**... Source is Nedeltcheva AV, Kilkus JM, Imperial J, Kasza K, Schoeller DA, Penev PD. Sleep curtailment is accompanied by increased intake of calories from snacks. *Am J Clin Nutr* 2009 Jan;89(1):126-33.

- **Circumstantial evidence, most of it from long-term observational studies, indicates that there is a consistent relationship between sleeping fewer hours and increased weight**... For further reading on associations between sleep duration and weight we recommend reading some of these articles:

  - Asplund R. Obesity in elderly people with nocturia: cause or consequence? *Can J Urol* 2007 Feb;14(1):3424-8.
  - Bjorvatn B, Sagen IM, Oyane N, et al. The association between sleep duration, body mass index and metabolic measures in the Hordaland Health Study. *J Sleep Res* 2007 Mar;16(1):66-76.
  - Brotman DJ. "Regression" of adiposity with more sleep. *Arch Intern Med* 2005 Jun 13;165(11):1314-5; author reply 1315.
  - Buscemi D, Kumar A, Nugent R, Nugent K. Short sleep times predict obesity in internal medicine clinic patients. *J Clin Sleep Med* 2007 Dec 15;3(7):681-8.
  - Cappuccio FP, Taggart FM, Kandala NB, et al. Meta-analysis of short sleep duration and obesity in children and adults. *Sleep* 2008 May 1;31(5):619-26.
  - Chaput JP, Després JP, Bouchard C, Tremblay A. The association between sleep duration and weight gain in adults: a 6-year prospective study from the Quebec Family Study. *Sleep* 2008 Apr 1;31(4):517-23.
  - Kronholm E, Aunola S, Hyyppa MT, et al. Sleep in monozygotic twin pairs discordant for obesity. *J Appl Physiol* 1996 Jan;80(1):14-9.

- Lumeng JC, Somashekar D, Appugliese D, et al. Shorter sleep duration is associated with increased risk for being overweight at ages 9 to 12 years. *Pediatrics* 2007 Nov;120(5):1020-9.
- Marniemi J, Kronholm E, Aunola S, et al. Visceral fat and psychosocial stress in identical twins discordant for obesity. *J Intern Med* 2002 Jan;251(1):35-43
- Moreno CR, Louzada FM, Teixeira LR, et al. Short sleep is associated with obesity among truck drivers. *Chronobiol Int* 2006;23(6):1295-303.
- Patel SR, Blackwell T, Redline S, et al. The association between sleep duration and obesity in older adults. *Int J Obes (Lond)* 2008 Oct 21
- Patel SR, Malhotra A, White DP, et al. Association between reduced sleep and weight gain in women. *Am J Epidemiol* 2006 Nov 15;164(10):947-54.
- Patel SR, Redline S. Two epidemics: are we getting fatter as we sleep less? *Sleep* 2004 Jun 15;27(4):602-3.
- Snell EK, Adam EK, Duncan GJ. Sleep and the body mass index and overweight status of children and adolescents. *Child Dev* 2007 Jan-Feb;78(1):309-23.
- Touchette E, Petit D, Sekine M, et al. A dose-response relationship between short sleeping hours and childhood obesity: results of the Toyama Birth Cohort Study. *Child Care Health Dev* 2002 Mar;28(2):163-70.
- Tremblay RE, Boivin M, Falissard B, et al. Associations between sleep duration patterns and overweight/obesity at age 6. *Sleep* 2008 Nov 1;31(11):1507-14.
- van den Berg JF, Knvistingh Neven A, Tulen JH, et al. Actigraphic sleep duration and fragmentation are related to obesity in the elderly: the Rotterdam Study. *Int J Obes (Lond)* 2008 Jul;32(7):1083-90.
- von Kries R, Toschke AM, Wurmser H, et al. Reduced risk for overweight and obesity in 5- and 6-y-old children by duration of sleep--a cross-sectional study. *Int J Obes Relat Metab Disord* 2002 May;26(5):710-6
- Vorona RD, Winn MP, Babineau TW, et al. Overweight and obese patients in a primary care population report less sleep than patients with a normal body mass index. *Arch Intern Med* 2005 Jan 10;165(1):25-30.

- **Sleep Self-Regulation and Sleep**... The best resource for gaining further understanding about sleep self-regulation is the book *Promise of Sleep* by William Dement, MD founder and director of the Stanford University Sleep Research Center.
- **Microsleep**... Wikipedia has a "Microsleep" page that provides a good orientation to this non-volitional type of sleep.
- **Sleep Debt**... William Dement, MD, is a proponent of sleep debt. His book *Promise of Sleep* provides a good background on this concept. Additional reading n sleep debt can be found in the following references.

  - Bonnet MH, Arand DL. We are chronically sleep deprived. *Sleep* 1995 Dec;18(10):908-11.
  - Carter N, Ulfberg J, Nyström B, Edling C. Sleep debt, sleepiness and accidents among males in the general population and male professional drivers. *Accid Anal Prev* 2003 Jul;35(4):613-7.
  - Dement WC. Sleep extension: getting as much extra sleep as possible. *Clin Sports Med* 2005 Apr;24(2):251-68, viii.
  - Kahn-Greene ET, Killgore DB, Kamimori GH, et al. The effects of sleep deprivation on symptoms of psychopathology in healthy adults. *Sleep Med* 2007 Mar 15.
  - Kivistö M, Härmä M, Sallinen M, Kalimo R. Work-related factors, sleep debt and insomnia in IT professionals. *Occup Med (Lond)* 2008 Mar;58(2):138-40.
  - Klerman EB, Dijk DJ. Interindividual variation in sleep duration and its association with sleep debt in young adults. *Sleep* 2005 Oct 1;28(10):1253-9.
  - Lucidi F, Devoto A, Bertini M, et al. The effects of sleep debt on vigilance in young drivers: an education/research project in high schools. *J Adolesc* 2002 Aug;25(4):405-14.
  - Prather AA, Marsland AL, Hall M, et al. Normative variation in self-reported sleep quality and sleep debt is associated with stimulated pro-inflammatory cytokine production. *Biol Psychol* 2009 Sep;82(1):12-7.
  - Regestein Q, Natarajan V, Pavlova M, et al. Sleep debt and depression in female college students. *Psychiatry Res* 2010 Mar 30;176(1):34-39.
  - Rupp TL, Wesensten NJ, Bliese PD, Balkin TJ. Banking sleep: realization of benefits during subsequent sleep restriction and recovery. *Sleep* 2009 Mar 1;32(3):311-21.
  - Spiegel K, Leproult R, Van Cauter E. Impact of sleep debt on metabolic and endocrine function. *Lancet* 1999 Oct 23;354(9188):1435-9.
  - Van Dongen HP, Maislin G, Mullington JM, Dinges DF. The cumulative cost of additional wakefulness: dose-response effects on neurobehavioral functions and sleep physiology from chronic sleep restriction and total sleep deprivation. *Sleep* 2003 Mar 15;26(2):117-26.
  - [No Authors]. Repaying your sleep debt. If sleep were a credit card company, many of us would be in deep trouble. *Harv Womens Health Watch* 2007 Jul;14(11):1-3.

- [No authors listed]. The national sleep debt. Too many get too little. *Mayo Clin Health Lett* 2006 Aug;24(8):1-3.

- **The Case of Hibernation…** An article called *Tired, hungry and sad? Relax, you're hibernating* by Catherine Zandonella of the Daily Mail is a good place to begin to better understand concepts introduced in this section. It can be found at www.dailymail.co.uk/health/article-94678/Tired-hungry-sad-Relax-youre-hibernating.html. The article *Gene research scientists close to human hibernation breakthrough* by Jonathan Thompson (www.independent.co.uk/news/science/gene-research-scientists-close-to-human-hibernation-breakthrough-626287.html) discusses the first hibernator genes found in humans. Punctuated sleep and quiet rest—polyphasic sleep—is discussed in *Awakening to Sleep* by Verlyn Klinkenborg (http://www.nytimes.com/1997/01/05/magazine/awakening-to-sleep.html?sec=health&pagewanted=all). *Lights Out: Sleep, Sugar, and Survival* by T. S. Wiley (ISBN-10: 0671038680) is the best book on the evolutionary need for winter darkness and sleep. Other sources used for this section include:

  - Berger RJ. Slow wave sleep, shallow torpor and hibernation: homologous states of diminished metabolism and body temperature. *Biol Psychol* 1984;19:305-26
  - Dark J, Forger NG, Stern JS, Zucker I. Recovery of lipid mass after removal of adipose tissue in ground squirrels. *Am J Physiol* 1985 Jul;249(1 Pt 2):R73-8.
  - Dark J. Seasonal weight gain is attenuated in food-restricted ground squirrels with lesions of the suprachiasmatic nuclei. *Behav Neurosci* 1984 Oct;98(5):830-5.
  - Dark J, Forger NG, Zucker I. Rapid recovery of body mass after surgical removal of adipose tissue in ground squirrels. *Proc Natl Acad Sci U S A* 1984 Apr;81(7):2270-2.
  - Dark J, Stern JS, Zucker I. Adipose tissue dynamics during cyclic weight loss and weight gain of ground squirrels. *Am J Physiol* 1989 Jun;256(6 Pt 2):R1286-92.
  - Dark J, Forger NG, Zucker I. Regulation and function of lipid mass during the annual cycle of the golden-mantled squirrel. In Heller HC, Musacchia XJ, and Wand LCH (eds.). *Living in the Cold: Physiological and Biochemical Adaptations.* Elsevier, New York 1986;445-451.
  - Duncan WC, Barbato G, Fagioli I, et al. A biphasic daily pattern of slow wave activity during a two-day 90-minute sleep wake schedule. *Arch Ital Biol* 2009 Dec;147(4):117-30.
  - Ebling FJ, Barrett P. The regulation of seasonal changes in food intake and body weight. *J Neuroendocrinol* 2008 Jun;20(6):827-33.
  - Forger NG, Dark J, Barnes BM, Zucker I. Fat ablation and food restriction influence reproductive development and hibernation in ground squirrels. *Biol Reprod* 1986 Jun;34(5):831-40.
  - Heldmaier G, Ortmann S, Elvert R. Natural hypometabolism during hibernation and daily torpor in mammals. *Respir Physiol Neurobiol* 2004 Aug 12;141(3):317-29.
  - Martin SL. Mammalian hibernation: a naturally reversible model for insulin resistance in man? *Diab Vasc Dis Res* 2008 Jun;5(2):76-81.
  - Mercer JG. Regulation of appetite and body weight in seasonal mammals. *Comp Biochem Physiol C Pharmacol Toxicol Endocrinol* 1998 Jun;119(3):295-303
  - Morgan PJ, Ross AW, Mercer JG, Barrett P. Chapter 19: What can we learn from seasonal animals about the regulation of energy balance? *Prog Brain Res* 2006;153:325-37.
  - Mrosovsky N. The amplitude and period of circannual cycles of body weight in golden-mantled ground squirrels with medial hypothalamic lesions. *Brain Res* 1975 Nov 28;99(1):97-116.
  - Shavlakadze T, Grounds M. Of bears, frogs, meat, mice and men: complexity of factors affecting skeletal muscle mass and fat. *Bioessays* 2006 Oct;28(10):994-1009.
  - Walford RL, Spindler SR. The response to calorie restriction in mammals shows features also common to hibernation: a cross-adaptation hypothesis. *J Gerontol A Biol Sci Med Sci* 1997 Jul;52(4):B179-83
  - Wehr TA, Giesen HA, Moul DE, et al. Suppression of men's responses to seasonal changes in day length by modern artificial lighting. *Am J Physiol* 1995;269:R173-8.
  - Wehr TA, Moul DE, Barbato G, et al. Conservation of photoperiod-responsive mechanisms in humans. *Am J Physiol* 1993 Oct;265(4 Pt 2):R846-57.
  - Zahorska-Markiewicz B. Weight reduction and seasonal variation. *Int J Obes* 1980;4:139-43.

- **The Case of Post-pregnancy Weight Retention…** William Dement, MD, estimates sleep debt in pregnancy and post-pregnancy in *Promise of Sleep.* Other references used for this section are:

  - Gay CL, Lee KA, Lee SY. Sleep patterns and fatigue in new mothers and fathers. *Biol Res Nurs* 2004 Apr;5(4):311-8.
  - Gunderson EP, Rifas-Shiman SL, Oken E, et al. Association of fewer hours of sleep at 6 months postpartum with substantial weight retention at 1 year postpartum. *Am J Epidemiol* 2008 Jan 15;167(2):178-87.
  - Huang CM, Carter PA, Guo JL. A comparison of sleep and daytime sleepiness in depressed and non-depressed mothers during the early postpartum period. *J Nurs Res* 2004 Dec;12(4):287-96.

- Yamazaki A, Lee KA, Kennedy HP, Weiss SJ. Sleep-wake cycles, social rhythms, and sleeping arrangement during Japanese childbearing family transition. *J Obstet Gynecol Neonatal Nurs* 2005 May-Jun;34(3):342-8.

- **The Case of Sleep Apnea… Sources for this section include:**
  - Berger G, Berger R, Oksenberg A. Progression of snoring and obstructive sleep apnoea: the role of increasing weight and time. *Eur Respir J* 2008 Nov 14. [Epub ahead of print]
  - Carter R 3rd, Watenpaugh DE. Obesity and obstructive sleep apnea: Or is it OSA and obesity? *Pathophysiology* 2008 Aug;15(2):71-7.
  - Chin K, Shimizu K, Nakamura T, et al. Changes in intra-abdominal visceral fat and serum leptin levels in patients with obstructive sleep apnea syndrome following nasal continuous positive airway pressure therapy. *Circulation* 1999 Aug 17;100(7):706-12
  - Major GC, Sériès F, Tremblay A. Does the energy expenditure status in obstructive sleep apnea favour a positive energy balance? *Clin Invest Med* 2007;30(6):E262-8.
  - Oretmenolu O, Süslü AE, Yücel OT, et al. Body fat composition: a predictive factor for obstructive sleep apnea. *Laryngoscope* 2005 Aug;115(8):1493-8.
  - Phillips BG, Hisel TM, Kato M, et al. Recent weight gain in patients with newly diagnosed obstructive sleep apnea. *J Hypertens* 1999;17:1297-300
  - Pillar G, Shehadeh N. Abdominal fat and sleep apnea: the chicken or the egg? *Diabetes Care* 2008 Feb;31 Suppl 2:S303-9.
  - Sakkas GK, Karatzaferi C, Liakopoulos et al. Polysomnographic evidence of sleep apnoea disorders in lean and overweight haemodialysis patients. *J Ren Care* 2007 Oct-Dec;33(4):159-64.
  - Shinohara E, Kihara S, Yamashita S, et al. Visceral fat accumulation as an important risk factor for obstructive sleep apnoea syndrome in obese subjects. *J Intern Med* 1997 Jan;241(1):11-8.
  - Tatsumi K, Saibara T. Effects of obstructive sleep apnea syndrome on hepatic steatosis and nonalcoholic steatohepatitis. *Hepatol Res* 2005 Oct;33(2):100-4. Epub 2005 Oct 7.
  - Trenell MI, Ward JA, Yee BJ, et al. Influence of constant positive airway pressure therapy on lipid storage, muscle metabolism and insulin action in obese patients with severe obstructive sleep apnoea syndrome. *Diabetes Obes Metab* 2007 Sep;9(5):679-87.
  - Vgontzas AN, Papanicolaou DA, Bixler EO, et al. Sleep apnea and daytime sleepiness and fatigue: relation to visceral obesity, insulin resistance, and hypercytokinemia. *J Clin Endocrinol Metab* 2000 Mar;85(3):1151-8

- **Cases of Intentional Sleep Deprivation**… The online article (http://news.yahoo.com/s/nm/20090610/hl_nm/us_sleep_gain_1) **Sleep deprivation tied to weight gain by** Karla Gale Karla Gale provides a good overview of the effects sleep deprivation has on shape. *Sleep May Be Factor In Weight Control* (http://www.sciencedaily.com /releases/2009/05/090517143222.htm) also provides a good overview. Glamour magazine article— *Lose Weight While You Sleep!*— by Jenny Stamos Kovacs is available online (http://www.glamour.com/magazine/2009/02/lose-weight-while-you-sleep). Other references used in this section are:
  - Gonzalez-Ortiz M, Martinez-Abundis E, Balcazar-Munoz BR, Pascoe-Gonzalez S. Effect of sleep deprivation on insulin sensitivity and cortisol concentration in healthy subjects. *Diabetes Nutr Metab* 2000;13:80-3.
  - Laposky AD, Bass J, Kohsaka A, Turek FW. Sleep and circadian rhythms: key components in the regulation of energy metabolism. *FEBS Lett* 2008 Jan 9;582(1):142-51.
  - Schmid SM, Hallschmid M, Jauch-Chara K, et al. A single night of sleep deprivation increases ghrelin levels and feelings of hunger in normal-weight healthy men. *J Sleep Res* 2008 Sep;17(3):331-4.
  - Spiegel K, Tasali E, Penev P, Van Cauter E. Brief communication: Sleep curtailment in healthy young men is associated with decreased leptin levels, elevated ghrelin levels, and increased hunger and appetite. *Ann Intern Med* 2004 Dec 7;141(11):846-50.
  - Spiegel K, Leproult R, Van Cauter E. Impact of sleep debt on metabolic and endocrine function. *Lancet* 1999 Oct 23;354(9188):1435-9.
  - Van Dongen HP, Maislin G, Mullington JM, Dinges DF. The cumulative cost of additional wakefulness: dose-response effects on neurobehavioral functions and sleep physiology from chronic sleep restriction and total sleep deprivation. *Sleep* 2003 Mar 15;26(2):117-26.
  - Vanitallie TB. Sleep and energy balance: Interactive homeostatic systems. *Metabolism* 2006 Oct;55(10 Suppl 2):S30-5.
  - Voderholzer U, Hohagen F, Klein T, et al. Impact of sleep deprivation and subsequent recovery sleep on cortisol in unmedicated depressed patients. *Am J Psychiatry* 2004 Aug;161(8):1404-10.

Chapter 12

- **Our weight does not stay constant; it constantly fluctuates**... For further reading in this area (daily, monthly, and seasonal weight change), including how daily weight fluctuations might be a clue to whether or not a person is at or below natural weight, we recommend reading:
  - Cugini P, Salandri A, Celli Vet al. Circadian rhythm of some parameters of body composition in the elderly investigated by means of bioelectrical impedance analysis. *Eat Weight Disord* 2002 Sep;7(3):182-9.
  - Cugini P, Salandri A, Cilli M, et al. Daily hunger sensation and body composition: I. Their relationships in clinically healthy subjects. *Eat Weight Disord* 1998 Dec;3(4):168-72.
  - Cugini P, Salandri A, Petrangeli CM, et al. Circadian rhythms in human body composition. *Chronobiol Int* 1996 Nov;13(5):359-71.
  - Ebling FJ, Barrett P. The regulation of seasonal changes in food intake and body weight. *J Neuroendocrinol* 2008 Jun;20(6):827-33.
  - Heatherton TF, Polivy J, Herman CP. Restraint, weight loss, and variability of body weight. *J Abnorm Psychol* 1991 Feb;100(1):78-83.
  - Morgan PJ, Ross AW, Mercer JG, Barrett P. Chapter 19: What can we learn from seasonal animals about the regulation of energy balance? *Prog Brain Res* 2006;153:325-37.
  - Rodriguez G, Moreno LA, Sarria A, et al. Assessment of nutritional status and body composition in children using physical anthropometry and bioelectrical impedance: influence of diurnal variations. *J Pediatr Gastroenterol Nutr* 2000 Mar;30(3):305-9.
  - Svartberg J, Jorde R, Sundsfjord J, et al. Seasonal variation of testosterone and waist to hip ratio in men: the Tromso study. *J Clin Endocrinol Metab* 2003 Jul;88(7):3099-104.
  - Tanaka M, Itoh K, Abe S, et al. Irregular patterns in the daily weight chart at night predict body weight regain. *Exp Biol Med (Maywood)* 2004 Oct;229(9):940-5.
- **Figuratively speaking, we are clocks and calendars**... A very good introductory book on body clocks and calendars is *The Body Clock Guide to Better Health: How to Use Your Body's Natural Clock to Fight Illness and Achieve Maximum Health* by Michael Smolensky (ISBN-10: 0805056629).
- **Body clock research reveals that some people are morning people**... This is referred to as a person's chronotype. It is usually assessed using a morningness/eveningness questionnaire, with morning people referred to as larks and night people as owls. The source for the link to shape and bipolar disease is Soreca I, Fagiolini A, Frank E, Goodpaster BH, Kupfer DJ. Chronotype and body composition in bipolar disorder. *Chronobiol Int* 2009 May;26(4):780-8.
- **The *Case of Polycystic Ovarian Syndrome*...** The sources for lights effects on producing this syndrome in animals are:
  - Bacon WL, Liu HK. Influence of photoperiod and age of photostimulation on the incidence of polycystic ovarian follicle syndrome in turkey breeder hens. *Poult Sci* 2003 Dec;82(12):1985-9.
  - Barron ML. Light exposure, melatonin secretion, and menstrual cycle parameters: an integrative review. *Biol Res Nurs* 2007 Jul;9(1):49-69.
  - Ferrari E, Bossolo PA, Foppa S, et al. Prolactin secretion in polycystic ovary syndrome: circadian rhythmicity and dynamic aspects. *Gynecol Endocrinol* 1988 Jun;2(2):101-11.
  - Hamilton-Fairley D, White D, Griffiths M, et al. Diurnal variation of sex hormone binding globulin and insulin-like growth factor binding protein-1 in women with polycystic ovary syndrome. *Clin Endocrinol (Oxf)* 1995 Aug;43(2):159-65.
  - Ortega HH, Lorente JA, Mira GA, et al. Constant light exposure causes dissociation in gonadotrophin secretion and inhibits partially neuroendocrine differentiation of Leydig cells in adult rats. *Reprod Domest Anim* 2004 Dec;39(6):417-23.
  - Prata Lima MF, Baracat EC, Simoes MJ. Effects of melatonin on the ovarian response to pinealectomy or continuous light in female rats: similarity with polycystic ovary syndrome. *Braz J Med Biol Res* 2004 Jul;37(7):987-95.
  - Veldhuis JD, Pincus SM, Garcia-Rudaz MC, et al. Disruption of the joint synchrony of luteinizing hormone, testosterone, and androstenedione secretion in adolescents with polycystic ovarian syndrome. *J Clin Endocrinol Metab* 2001 Jan;86(1):72-9.
  - Zumoff B, Freeman R, Coupey S, et al. A chronobiologic abnormality in luteinizing hormone secretion in teenage girls with the polycystic-ovary syndrome. *N Engl J Med* 1983 Nov 17;309(20):1206-9.
- **The *Cases of the Implanted Cancer*...** Sources for this case are:
  - Dauchy RT, Sauer LA, Blask DE, Vaughan GM. Light contamination during the dark phase in "photoperiodically controlled" animal rooms: effect on tumor growth and metabolism in rats. *Lab Anim Sci* 1997 Oct;47(5):511-8.
  - Filipski E, King VM, Li XM, et al. Host Circadian Clock as a Control Point in Tumor Progression. *J Natl Cancer Inst* 2002;94:690-697
  - Filipski E, Innominato PF, Wu M, et al. Effects of light and food schedules on liver and tumor molecular clocks in mice. *J Natl Cancer Inst* 2005 Apr 6;97(7):507-17.

- Wu MW, Li XM, Xian LJ, Levi F. Effects of meal timing on tumor progression in mice. *Life Sci* 2004 Jul 23;75(10):1181-93.
- The *Cases of Digestion*... Sources for this case are:
    - Hirota N, Sone Y, Tokura H. Effect of evening exposure to dim or bright light on the digestion of carbohydrate in the supper meal. *Chronobiol Int* 2003 Sep;20(5):853-62.
    - Sone Y, Hyun KJ, Nishimura S, Lee YA, Tokura H. Effects of dim or bright-light exposure during the daytime on human gastrointestinal activity. *Chronobiol Int* 2003 Jan;20(1):123-33.
- The *Case of the Timed Hormones*... Source for this case is Cincotta AH, Wilson JM, deSouza CJ, Meier AH. Properly timed injections of cortisol and prolactin produce long-term reductions in obesity, hyperinsulinaemia and insulin resistance in the Syrian hamster (Mesocricetus auratus). *J Endocrinol* 1989 Mar;120(3):385-91.
- The *Case of Intentionally Disrupting Timing*... Source for this case is Scheer FA, Hilton MF, Mantzoros CS, Shea SA. Adverse metabolic and cardiovascular consequences of circadian misalignment. *Proc Natl Acad Sci* 2009 Mar 17;106(11):4453-8.
- **Internal desynchronization**... For more reading about possible shape consequences we suggest beginning with:
    - Ferrari E, Magri F, Pontiggia B, et al. Circadian neuroendocrine functions in disorders of eating behavior. *Eat Weight Disord* 1997 Dec;2(4):196-202.
    - Mishra A, Cheng CH, Lee WC, Tsai LL. Proteomic changes in the hypothalamus and retroperitoneal fat from male F344 rats subjected to repeated light-dark shifts. *Proteomics* 2009 Aug 5.
    - Preuss F, Tang Y, Laposky AD, et al. Adverse effects of chronic circadian desynchronization in animals in a "challenging" environment. *Am J Physiol Regul Integr Comp Physiol* 2008 Oct 8.
    - Scheer FA, Hilton MF, Mantzoros CS, Shea SA. Adverse metabolic and cardiovascular consequences of circadian misalignment. *Proc Natl Acad Sci* 2009 Mar 17;106(11):4453-8.
    - Tsai LL, Tsai YC, Hwang K, et al. Repeated light-dark shifts speed up body weight gain in male F344 rats. *Am J Physiol Endocrinol Metab* 2005 Aug;289(2):E212-7.
    - Tsai YC. The effect of scheduled forced wheel activity on body weight in male F344 rats undergoing chronic circadian desynchronization. *Int J Obes (Lond)* 2007 Mar 13.
- **Rats are nocturnal (night) animals. Cattle, like humans, are diurnal (day) creatures**... There is a great deal of research on photoperiod and shape in animals. Sources used to make this statement are:
    - Boon P, Visser H, Daan S. Effect of photoperiod on body mass, and daily energy intake and energy expenditure in young rats. *Physiol Behav* 1997 Oct;62(4):913-9.
    - Larkin LM, Moore BJ, Stern JS, Horwitz BA. Effect of photoperiod on body weight and food intake of obese and lean Zucker rats. *Life Sci* 1991;49(10):735-45.
    - Tucker HA, Petitclerc D, Zinn SA. The influence of photoperiod on body weight gain, body composition, nutrient intake and hormone secretion. *J Anim Sci* 1984 Dec;59(6):1610-20.
    - Wideman CH, Murphy HM. Constant light induces alterations in melatonin levels, food intake, feed efficiency, visceral adiposity, and circadian rhythms in rats. *Nutr Neurosci.* 2009 Oct;12(5):233-40.
- **Body clock orientation in time has a pronounced effect on shape and metabolism**... Some good articles on this topic include:
    - Bechtold DA. Energy-responsive timekeeping. *J Genet* 2008 Dec;87(5):447-58.
    - Block G. Keep time, stay healthy. *Sci Aging Knowledge Environ* 2005 May 11;2005(19):pe13.
    - Kohsaka A, Bass J. A sense of time: how molecular clocks organize metabolism. *Trends Endocrinol Metab* 2006 Nov 29.
    - Staels B. When the Clock stops ticking, metabolic syndrome explodes. *Nat Med* 2006 Jan;12(1):54-5.
    - Zvonic S, Ptitsyn AA, Conrad SA, et al. Characterization of peripheral circadian clocks in adipose tissues. *Diabetes* 2006 Apr;55(4):962-70.
- The *Case of Clock Mutant Mice*... Sources for this case are:
    - Oishi K, Atsumi G, Sugiyama S, et al. Disrupted fat absorption attenuates obesity induced by a high-fat diet in Clock mutant mice. *FEBS Lett* 2006 Jan 9;580(1):127-30.
    - Turek FW, Joshu C, Kohsaka A, et al. Obesity and metabolic syndrome in circadian Clock mutant mice. *Science* 2005 May 13;308(5724):1043-5.
    - Williams DL, Schwartz MW. Out of synch: Clock mutation causes obesity in mice. *Cell Metab* 2005 Jun;1(6):355-6.
- **Shift work**... Many studies have reported an association between shift work and shape. We suggest the following references for more reading on this topic.
    - Boyce RW, Boone EL, Cioci BW, Lee AH. Physical activity, weight gain and occupational health among call centre employees. *Occup Med (Lond)* 2008 Jun;58(4):238-44.

- Di Lorenzo L, De Pergola G, Zocchetti C, et al. Effect of shift work on body mass index: results of a study performed in 319 glucose-tolerant men working in a Southern Italian industry. *Int J Obes Relat Metab Disord* 2003 Nov;27(11):1353-8.
- Ekmekcioglu C, Touitou Y. Chronobiological aspects of food intake and metabolism and their relevance on energy balance and weight regulation. *Obes Rev.* 2010 Jan 27.
- Geliebter A, Gluck ME, Tanowitz M, et al. Work-shift period and weight change. *Nutrition* 2000 Jan;16(1):27-9.
- Ketchum ES, Morton JM. Disappointing weight loss among shift workers after laparoscopic gastric bypass surgery. *Obes Surg* 2007 May;17(5):581-4.
- Suwazono Y, Dochi M, Sakata K, et al. A longitudinal study on the effect of shift work on weight gain in male Japanese workers. *Obesity (Silver Spring)* 2008 Aug;16(8):1887-93.
- Yamada Y, Kameda M, Noborisaka Y, et al. Excessive fatigue and weight gain among cleanroom workers after changing from an 8-hour to a 12-hour shift. *Scand J Work Environ Health* 2001 Oct;27(5):318-26.

- The *Case of Freshman Weight Gain*… Sources for this case are:
  - Anderson DA, Shapiro JR, Lundgren JD. The freshman year of college as a critical period for weight gain: an initial evaluation. *Eat Behav* 2003 Nov;4(4):363-7.
  - Crombie AP, Ilich JZ, Dutton GR, et al. The freshman weight gain phenomenon revisited. *Nutr Rev* 2009 Feb;67(2):83-94.
  - Delinsky SS, Wilson GT. Weight gain, dietary restraint, and disordered eating in the freshman year of college. *Eat Behav* 2008 Jan;9(1):82-90.
  - Edmonds MJ, Ferreira KJ, Nikiforuk EA, et al. Body weight and percent body fat increase during the transition from high school to university in females. *J Am Diet Assoc* 2008 Jun;108(6):1033-7.
  - Holm-Denoma JM, Joiner TE, Vohs KD, Heatherton TF. The "freshman fifteen" (the "freshman five" actually): predictors and possible explanations. *Health Psychol* 2008 Jan;27(1 Suppl):S3-9.
  - Hoffman DJ, Policastro P, Quick V, Lee SK. Changes in body weight and fat mass of men and women in the first year of college: A study of the "freshman 15". *J Am Coll Health* 2006 Jul-Aug;55(1):41-5.
  - Levitsky DA, Halbmaier CA, Mrdjenovic G. The freshman weight gain: a model for the study of the epidemic of obesity. *Int J Obes Relat Metab Disord* 2004 Nov;28(11):1435-42.
  - Mihalopoulos NL, Auinger P, Klein JD. The Freshman 15: is it real? *J Am Coll Health.* 2008 Mar-Apr;56(5):531-3.
  - Morrow ML, Heesch KC, Dinger MK, et al. Freshman 15: fact or fiction? *Obesity (Silver Spring)* 2006 Aug;14(8):1438-43.
  - Pliner P, Saunders T. Vulnerability to freshman weight gain as a function of dietary restraint and residence. *Physiol Behav* 2008 Jan 28;93(1-2):76-82.
  - Qin LQ, Li J, Wang Y, et al. The effects of nocturnal life on endocrine circadian patterns in healthy adults. *Life Sci* 2003 Sep 26;73(19):2467-75.
  - Racette SB, Deusinger SS, Strube MJ, et al. Changes in weight and health behaviors from freshman through senior year of college. *J Nutr Educ Behav* 2008 Jan-Feb;40(1):39-42.

- The *Case of Night Eating*… Source for this case is Friedman S, Even C, Dardennes R, Guelfi JD. Light Therapy, Obesity, and Night-Eating Syndrome. *Am J Psychiatry* 159:875-876, May 2002 (letter)
  The *Case of Phototherapy and Weight*… Source for this case is Bylesjo EI, Boman K, Wetterberg L. Obesity treated with phototherapy: four case studies. *Int J Eat Disord* 1996 Dec;20(4):443-46.

- The *Case of Light Therapy and Exercise*… Source for this case is Dunai A, Novak M. Chung SM, et al. Moderate Exercise and Bright Light Treatment in Overweight and Obese Individuals. *Obesity* 15:1749-1757 (2007).

- **An eight percent increase in meal size has been observed at the time of the full moon**… Source is de Castro JM, Pearcey SM. Lunar rhythms of the meal and alcohol intake of humans. *Physiol Behav* 1995 Mar;57(3):439-44.

- **Calendar functions shift the shape of many animals**… For further reading on seasonal and photoperiod effects on the shape of animals we recommend reading the following:
  - Bartness TJ, Wade GN. Photoperiodic control of seasonal body weight cycles in hamsters. *Neurosci Biobehav Rev* 1985 Winter;9(4):599-612.
  - Bartness TJ, Demas GE, Song CK. Seasonal changes in adiposity: the roles of the photoperiod, melatonin and other hormones, and sympathetic nervous system. *Exp Biol Med (Maywood)* 2002 Jun;227(6):363-76.
  - Bartness TJ. Photoperiod, sex, gonadal steroids, and housing density affect body fat in hamsters. *Physiol Behav* 1996 Aug;60(2):517-29.
  - Bartness TJ. Short day-induced depletion of lipid stores is fat pad- and gender-specific in Siberian hamsters. *Physiol Behav* 1995 Sep;58(3):539-50.
  - Boon P, Visser H, Daan S. Effect of photoperiod on body mass, and daily energy intake and energy expenditure in young rats. *Physiol Behav* 1997 Oct;62(4):913-9.

- Clarke IJ, Rao A, Chilliard Y, et al. Photoperiod effects on gene expression for hypothalamic appetite-regulating peptides and food intake in the ram. *Am J Physiol Regul Integr Comp Physiol* 2003 Jan;284(1):R101-15.
- Dark J, Forger NG, Stern JS, Zucker I. Recovery of lipid mass after removal of adipose tissue in ground squirrels. *Am J Physiol* 1985 Jul;249(1 Pt 2):R73-8.
- Dark J. Seasonal weight gain is attenuated in food-restricted ground squirrels with lesions of the suprachiasmatic nuclei. *Behav Neurosci* 1984 Oct;98(5):830-5.
- Dark J, Forger NG, Zucker I. Rapid recovery of body mass after surgical removal of adipose tissue in ground squirrels. *Proc Natl Acad Sci U S A* 1984 Apr;81(7):2270-2.
- Dark J, Stern JS, Zucker I. Adipose tissue dynamics during cyclic weight loss and weight gain of ground squirrels. *Am J Physiol* 1989 Jun;256(6 Pt 2):R1286-92.
- Dark J, Wade GN, Zucker I. Short day lengths decrease body mass of overweight female meadow voles. *Physiol Behav* 1986;38(3):381-4.
- El-Bakry HA, Plunkett SS, Bartness TJ. Photoperiod, but not a high-fat diet, alters body fat in Shaw's jird. *Physiol Behav* 1999 Dec 1-15;68(1-2):87-91.
- Hunter HL, Nagy TR. Body composition in a seasonal model of obesity: longitudinal measures and validation of DXA. *Obes Res* 2002 Nov;10(11):1180-7.
- Karpouzos H, Hernandez AM, MacDougall-Shackleton EA, MacDougall-Shackleton SA. Effects of day-length and food availability on food caching, mass and fat reserves in black-capped chickadees (Poecile atricapillus). *Physiol Behav* 2005 Mar 16;84(3):465-9.
- Krol E, Redman P, Thomson PJ, et al. Effect of photoperiod on body mass, food intake and body composition in the field vole, Microtus agrestis. *J Exp Biol* 2005 Feb;208(Pt 3):571-84.
- Larkin LM, Moore BJ, Stern JS, Horwitz BA. Effect of photoperiod on body weight and food intake of obese and lean Zucker rats. *Life Sci* 1991;49(10):735-45.
- Peacock WL, Krol E, Moar KM, et al. Photoperiodic effects on body mass, energy balance and hypothalamic gene expression in the bank vole. *J Exp Biol* 2004 Jan;207(Pt 1):165-77.
- Plunkett SS, Fine JB, Bartness TJ. Photoperiod and gender affect adipose tissue growth and cellularity in juvenile Syrian hamsters. *Physiol Behav* 2000 Dec;71(5):493-501.
- Tucker HA, Petitclerc D, Zinn SA. The influence of photoperiod on body weight gain, body composition, nutrient intake and hormone secretion. *J Anim Sci* 1984 Dec;59(6):1610-20.
- Wade GN. Dietary obesity in golden hamsters: reversibility and effects of sex and photoperiod. *Physiol Behav* 1983 Jan;30(1):131-7.
- Zhao ZJ, Wang DH. Short photoperiod influences energy intake and serum leptin level in Brandt's voles (Microtus brandtii). *Horm Behav* 2006 Apr;49(4):463-9.

- **The *Case of Holiday Weight Gain*...** Sources for this case are:
  - Adam CL, Mercer JG. Appetite regulation and seasonality: implications for obesity. *Proc Nutr Soc* 2004 Aug;63(3):413-9.
  - Hull HR, Morrow ML, Heesch KC, et al. Effect of the summer months on body weight and composition in college women. *J Womens Health (Larchmt)* 2007 Dec;16(10):1510-5.
  - Hull HR, Hester CN, Fields DA. The effect of the holiday season on body weight and composition in college students. *Nutr Metab (Lond)* 2006 Dec 28;3:44.
  - Hull HR, Radley D, Dinger MK, Fields DA. The effect of the Thanksgiving holiday on weight gain. *Nutr J* 2006 Nov 21;5:29.
  - Yanovski JA, Yanovski SZ, Sovik KN, et al. A prospective study of holiday weight gain. *N Engl J Med* 2000;342:861-7
  - Zahorska-Markiewicz B. Weight reduction and seasonal variation. *Int J Obes* 1980;4(2):139-43.

- **In a study of office workers during the winter...** Source is Partonen T, Lonnqvist J. Bright light improves vitality and alleviates distress in healthy people. *J Affect Disord* 2000 Jan-Mar;57(1-3):55-61.
- **The *Case of Seasonally Affective Disorder*...** Sources for this case are:
  - Cizza G, Romagni P, Lotsikas A, et al. Plasma leptin in men and women with seasonal affective disorder and in healthy matched controls. *Horm Metab Res* 2005 Jan;37(1):45-8.
  - Cugini P, Passynkova NR, Di Cristofano F, et al. Daily sensation of hunger, before and after phototherapy, in subjects with depression-type seasonal affective disorder. *Clin Ter* 2001 Nov-Dec;152(6):353-62.
  - Lam RW, Lee SK, Tam EM, et al. An open trial of light therapy for women with seasonal affective disorder and comorbid bulimia nervosa. *J Clin Psychiatry* 2001 Mar;62(3):164-8.

- **The *Case of Bulimia*...** Sources for this case are:
  - Blouin A, Blouin J, Aubin P, et al. Seasonal patterns of bulimia nervosa. *Am J Psychiatry* 1992 Jan;149(1):73-81.
  - Blouin AG, Blouin JH, Iversen H, et al. Light therapy in bulimia nervosa: a double-blind, placebo-controlled study. *Psychiatry Res* 1996 Feb 28;60(1):1-9.

- Gaist PA, Obarzanek E, Skwerer RG, et al. Effects of bright light on resting metabolic rate in patients with seasonal affective disorder and control subjects. *Biol Psychiatry* 1990 Dec 1;28(11):989-96.
- Lam RW, Lee SK, Tam EM, et al. An open trial of light therapy for women with seasonal affective disorder and comorbid bulimia nervosa. *J Clin Psychiatry* 2001 Mar;62(3):164-8.

- **The duration of the photoperiod appears to have a strong impact on shape**... To read more about the hypothesis that photoperiod might influence human shape we suggest reading:
  - Bronson FH. Are humans seasonally photoperiodic? *J Biol Rhythms* 2004 Jun;19(3):180-92.
  - Vondrasova D, Hajek I, Illnerova H. Exposure to long summer days affects the human melatonin and cortisol rhythms. *Brain Res* 1997 Jun 6;759(1):166-70.
  - Wehr TA. Photoperiodism in humans and other primates: evidence and implications. *J Biol Rhythms* 2001 Aug;16(4):348-64.
  - Wehr TA, Moul DE, Barbato G, et al. Conservation of photoperiod-responsive mechanisms in humans. *Am J Physiol* 1993 Oct;265(4 Pt 2):R846-57.
  - Wehr TA. In short photoperiods, human sleep is biphasic. *J Sleep Res* 1992 Jun;1(2):103-107.

- **The Solution: Naturalistic Lighting**... For further reading in the therapeutic use of light and darkness we suggest reading:
  - Anderson DJ, Legg NJ, Ridout DA. Preliminary trial of photic stimulation for premenstrual syndrome. *J Obstet Gynaecol* 1997 Jan;17(1):76-9.
  - Avery DH, Eder DN, Bolte MA, et al. Dawn simulation and bright light in the treatment of SAD: a controlled study. *Biol Psychiatry* 2001 Aug 1;50(3):205-16.
  - Avery DH, Bolte MA, Ries R. Dawn simulation treatment of abstinent alcoholics with winter depression. *J Clin Psychiatry* 1998 Jan;59(1):36-42.
  - Avery DH, Bolte MA, Wolfson JK, Kazaras AL. Dawn simulation compared with a dim red signal in the treatment of winter depression. *Biol Psychiatry* 1994 Aug 1;36(3):180-8.
  - Barbini B, Benedetti F, Colombo C, et al. Dark therapy for mania: a pilot study. *Bipolar Disord* 2005 Feb;7(1):98-101.
  - Boivin DB, James FO. Circadian adaptation to night-shift work by judicious light and darkness exposure. *J Biol Rhythms* 2002 Dec;17(6):556-67.
  - Cajochen C, Jud C, Munch M, et al. Evening exposure to blue light stimulates the expression of the clock gene PER2 in humans. *Eur J Neurosci* 2006 Feb;23(4):1082-6.
  - Crowley SJ, Lee C, Tseng CY, et al. Combinations of bright light, scheduled dark, sunglasses, and melatonin to facilitate circadian entrainment to night shift work. *J Biol Rhythms* 2003 Dec;18(6):513-23.
  - Doljansky JT, Kannety H, Dagan Y. Working under daylight intensity lamp: an occupational risk for developing circadian rhythm sleep disorder? *Chronobiol Int* 2005;22(3):597-605.
  - Eastman CI, Boulos Z, Terman M, et al. Light treatment for sleep disorders: consensus report. VI. Shift work. *J Biol Rhythms* 1995 Jun;10(2):157-64.
  - Evans JA, Elliott JA, Gorman MR. Circadian entrainment and phase resetting differ markedly under dimly illuminated versus completely dark nights. *Behav Brain Res* 2005 Jul 1;162(1):116-26.
  - Fontana Gasio P, Krauchi K, Cajochen C, et al. Dawn-dusk simulation light therapy of disturbed circadian rest-activity cycles in demented elderly. *Exp Gerontol* 2003 Jan-Feb;38(1-2):207-16.
  - Glickman G, Byrne B, Pineda C, et al. Light therapy for seasonal affective disorder with blue narrow-band light-emitting diodes (LEDs). *Biol Psychiatry* 2006 Mar 15;59(6):502-7.
  - Golden RN, Gaynes BN, Ekstrom RD, et al. The efficacy of light therapy in the treatment of mood disorders: a review and meta-analysis of the evidence. *Am J Psychiatry* 2005;162:656-662.
  - Kirisoglu C, Guilleminault C. Twenty minutes versus forty-five minutes morning bright light treatment on sleep onset insomnia in elderly subjects. *J Psychosom Res* 2004 May;56(5):537-42.
  - Leppamaki S, Meesters Y, Haukka J, et al. Effect of simulated dawn on quality of sleep--a community-based trial. *BMC Psychiatry* 2003 Oct 27;3(1):14.
  - Lingjaerde O, Foreland AR, Dankertsen J. Dawn simulation vs. lightbox treatment in winter depression: a comparative study. *Acta Psychiatr Scand* 1998 Jul;98(1):73-80
  - McEnany GW, Lee KA. Effects of light therapy on sleep, mood, and temperature in women with nonseasonal major depression. *Issues Ment Health Nurs* 2005 Aug-Sep;26(7):781-94.
  - Morita T, Tokura H. The influence of different wavelengths of light on human biological rhythms. *Appl Human Sci* 1998 May;17(3):91-6.

- Munch M, Kobialka S, Steiner R, et al. Wavelength-dependent effects of evening light exposure on sleep architecture and sleep EEG power density in men. *Am J Physiol Regul Integr Comp Physiol* 2006 May;290(5):R1421-8.
- Norden MJ, Avery DH. A controlled study of dawn simulation in subsyndromal winter depression. *Acta Psychiatr Scand* 1993 Jul;88(1):67-71
- Park SJ, Tokura H. Bright light exposure during the daytime affects circadian rhythms of urinary melatonin and salivary immunoglobulin A. *Chronobiol Int* 1999 May;16(3):359-71
- Rybak YE, McNeely HE, Mackenzie BE, et al. An open trial of light therapy in adult attention-deficit/hyperactivity disorder. *J Clin Psychiatry* 2006 Oct;67(10):1527-35.
- Sasseville A, Paquet N, Sevigny J, Hebert M. Blue blocker glasses impede the capacity of bright light to suppress melatonin production. *J Pineal Res* 2006 Aug;41(1):73-8.
- Terman JS, Terman M, Lo ES, Cooper TB. Circadian time of morning light administration and therapeutic response in winter depression. *Arch Gen Psychiatry* 2001 Jan;58(1):69-75.
- Thorn L, Hucklebridge F, Esgate A, Evans P, Clow A. The effect of dawn simulation on the cortisol response to awakening in healthy participants. *Psychoneuroendocrinology* 2004 Aug;29(7):925-30.
- Wehr TA, Turner EH, Shimada JM, et al. Treatment of rapidly cycling bipolar patient by using extended bed rest and darkness to stabilize the timing and duration of sleep. *Biol Psychiatry* 1998 Jun 1;43(11):822-8.

Chapter 13

- **The Case of Food Sensitive Body Clocks**… For further reading about the effects of food timing on body clocks we recommend reading:

  - Apfelbaum M, Reinberg A, Lacatis D. Effects of meal timing on circadian rhythms in 9 physiologic variables of young healthy but obese women on a calorie restricted diet. *Int J Chronobiol* 1976;4(1):29-37.
  - Aschoff J, von Goetz C, Wildgruber C, Wever RA. Meal timing in humans during isolation without time cues. *J Biol Rhythms* 1986 Summer;1(2):151-62
  - Beebe CA, Van Cauter E, Shapiro ET, et al. Effect of temporal distribution of calories on diurnal patterns of glucose levels and insulin secretion in NIDDM. *Diabetes Care* 1990 Jul;13(7):748-55.
  - Boulos Z, Terman M. Food availability and daily biological rhythms. *Neurosci Biobehav Rev* 1980 Summer;4(2):119-31.
  - Davidson AJ, Poole AS, Yamazaki S, Menaker M. Is the food-entrainable circadian oscillator in the digestive system? *Genes Brain Behav* 2003 Feb;2(1):32-9.
  - Cella LK, Van Cauter E, Schoeller DA. Effect of meal timing on diurnal rhythm of human cholesterol synthesis. *Am J Physiol* 1995 Nov;269(5 Pt 1):E878-83.
  - Follenius M, Brandenberger G, Hietter B. Diurnal cortisol peaks and their relationships to meals. *J Clin Endocrinol Metab* 1982 Oct;55(4):757-61.
  - Goetz F, Bishop J, Halberg F, et al. Timing of single daily meal influences relations among human circadian rhythms in urinary cyclic AMP and hemic glucagon, insulin and iron. *Experientia* 1976 Aug 15;32(8):1081-4
  - Green J, Pollak CP, Smith GP. The effect of desynchronization on meal patterns of humans living in time isolation. *Physiol Behav* 1987;39(2):203-9.
  - Krieger DT, Hauser H. Comparison of synchronization of circadian corticosteroid rhythms by photoperiod and food. *Proc Natl Acad Sci U S A.* 1978 Mar;75(3):1577-81.
  - Lax P, Zamora S, Madrid JA. Food-entrained feeding and locomotor circadian rhythms in rats under different lighting conditions. *Chronobiol Int* 1999 May;16(3):281-91.
  - Mendoza J. Circadian clocks: setting time by food. *J Neuroendocrinol* 2007 Feb;19(2):127-37.
  - Mistlberger RE. Circadian rhythms: perturbing a food-entrained clock. *Curr Biol* 2006 Nov 21;16(22):R968-9.
  - Mistlberger RE, Houpt TA, Moore-Ede MC. Characteristics of food-entrained circadian rhythms in rats during long-term exposure to constant light. *Chronobiol Int* 1990;7(5-6):383-91.
  - Russell JE, Simmons DJ, Huber B, Roos BA. Meal timing as a Zeitgeber for skeletal deoxyribonucleic acid and collagen synthesis rhythms. *Endocrinology* 1983 Dec;113(6):2035-42.
  - Satoh Y, Kawai H, Kudo N, et al. Time-restricted feeding entrains daily rhythms of energy metabolism in mice. *Am J Physiol Regul Integr Comp Physiol* 2006 May;290(5):R1276-83.
  - Schoeller DA, Cella LK, Sinha MK, Caro JF. Entrainment of the diurnal rhythm of plasma leptin to meal timing. *J Clin Invest* 1997 Oct 1;100(7):1882-7.
  - Stephan FK. The "other" circadian system: food as a Zeitgeber. *J Biol Rhythms* 2002 Aug;17(4):284-92.

- Stephan FK. Calories affect zeitgeber properties of the feeding entrained circadian oscillator. *Physiol Behav* 1997 Nov;62(5):995-1002.
- Strubbe JH, Woods SC. The timing of meals. *Psychol Rev* 2004 Jan;111(1):128-41.
- Strubbe JH, van Dijk G. The temporal organization of ingestive behaviour and its interaction with regulation of energy balance. *Neurosci Biobehav Rev* 2002 Jun;26(4):485-98.

- **The Cases of the Implanted Cancer**... Sources for this case are:
  - Filipski E, Innominato PF, Wu M, et al. Effects of light and food schedules on liver and tumor molecular clocks in mice. *J Natl Cancer Inst* 2005 Apr 6;97(7):507-17.
  - Wu MW, Li XM, Xian LJ, Levi F. Effects of meal timing on tumor progression in mice. *Life Sci* 2004 Jul 23;75(10):1181-93.

- **Limiting food access to a particular time of day (or night)**... Much of the human research on restricting food access to certain hours has been done on Ramadan. During Ramadan food can be eaten only between the hours of sunset and sunrise. This has profound effects on human behavior and biology. Suggested reading on limiting food access to certain time periods include:
  - Abe H, Honma S, Honma K. Daily restricted feeding resets the circadian clock in the suprachiasmatic nucleus of CS mice. *Am J Physiol Regul Integr Comp Physiol* 2007 Jan;292(1):R607-15.
  - Al-Naimi S, Hampton SM, Richard P, et al. Postprandial metabolic profiles following meals and snacks eaten during simulated night and day shift work. *Chronobiol Int* 2004;21(6):937-47.
  - Bogdan A, Bouchareb B, Touitou Y. Ramadan fasting alters endocrine and neuroendocrine circadian patterns. Meal-time as a synchronizer in humans? *Life Sci* 2001 Feb 23;68(14):1607-15.
  - Boulos Z, Terman M. Food availability and daily biological rhythms. *Neurosci Biobehav Rev* 1980 Summer;4(2):119-31.
  - Philippens KM, von Mayersbach H, Scheving LE. Effects of the scheduling of meal-feeding at different phases of the circadian system in rats. *J Nutr* 1977 Feb;107(2):176-93.
  - Satoh Y, Kawai H, Kudo N, et al. Time-restricted feeding entrains daily rhythms of energy metabolism in mice. *Am J Physiol Regul Integr Comp Physiol* 2006 May;290(5):R1276-83.
  - Sturtevant RP, Garber SL. Meal timing dominates the lighting regimen as a synchronizer of the circadian blood ethanol clearance rate rhythm in rats. *J Nutr* 1981 Nov;111(11):2000-5

- **The Case of Modifying the Time of Feeding**... The sources for this case are:
  - Arble DM, Bass J, Laposky AD, Vitaterna MH, Turek FW. Circadian Timing of Food Intake Contributes to Weight Gain. *Obesity* 2009:264.
  - Salgado-Delgado R, Angeles-Castellanos M, Saderi N, Buijs RM, Escobar C. Food intake during the normal activity phase prevents obesity and circadian desynchrony in a rat model of night work. *Endocrinology.* 2010 Mar;151(3):1019-29.

- **The Case of Ramadan**... Ramadan has been extensively studied. Listing all this research is impractical; however, suggested reading includes:
  - Bogdan A, Bouchareb B, Touitou Y. Ramadan fasting alters endocrine and neuroendocrine circadian patterns. Meal-time as a synchronizer in humans? *Life Sci* 2001 Feb 23;68(14):1607-15.
  - Iraki L, Bogdan A, Hakkou F, et al. Ramadan diet restrictions modify the circadian time structure in humans. A study on plasma gastrin, insulin, glucose, and calcium and on gastric pH. *J Clin Endocrinol Metab* 1997 Apr;82(4):1261-73.
  - Leiper JB, Molla AM, Molla AM. Effects on health of fluid restriction during fasting in Ramadan. *Eur J Clin Nutr* 2003 Dec;57 Suppl 2:S30-8.
  - Roky R, Iraki L, HajKhlifa R, et al. Daytime alertness, mood, psychomotor performances, and oral temperature during Ramadan intermittent fasting. *Ann Nutr Metab* 2000;44(3):101-7.
  - Roky R, Houti I, Moussamih S, et al. Physiological and chronobiological changes during Ramadan intermittent fasting. *Ann Nutr Metab* 2004;48(4):296-303.
  - Shariatpanahi ZV, Shariatpanahi MV, Shahbazi S, et al. Effect of Ramadan fasting on some indices of insulin resistance and components of the metabolic syndrome in healthy male adults. *Br J Nutr* 2008 Jul;100(1):147-51.
  - Waterhouse J, Alkib L, Reilly T. Effects of Ramadan upon fluid and food intake, fatigue, and physical, mental, and social activities: a comparison between the UK and Libya. *Chronobiol Int* 2008 Sep;25(5):697-724.

- **The Case of Breakfast**... Sources for this case are:
  - Berkey CS, Rockett HR, Gillman MW, et al. Longitudinal study of skipping breakfast and weight change in adolescents. *Int J Obes Relat Metab Disord* 2003 Oct;27(10):1258-66.
  - Dubois L, Girard M, Potvin Kent M, et al. Breakfast skipping is associated with differences in meal patterns, macronutrient intakes and overweight among pre-school children. *Public Health Nutr* 2008 Mar 18:1-10.

- Dubois L, Girard M, Potvin Kent M. Breakfast eating and overweight in a pre-school population: is there a link? *Public Health Nutr* 2006 Jun;9(4):436-42.
- Farshchi HR, Taylor MA, Macdonald IA. Deleterious effects of omitting breakfast on insulin sensitivity and fasting lipid profiles in healthy lean women. *Am J Clin Nutr* 2005 Feb;81(2):388-96.
- Haines PS, Guilkey DK, Popkin BM. Trends in breakfast consumption of US adults between 1965 and 1991. *J Am Diet Assoc* 1996 May;96(5):464-70.
- Halberg F, Haus E, Cornélissen G. From Biologic Rhythms to Chronomes Relevant for Nutrition. From: *Not Eating Enough*, 1995:361–372. Washington, D.C. National Academy Press
- Halberg F. Some Aspects of the Chronobiology of Nutrition: More Work is Needed on "When to Eat". *J Nutr* 1989;119:333-343.
- Masheb RM, Grilo CM. Eating patterns and breakfast consumption in obese patients with binge eating disorder. *Behav Res Ther* 2006 Nov;44(11):1545-53.
- Nicklas TA, Morales M, Linares A, et al. Children's meal patterns have changed over a 21-year period: the Bogalusa Heart Study. *J Am Diet Assoc* 2004 May;104(5):753-61.
- Niemeier HM, Raynor HA, Lloyd-Richardson EE, et al. Fast food consumption and breakfast skipping: predictors of weight gain from adolescence to adulthood in a nationally representative sample. *J Adolesc Health* 2006 Dec;39(6):842-9.
- Ortega RM, Requejo AM, Lopez-Sobaler AM, et al. Difference in the breakfast habits of overweight/obese and normal weight schoolchildren. *Int J Vitam Nutr Res* 1998;68(2):125-32.
- Panagiotakos DB, Antonogeorgos G, Papadimitriou A, et al. Breakfast cereal is associated with a lower prevalence of obesity among 10-12-year-old children: The PANACEA study. *Nutr Metab Cardiovasc Dis* 2008 May 22.
- Purslow LR, Sandhu MS, Forouhi N, et al. Energy intake at breakfast and weight change: prospective study of 6,764 middle-aged men and women. *Am J Epidemiol* 2008 Jan 15;167(2):188-92.
- Rampersaud GC, Pereira MA, Girard BL, et al. Breakfast habits, nutritional status, body weight, and academic performance in children and adolescents. *J Am Diet Assoc* 2005 May;105(5):743-60.
- Siega-Riz AM, Popkin BM, Carson T. Trends in breakfast consumption for children in the United States from 1965-1991. *Am J Clin Nutr* 1998 Apr;67(4):748S-756S.
- Smith AP. Breakfast cereal consumption and subjective reports of health by young adults. *Nutr Neurosci* 2003 Feb;6(1):59-61.
- Timlin MT, Pereira MA, Story M, Neumark-Sztainer D. Breakfast eating and weight change in a 5-year prospective analysis of adolescents: Project EAT (Eating Among Teens). *Pediatrics* 2008 Mar;121(3):e638-45.
- Vagstrand K, Barkeling B, Forslund HB, et al. Eating habits in relation to body fatness and gender in adolescents – results from the 'SWEDES' study. *Eur J Clin Nutr* 2006 Sep 27
- van der Heijden AA, Hu FB, Rimm EB, van Dam RM. A prospective study of breakfast consumption and weight gain among U.S. men. *Obesity (Silver Spring)* 2007 Oct;15(10):2463-9.
- Wyatt HR, Grunwald GK, Mosca CL, et al. Long-term weight loss and breakfast in subjects in the National Weight Control Registry. *Obes Res* 2002 Feb;10(2):78-82.
- **The Case of Night Eating**... Sources for this case are:
  - Adami GF, Campostano A, Marinari GM, et al. Night eating in obesity: a descriptive study. *Nutrition* 2002 Jul;18(7-8):587-9.
  - Andersen GS, Stunkard AJ, Sorensen TI, et al. Night eating and weight change in middle-aged men and women. *Int J Obes Relat Metab Disord* 2004 Oct;28(10):1338-43.
  - Friedman S, Even C, Dardennes R, Guelfi JD. Light therapy, obesity, and night-eating syndrome. *Am J Psychiatry* 2002 May;159(5):875-6.
  - Gluck ME, Venti CA, Salbe AD, Krakoff J. Nighttime eating: commonly observed and related to weight gain in an inpatient food intake study. *Am J Clin Nutr* 2008 Oct;88(4):900-5.
  - Gluck ME, Geliebter A, Satov T. Night eating syndrome is associated with depression, low self-esteem, reduced daytime hunger, and less weight loss in obese outpatients. *Obes Res* 2001 Apr;9(4):264-7.
  - Goel N, Stunkard AJ, Rogers NL, et al. Circadian rhythm profiles in women with night eating syndrome. *J Biol Rhythms* 2009 Feb;24(1):85-94.
  - Harris RB, Zhou J, Mitchell T, et al. Rats fed only during the light period are resistant to stress-induced weight loss. *Physiol Behav* 2002 Aug;76(4-5):543-50.
  - Lundgren JD, Allison KC, O'Reardon JP, Stunkard AJ. A descriptive study of non-obese persons with night eating syndrome and a weight-matched comparison group. *Eat Behav* 2008 Aug;9(3):343-51.

- Morse SA, Ciechanowski PS, Katon WJ, Hirsch IB. Isn't this just bedtime snacking? The potential adverse effects of night-eating symptoms on treatment adherence and outcomes in patients with diabetes. *Diabetes Care* 2006 Aug;29(8):1800-4.
- Qin LQ, Li J, Wang Y, et al. The effects of nocturnal life on endocrine circadian patterns in healthy adults. Circadian eating and sleeping patterns in the night eating syndrome. *Obes Res* 2004 Nov;12(11):1789-96.
- Sanchez-Alavez M, Klein I, Brownell SE, et al. Night eating and obesity in the EP3R-deficient mouse. *Proc Natl Acad Sci U S A.* 2007 Feb 20;104(8):3009-14.
- Stunkard AJ, Grace WJ, Wolff HG. The night-eating syndrome; a pattern of food intake among certain obese patients. *Am J Med* 1955 Jul;19(1):78-86.
- Tholin S, Lindroos A, Tynelius P, et al. Prevalence of night eating in obese and nonobese twins. *Obesity (Silver Spring)* 2009 May;17(5):1050-5.

- **Adventures in Meal Frequency**... Sources include:
  - Andersson I, Lennernas M, Rossner S. Meal pattern and risk factor evaluation in one-year completers of a weight reduction program for obese men - the 'Gustaf' study. *J Intern Med* 2000 Jan;247(1):30-8.
  - Antoine JM, Rohr R, Gagey MJ, et al. Feeding frequency and nitrogen balance in weight-reducing obese women. *Hum Nutr Clin Nutr* 1984 Jan;38(1):31-8.
  - Bellisle F, McDevitt R, Prentice AM. Meal frequency and energy balance. *Br J Nutr* 1997 Apr;77 Suppl 1:S57-70
  - Bertelsen J, Christiansen C, Thomsen C, et al. Effect of meal frequency on blood glucose, insulin, and free fatty acids in NIDDM subjects. *Diabetes Care* 1993 Jan;16(1):4-7.
  - Carlson O, Martin B, Stote KS, et al. Impact of reduced meal frequency without caloric restriction on glucose regulation in healthy, normal-weight middle-aged men and women. *Metabolism* 2007 Dec;56(12):1729-34.
  - Chapelot D, Marmonier C, Aubert R, et al. Consequence of omitting or adding a meal in man on body composition, food intake, and metabolism. *Obesity (Silver Spring)* 2006 Feb;14(2):215-27.
  - Cohn C. Feeding Frequency and Body Composition. *Ann N Y Acad Sci* 1963 Sep 26;110:395-409.
  - Cohn C, Joseph D, Bell L, Allweiss MD. Studies on the effects of feeding frequency and dietary composition on fat deposition. *Ann N Y Acad Sci* 1965 Oct 8;131(1):507-18.
  - Cohn C, Joseph D. Caloric intake, weight loss and changes in body composition of rats as influenced by feeding frequency. *J Nutr* 1968;96:94–100.
  - Dallosso HM, Murgatroyd PR, James WP. Feeding frequency and energy balance in adult males. *Hum Nutr Clin Nutr* 1982;36C(1):25-39.
  - Farshchi HR, Taylor MA, Macdonald IA. Regular meal frequency creates more appropriate insulin sensitivity and lipid profiles compared with irregular meal frequency in healthy lean women. *Eur J Clin Nutr* 2004 Jul;58(7):1071-7.
  - Farshchi HR, Taylor MA, Macdonald IA. Beneficial metabolic effects of regular meal frequency on dietary thermogenesis, insulin sensitivity, and fasting lipid profiles in healthy obese women. *Am J Clin Nutr* 2005 Jan;81(1):16-24.
  - Franko DL, Striegel-Moore RH, Thompson D, et al. The relationship between meal frequency and body mass index in black and white adolescent girls: more is less. *Int J Obes (Lond)* 2008 Jan;32(1):23-9.
  - Garrow JS, Durrant M, Blaza S, et al. The effect of meal frequency and protein concentration on the composition of the weight lost by obese subjects. *Br J Nutr* 1981 Jan;45(1):5-15.
  - Jenkins DJ, Jenkins AL, Wolever TM, et al. Low glycemic index: lente carbohydrates and physiological effects of altered food frequency. *Am J Clin Nutr* 1994 Mar;59(3 Suppl):706S-709S.
  - Jones PJ, Leitch CA, Pederson RA. Meal-frequency effects on plasma hormone concentrations and cholesterol synthesis in humans. *Am J Clin Nutr* 1993 Jun;57(6):868-74.
  - Levitsky DA, Halbmaier CA, Mrdjenovic G. The freshman weight gain: a model for the study of the epidemic of obesity. *Int J Obes Relat Metab Disord* 2004 Nov;28(11):1435-42.
  - Louis-Sylvestre J, Lluch A, Neant F, Blundell JE. Highlighting the positive impact of increasing feeding frequency on metabolism and weight management. *Forum Nutr* 2003;56:126-8.
  - McGrath SA, Gibney MJ. The effects of altered frequency of eating on plasma lipids in free-living healthy males on normal self-selected diets. *Eur J Clin Nutr* 1994 Jun;48(6):402-7.
  - Mota J, Fidalgo F, Silva R, et al. Relationships between physical activity, obesity and meal frequency in adolescents. *Ann Hum Biol* 2008 Jan-Feb;35(1):1-10.
  - Ruidavets JB, Bongard V, Bataille V, et al. Eating frequency and body fatness in middle-aged men. *Int J Obes Relat Metab Disord* 2002 Nov;26(11):1476-83.

- Smeets AJ, Westerterp-Plantenga MS. Acute effects on metabolism and appetite profile of one meal difference in the lower range of meal frequency. *Br J Nutr* 2008 Jun;99(6):1316-21.
- Solomon TP, Chambers ES, Jeukendrup AE, et al. The effect of feeding frequency on insulin and ghrelin responses in human subjects. *Br J Nutr* 2008 Oct;100(4):810-9.
- Speechly DP, Rogers GG, Buffenstein R. Acute appetite reduction associated with an increased frequency of eating in obese males. *Int J Obes Relat Metab Disord* 1999 Nov;23(11):1151-9.
- Speechly DP, Buffenstein R. Greater appetite control associated with an increased frequency of eating in lean males. *Appetite* 1999 Dec;33(3):285-97.
- Toschke AM, Kuchenhoff H, Koletzko B, von Kries R. Meal frequency and childhood obesity. *Obes Res* 2005 Nov;13(11):1932-8.
- Wardlaw JM, Hennyey DJ, Clarke RH. The effect of decreased feeding frequency on body composition in mature and immature male and female rats. *Can J Physiol Pharmacol* 1969;47:47–52.
- Zizza C, Siega-Riz AM, Popkin BM. Significant increase in young adults' snacking between 1977–1978 and 1994-1996 represents a cause for concern! *Prev Med* 2001;32:303-10.

- **The Case of Starved Boxers**… Sources for this case are:
    - Garrow JS, Durrant M, Blaza S, et al. The effect of meal frequency and protein concentration on the composition of the weight lost by obese subjects. *Br J Nutr* 1981;45:5–15.
    - Iwao S, Mori K, Sato Y. Effects of meal frequency on body composition during weight control in boxers. *Scand J Med Sci Sports* 1996 Oct;6(5):265-72.
- **The Case of 7, 5 or 3**… Source for this case is Fabry P, Hejda S, Cerny K, et al. Effect of meal frequency in schoolchildren: changes in weight-height proportion and skinfold thickness. *Am J Clin Nutr* 1966;18: 358–61.

Chapter 14

- **The Case of Manned Space Stations**… Wikipedia has a page dedicated to the International Space Station. It serves as a research laboratory for studying the effects of microgravity. For further reading into the effects of gravity on shape we suggest starting with the following:
    - Da Silva MS, Zimmerman PM, Meguid MM, et al. Anorexia in space and possible etiologies: an overview. *Nutrition* 2002 Oct;18(10):805-13.
    - Gazenko OG, Gurjian AA. On the biological role of gravity. *Life Sci Space Res* 1965;3:241-57.
    - Gould SJ. Weight and shape. *Life Sci Space Res* 1976;14:57-68.
    - Lane HW, Smith SM. Physiological adaptations to space flight. *Life Support Biosph Sci* 1999;6(1):13-8.
    - Leach CS, Inners LD, Charles JB. Changes in total body water during spaceflight. *J Clin Pharmacol* 1991 Oct;31(10):1001-6.
    - McCarthy ID. Fluid shifts due to microgravity and their effects on bone: a review of current knowledge. *Ann Biomed Eng* 2005 Jan;33(1):95-103.
    - Rambaut PC, Leach CS, Leonard JI. Observations in energy balance in man during spaceflight. *Am J Physiol* 1977 Nov;233(5):R208-12.
    - Stein TP, Leskiw MJ, Schluter MD, et al. Energy expenditure and balance during spaceflight on the space shuttle. *Am J Physiol* 1999 Jun;276(6 Pt 2):R1739-48.
    - Tesch PA, Berg HE. Effects of spaceflight on muscle. *J Gravit Physiol* 1998 Jul;5(1):P19-22.
    - Thornton W, Ord J. Physiological mass measurements on Skylab 1/2 and 1/3. *Acta Astronaut* 1975 Jan-Feb;2(1-2):103-13.
    - Wade CE. Responses across the gravity continuum: hypergravity to microgravity. *Adv Space Biol Med* 2005;10:225-45.
    - Wade CE, Miller MM, Baer LA, et al. Body mass, energy intake, and water consumption of rats and humans during space flight. *Nutrition* 2002 Oct;18(10):829-36.
    - Webb P. Weight loss in men in space. *Science* 1967 Feb 3;155(762):558-60.
- **If a rat is taken from a normal environment and placed in an extremely frigid one**… The original experiments done on subjecting rats to cold stress was conducted by Hans Selye. For further reading about these and other findings we recommend his book *The Stress of Life* (ISBN-10: 0070562121).
- **Circumstantial and direct evidence indicates that stress and shape are interrelated**… For further reading we recommend:
    - Branth S, Ronquist G, Stridsberg M, et al. Development of abdominal fat and incipient metabolic syndrome in young healthy men exposed to long-term stress. *Nutr Metab Cardiovasc Dis* 2006 Jun 27.

- Brunner EJ, Chandola T, Marmot MG. Prospective Effect of Job Strain on General and Central Obesity in the Whitehall II Study. *Am J Epidemiol* 2007 Apr 1;165(7):828-37.
- Fogel CI. Hard time: the stressful nature of incarceration for women. *Issues Ment Health Nurs* 1993 Oct-Dec;14(4):367-77.
- Gluck ME, Geliebter A, Lorence M. Cortisol stress response is positively correlated with central obesity in obese women with binge eating disorder (BED) before and after cognitive-behavioral treatment. *Ann N Y Acad Sci* 2004 Dec;1032:202-7.
- Kivimäki M, Head J, Ferrie JE, et al. Work stress, weight gain and weight loss: evidence for bidirectional effects of job strain on body mass index in the Whitehall II study. *Int J Obes (Lond)* 2006 Jun;30(6):982-7.
- Kouvonen A, Kivimaki M, Cox SJ, et al. Relationship between work stress and body mass index among 45,810 female and male employees. *Psychosom Med* 2005 Jul-Aug;67(4):577-83.
- Lallukka T, Laaksonen M, Martikainen P, et al. Psychosocial working conditions and weight gain among employees. *Int J Obes (Lond)* 2005 Aug;29(8):909-15.
- Marniemi J, Kronholm E, Aunola S, et al. Visceral fat and psychosocial stress in identical twins discordant for obesity. *J Intern Med* 2002 Jan;251(1):35-43.
- Mellbin T, Vuille JC. Rapidly developing overweight in school children as an indicator of psychosocial stress. *Acta Paediatr Scand* 1989 Jul;78(4):568-75.
- Overgaard D, Gamborg M, Gyntelberg F, Heitmann BL. Psychological workload and weight gain among women with and without familial obesity. *Obesity (Silver Spring)* 2006 Mar;14(3):458-63.
- Raikkonen K, Hautanen A, Keltikangas-Jarvinen L. Association of stress and depression with regional fat distribution in healthy middle-aged men. *J Behav Med* 1994 Dec;17(6):605-16.
- Roberts C, Troop N, Connan F, et al. The effects of stress on body weight: biological and psychological predictors of change in BMI. *Obesity (Silver Spring)* 2007 Dec;15(12):3045-55.
- Rookus MA, Burema J, Frijters JE. Changes in body mass index in young adults in relation to number of life events experienced. *Int J Obes* 1988;12(1):29-39.
- Vieweg WV, Julius DA, Bates J, et al. Posttraumatic stress disorder as a risk factor for obesity among male military veterans. *Acta Psychiatr Scand* 2007 Dec;116(6):483-7.
- Vines AI, Baird DD, Stevens J, et al. Associations of abdominal fat with perceived racism and passive emotional responses to racism in African American women. *Am J Public Health* 2007 Mar;97(3):526-30.
- Yamada Y, Kameda M, Noborisaka Y, et al. Excessive fatigue and weight gain among cleanroom workers after changing from an 8-hour to a 12-hour shift. *Scand J Work Environ Health* 2001 Oct;27(5):318-26.

• **The Case of Voluntary Caregivers**… Sources are:
- Smith AW, Baum A, Wing RR. Stress and weight gain in parents of cancer patients. *Int J Obes (Lond)* 2005 Feb;29(2):244-50.
- Vitaliano PP, Russo J, Scanlan JM, Greeno CG. Weight changes in caregivers of Alzheimer's care recipients: psychobehavioral predictors. *Psychol Aging* 1996 Mar;11(1):155-63.

• **The Case of Sexual Abuse**… Sources for this case are:
- Aaron DJ, Hughes TL. Association of childhood sexual abuse with obesity in a community sample of lesbians. *Obesity (Silver Spring)* 2007 Apr;15(4):1023-8.
- Buser A, Dymek-Valentine M, et al. Outcome following gastric bypass surgery: impact of past sexual abuse. *Obes Surg* 2004 Feb;14(2):170-4.
- Gruber AJ, Pope HG Jr. Compulsive weight lifting and anabolic drug abuse among women rape victims. *Compr Psychiatry* 1999 Jul-Aug;40(4):273-7.
- Johnson JG, Cohen P, Kasen S, Brook JS. Childhood adversities associated with risk for eating disorders or weight problems during adolescence or early adulthood. *Am J Psychiatry* 2002 Mar;159(3):394-400.
- Jia H, Li JZ, Leserman J, Hu Y, Drossman DA. Relationship of abuse history and other risk factors with obesity among female gastrointestinal patients. *Dig Dis Sci* 2004 May;49(5):872-7.
- Johnson PJ, Hellerstedt WL, Pirie PL. Abuse history and nonoptimal prenatal weight gain. *Public Health Rep* 2002 Mar-Apr;117(2):148-56.
- King TK, Clark MM, Pera V. History of sexual abuse and obesity treatment outcome. *Addict Behav* 1996 May-Jun;21(3):283-90.
- Larsen JK, Geenen R. Childhood sexual abuse is not associated with a poor outcome after gastric banding for severe obesity. *Obes Surg* 2005 Apr;15(4):534-7.
- Lissau I, Sorensen TI. Parental neglect during childhood and increased risk of obesity in young adulthood. *Lancet* 1994 Feb 5;343(8893):324-7.
- Ray EC, Nickels MW, Sayeed S, Sax HC. Predicting success after gastric bypass: the role of psychosocial and behavioral factors. *Surgery* 2003 Oct;134(4):555-63; discussion 563-4.

- Rayworth BB, Wise LA, Harlow BL. Childhood abuse and risk of eating disorders in women. *Epidemiology* 2004 May;15(3):271-8.
- Thompson KM, Wonderlich SA, Crosby RD, Mitchell JE. Sexual violence and weight control techniques among adolescent girls. *Int J Eat Disord* 2001 Mar;29(2):166-76.
- Williamson DF, Thompson TJ, Anda RF, et al. Body weight and obesity in adults and self-reported abuse in childhood. *Int J Obes Relat Metab Disord* 2002 Aug;26(8):1075-82
- Wonderlich SA, Crosby RD, Mitchell JE, et al. Relationship of childhood sexual abuse and eating disturbance in children. *J Am Acad Child Adolesc Psychiatry* 2000 Oct;39(10):1277-83.
- Wiederman MW, Sansone RA, Sansone LA. Obesity among sexually abused women: an adaptive function for some? *Women Health* 1999;29(1):89-100.

- **The Case of Social Stress…** Robert M. Sapolsky writes about the role of social stress, based in large part on his observations of primates, in his book *Why Zebras Don't Get Ulcers* (ISBN-10: 0716732106). Sources for this case are:
  - Foster MT, Solomon MB, Huhman KL, Bartness TJ. Social defeat increases food intake, body mass, and adiposity in Syrian hamsters. *Am J Physiol Regul Integr* Comp Physiol 2006 May;290(5):R1284-93.
  - Lemeshow AR, Fisher L, Goodman E, et al. Subjective social status in the school and change in adiposity in female adolescents: findings from a prospective cohort study. *Arch Pediatr Adolesc Med* 2008 Jan;162(1):23-8.
  - Moles A, Bartolomucci A, Garbugino L, et al. Psychosocial stress affects energy balance in mice: modulation by social status. *Psychoneuroendocrinology* 2006 Jun;31(5):623-33.
  - Shively CA, Register TC, Clarkson TB. Social stress, visceral obesity, and coronary artery atherosclerosis in female primates. *Obesity (Silver Spring)* 2009 Aug;17(8):1513-20.
  - Shively CA, Register TC, Clarkson TB. Social stress, visceral obesity, and coronary artery atherosclerosis: product of a primate adaptation. *Am J Primatol* 2009 Sep;71(9):742-51.
  - Solomon MB, Foster MT, Bartness TJ, Huhman KL. Social defeat and footshock increase body mass and adiposity in male Syrian hamsters. *Am J Physiol Regul Integr Comp Physiol* 2007 Jan;292(1):R283-90.
  - Strickland OL, Giger JN, Nelson MA, Davis CM. The relationships among stress, coping, social support, and weight class in premenopausal African American women at risk for coronary heart disease. *J Cardiovasc Nurs* 2007 Jul-Aug;22(4):272-8.
  - Tamashiro KL, Hegeman MA, Nguyen MM, et al. Dynamic body weight and body composition changes in response to subordination stress. *Physiol Behav* 2007 Jul 24;91(4):440-8.
  - Tamashiro KL, Nguyen MM, Ostrander MM, et al. Social stress and recovery: implications for body weight and body composition. *Am J Physiol Regul Integr Comp Physiol* 2007 Nov;293(5):R1864-74.
  - Tamashiro KL, Hegeman MA, Sakai RR. Chronic social stress in a changing dietary environment. *Physiol Behav* 2006 Nov 30;89(4):536-42.
  - Wallace JM, Shively CA, Clarkson TB. Effects of hormone replacement therapy and social stress on body fat distribution in surgically postmenopausal monkeys. *Int J Obes Relat Metab Disord* 1999 May;23(5):518-27.

- **In a study of adolescent girls…** Source is Lemeshow AR, Fisher L, Goodman E, et al. Subjective social status in the school and change in adiposity in female adolescents: findings from a prospective cohort study. *Arch Pediatr Adolesc Med* 2008 Jan;162(1):23-8.
- **The Case of Identical Twins…** Source is Marniemi J, Kronholm E, Aunola S, et al. Visceral fat and psychosocial stress in identical twins discordant for obesity. *J Intern Med* 2002 Jan;251(1):35-43.
- **Big life events including…** Source is Rookus MA, Burema J, Frijters JE. Changes in body mass index in young adults in relation to number of life events experienced. *Int J Obes* 1988;12(1):29-39.
- **Because of the strong links between stress and belly fat…** For further reading on these links we recommend reading:
  - Bjorntorp P. Do stress reactions cause abdominal obesity and comorbidities? *Obes Rev* 2001 May;2(2):73-86.
  - Branth S, Ronquist G, Stridsberg M, et al. Development of abdominal fat and incipient metabolic syndrome in young healthy men exposed to long-term stress. *Nutr Metab Cardiovasc Dis* 2006 Jun 27.
  - Brydon L, Wright CE, O'Donnell K, et al. Stress-induced cytokine responses and central adiposity in young women. *Int J Obes (Lond)* 2007 Dec 4.
  - Drapeau V, Therrien F, Richard D, Tremblay A. Is visceral obesity a physiological adaptation to stress? *Panminerva Med* 2003 Sep;45(3):189-95.
  - Duclos M, Gatta B, Corcuff JB, et al. Fat distribution in obese women is associated with subtle alterations of the hypothalamic-pituitary-adrenal axis activity and sensitivity to glucocorticoids. *Clin Endocrinol (Oxf)* 2001 Oct;55(4):447-54.

- Epel ES, McEwen B, Seeman T, et al. Stress and body shape: stress-induced cortisol secretion is consistently greater among women with central fat. *Psychosom Med* 2000 Sep-Oct;62(5):623-32.
- Kyrou I, Chrousos GP, Tsigos C. Stress, visceral obesity, and metabolic complications. *Ann N Y Acad Sci* 2006 Nov;1083:77-110.
- Marin P, Darin N, Amemiya T, et al. Cortisol secretion in relation to body fat distribution in obese premenopausal women. *Metabolism* 1992 Aug;41(8):882-6.
- Rosmond R, Dallman MF, Bjorntorp P. Stress-related cortisol secretion in men: relationships with abdominal obesity and endocrine, metabolic and hemodynamic abnormalities. *J Clin Endocrinol Metab* 1998 Jun;83(6):1853-9.

- **People who effectively manage stress are far more likely to experience and keep positive shape changes**... Source is Ryden A, Karlsson J, Sullivan M, et al. Coping and distress: what happens after intervention? A 2-year follow-up from the Swedish Obese Subjects (SOS) study. *Psychosom Med* 2003 May-Jun;65(3):435-42.
- **Detecting Sources of Stress**... To gain a better understanding of stress and the stress response we suggest reading:
  - Hans Selye Hans Selye. *The Stress of Life* (ISBN-10: 0070562121).
  - Robert M. Sapolsky. *Why Zebras Don't Get Ulcers* (ISBN-10: 0716732106).

Chapter 15

- **Many man-made chemicals persist in the environment**... To read more about persistent organic pollutants we suggests you begin by reading the Wikipedia page dedicated to this topic (http://en.wikipedia.org/wiki/Persistent_organic_pollutant).
- **The 2005 *European Family Biomonitoring Survey***... A PDF version of this report can be downloaded at http://assets.panda.org/downloads/generationsx.pdf.
- **In 2009, the Environmental Working Group released the results**... This report can be found at the EWG website (http://www.ewg.org/minoritycordblood/home).
- **The last piece of evidence comes from the *Fourth National Report on Human Exposure to Environmental Chemicals***... This report can be found at the CDC website (http://www.cdc.gov/exposurereport/)
- **Estimates suggest that an average person might routinely come in contact with as many as six thousand different chemicals**... Source for this estimate is the *Fourth National Report on Human Exposure to Environmental Chemicals*.
- **The *Case of Chloroform***... To read more about chloroform we suggests you begin by reading the Wikipedia page (http://en.wikipedia.org/wiki/Chloroform) and the CDC ToxFAQs for chloroform (http://www.atsdr.cdc.gov/tfacts6.html).
- **Polychlorinated biphenyls (PCBs) were first made in**... To read more about PCBs we suggests you begin by reading the Wikipedia page (http://en.wikipedia.org/wiki/Polychlorinated_biphenyls) and the CDC ToxFAQs for chloroform (http://www.atsdr.cdc.gov/substances/toxsubstance.asp?toxid=26).
- **When the World Trade Center towers collapsed**... A good place to read more about "Ground Zero" illness is the Wikipedia page dedicated to this topic (http://en.wikipedia.org/wiki/Health_effects_arising_from_the_September_11_attacks). Other introductions to this topic include the *USA today* article *Health troubles persist for 9/11 rescue workers* (http://www.usatoday.com/money/industries/health/2006-06-25-911-health-usat_x.htm) and the *New York Times* article *What Was Found in the Dust* (http://www.nytimes.com/imagepages/2006/09/05/nyregion/20060905_HEALTH_GRAPHIC.htm)
- **The *Case of Running Behind Mosquito Spray Trucks***... To read more about DDT (the chemical that was sprayed in this mist) we suggest you begin by reading the Wikipedia page (http://en.wikipedia.org/wiki/Ddt) and the CDC ToxFAQs for DDT (http://www.atsdr.cdc.gov/substances/toxsubstance.asp?toxid=20).
- **BPA is used in polycarbonate bottles and in epoxy resins**... To read more about BPA we suggests you begin by reading the Wikipedia page (http://en.wikipedia.org/wiki/Bisphenol_a). To read about the newest FDA position on BPA we suggest you read the *New York Times* article *F.D.A. Concerned About Substance in Food Packaging* (http://www.nytimes.com/2010/01/16/health/16plastic.html?th&emc=th).
- **All else being equal, a person with more body fat is likely to have greater amounts of chemicals in their body, in general, and in adipose tissue, specifically**... Sources for this statement include:
  - Hatch EE, Nelson JW, Qureshi MM, et al. Association of urinary phthalate metabolite concentrations with body mass index and waist circumference: a cross-sectional study of NHANES data, 1999-2002. *Environ Health.* 2008 Jun 3;7:27.

- Johnson-Restrepo B, Kannan K, Rapaport DP, Rodan BD. Polybrominated diphenyl ethers and polychlorinated biphenyls in human adipose tissue from New York. *Environ Sci Technol*. 2005 Jul 15;39(14):5177-82.
- Müllerová D, Kopeck J. White Adipose Tissue: Storage and Effector Site for Environmental Pollutants. *Physiol. Res.* 56: 375-381, 2007
- Pelletier C, Després JP, Tremblay A. Plasma organochlorine concentrations in endurance athletes and obese individuals. *Med Sci Sports Exerc*. 2002 Dec;34(12):1971-5.
- Pierce CH, Tozer TN. Styrene in adipose tissue of nonoccupationally exposed persons. *Environ Res*. 1992 Aug;58(2):230-5.
- Stahlhut RW, van Wijngaarden E, Dye TD, et al. Concentrations of urinary phthalate metabolites are associated with increased waist circumference and insulin resistance in adult U.S. males. *Environ Health Perspect*. 2007 Jun;115(6):876-82.
- Takeuchi T, Tsutsumi O, Ikezuki Y, et al. Positive relationship between androgen and the endocrine disruptor, bisphenol A, in normal women and women with ovarian dysfunction. *Endocr J*. 2004 Apr;51(2):165-9.
- Tremblay A, Doucet E. Obesity: a disease or a biological adaptation? *Obes Rev*. 2000 May;1(1):27-35.

- **Circumstantial evidence links certain man-made chemicals with metabolic obesity**... Sources for this include:

  - Baccarelli A, Pesatori AC, Consonni D, et al. Health status and plasma dioxin levels in chloracne cases 20 years after the Seveso, Italy accident. *Br J Dermatol*. 2005 Mar;152(3):459-65.
  - Carpenter DO. Environmental contaminants as risk factors for developing diabetes. *Rev Environ Health*. 2008 Jan-Mar;23(1):59-74.
  - Cotrim HP, De Freitas LA, Freitas C, et al. Clinical and histopathological features of NASH in workers exposed to chemicals with or without associated metabolic conditions. *Liver Int*. 2004 Apr;24(2):131-5.
  - Cranmer M, Louie S, Kennedy RH, et al. Exposure to 2,3,7,8-tetrachlorodibenzo-p-dioxin (TCDD) is associated with hyperinsulinemia and insulin resistance. *Toxicol Sci* 2000 Aug;56(2):431-6
  - Henriksen GL, Ketchum NS, Michalek JE, Swaby JA. Serum dioxin and diabetes mellitus in veterans of Operation Ranch Hand. *Epidemiology*. 1997 May;8(3):252-8.
  - Huang X, Lessner L, Carpenter DO. Exposure to persistent organic pollutants and hypertensive disease. *Environ Res*. 2006 Sep;102(1):101-6.
  - Kern PA, Said S, Jackson WG Jr, Michalek JE. Insulin sensitivity following agent orange exposure in Vietnam veterans with high blood levels of 2,3,7,8-tetrachlorodibenzo-p-dioxin. *J Clin Endocrinol Metab*. 2004 Sep;89(9):4665-72.
  - Kreiss K, Zack MM, Kimbrough RD, et al. Association of blood pressure and polychlorinated biphenyl levels. *JAMA*. 1981 Jun 26;245(24):2505-9.
  - Lang IA, Galloway TS, Scarlett A, et al. Association of urinary bisphenol A concentration with medical disorders and laboratory abnormalities in adults. *JAMA*. 2008 Sep 17;300(11):1303-10.
  - Lee DH, Lee IK, Song K, et al. A strong dose-response relation between serum concentrations of persistent organic pollutants and diabetes: results from the National Health and Examination Survey 1999-2002. *Diabetes Care*. 2006 Jul;29(7):1638-44.
  - Lee DH, Lee IK, Jin SH, et al. Association between serum concentrations of persistent organic pollutants and insulin resistance among nondiabetic adults: results from the National Health and Nutrition Examination Survey 1999-2002. *Diabetes Care*. 2007 Mar;30(3):622-8.
  - Lim JS, Lee DH, Jacobs DR Jr. Association of Brominated Flame Retardants with Diabetes and Metabolic syndrome in the United States Population: 2003-2004. *Diabetes Care*. 2008 Jun 16.
  - Lundqvist G, Flodin U, Axelson O. A case-control study of fatty liver disease and organic solvent exposure. *Am J Ind Med* 1999 Feb;35(2):132-6
  - Pelletier C, Imbeault P, Tremblay A. Energy balance and pollution by organochlorines and polychlorinated biphenyls. *Obes Rev*. 2003 Feb;4(1):17-24.
  - Takeuchi T, Tsutsumi O, Ikezuki Y, et al. Positive relationship between androgen and the endocrine disruptor, bisphenol A, in normal women and women with ovarian dysfunction. *Endocr J*. 2004 Apr;51(2):165-9.
  - Vasiliu O, Cameron L, Gardiner J, et al. Polybrominated biphenyls, polychlorinated biphenyls, body weight, and incidence of adult-onset diabetes mellitus. *Epidemiology*. 2006 Jul;17(4):352-9.

- **The *Case of Fatty Liver Disease*...** Source is Cotrim HP, Andrade ZA, Parana R, et al. Nonalcoholic steatohepatitis: a toxic liver disease in industrial workers. *Liver* 1999 Aug;19(4):299-304

- **Thirty-nine obese individuals dieted for 15 weeks**… Source for information in this HSI clue is Chevrier J, Dewailly E, Ayotte P, et al. Body weight loss increases plasma and adipose tissue concentrations of potentially toxic pollutants in obese individuals. *Int J Obes Relat Metab Disord.* 2000 Oct;24(10):1272-8.
- **One of these theories is the *Environmental Obesogen Hypothesis*…** A good starting place to read about the notion that man-made chemicals might be making us fat is the article *Born to be Big: Early exposure to common chemicals may be programming kids to be fat.* This article was written by Sharon Begley and appeared in the September 11, 2009 issue of *Newsweek*.

  Other sources for this notion include:
  - Casals-Casas C, Feige JN, Desvergne B. Interference of pollutants with PPARs: endocrine disruption meets metabolism. *Int J Obes (Lond).* 2008 Dec;32 Suppl 6:S53-61.
  - Grun F, Blumberg B. Environmental obesogens: organotins and endocrine disruption via nuclear receptor signaling. *Endocrinology.* 2006 Jun;147(6 Suppl):S50-5.
  - Grün F, Blumberg B. Perturbed nuclear receptor signaling by environmental obesogens as emerging factors in the obesity crisis. *Rev Endocr Metab Disord.* 2007 Jun;8(2):161-71.
  - Heindel JJ, vom Saal FS. Role of nutrition and environmental endocrine disrupting chemicals during the perinatal period on the aetiology of obesity. *Mol Cell Endocrinol.* 2009 May 25;304(1-2):90-6.
  - Hoppe AA, Carey GB. Polybrominated diphenyl ethers as endocrine disruptors of adipocyte metabolism. *Obesity (Silver Spring).* 2007 Dec;15(12):2942-50.
  - Pelletier C, Imbeault P, Tremblay A. Energy balance and pollution by organochlorines and polychlorinated biphenyls. *Obes Rev.* 2003 Feb;4(1):17-24.
  - Tabb MM, Blumberg B. New modes of action for endocrine-disrupting chemicals. *Mol Endocrinol.* 2006 Mar;20(3):475-82.
  - Tremblay A, Chaput JP. About unsuspected potential determinants of obesity. *Appl Physiol Nutr Metab.* 2008 Aug;33(4):791-6.
  - Tremblay A, Pelletier C, Doucet E, Imbeault P. Thermogenesis and weight loss in obese individuals: a primary association with organochlorine pollution. *Int J Obes Relat Metab Disord.* 2004 Jul;28(7):936-9.
  - Weinhold B. Obesity: pollutants may put on the pounds. *Environ Health Perspect.* 2006 Dec;114(12):A692.
  - Wolff MS. Endocrine disruptors: challenges for environmental research in the 21st century. *Ann N Y Acad Sci.* 2006 Sep;1076:228-38.
- **Based on existing scientific evidence chemical candidates include…** In addition to the sources listed above, other sources include:
  - Arsenescu V, Arsenescu RI, King V, et al. Polychlorinated biphenyl-77 induces adipocyte differentiation and proinflammatory adipokines and promotes obesity and atherosclerosis. *Environ Health Perspect.* 2008 Jun;116(6):761-8.
  - Boberg J, Metzdorff S, Wortziger R, et al. Impact of diisobutyl phthalate and other PPAR agonists on steroidogenesis and plasma insulin and leptin levels in fetal rats. *Toxicology.* 2008 Jun 17.
  - Lim S, Ahn SY, Song IC, et al. Chronic Exposure to the Herbicide, Atrazine, Causes Mitochondrial Dysfunction and Insulin Resistance. *PLoS ONE* 2009:4(4): e5186.
  - Obesity In Men Linked To Common Chemical Found In Plastic And Soap (http://www.sciencedaily.com/releases/2007/03/070314110441.htm)
- **The *Case of Tributyltin Chloride*…** Sources include:
  - Grun F, Watanabe H, Zamanian Z, et al. Endocrine-disrupting organotin compounds are potent inducers of adipogenesis in vertebrates. *Mol Endocrinol.* 2006 Sep;20(9):2141-55.
  - Inadera H, Shimomura A. Environmental chemical tributyltin augments adipocyte differentiation. *Toxicol Lett.* 2005 Dec 15;159(3):226-34.
  - Si J, Wu X, Wan C, et al. Peripubertal exposure to low doses of tributyltin chloride affects the homeostasis of serum T, E2, LH, and body weight of male mice. *Environ Toxicol.* 2010 Jan 5.
  - Zuo Z, Chen S, Wu T, et al. Tributyltin causes obesity and hepatic steatosis in male mice. *Environ Toxicol.* 2009 Sep 16.
- **The *Case of Benzo[a]pyrene*…** Source for this case is Irigaray P, Ogier V, Jacquenet S, et al. Benzo[a]pyrene impairs beta-adrenergic stimulation of adipose tissue lipolysis and causes weight gain in mice. A novel molecular mechanism of toxicity for a common food pollutant. *FEBS J.* 2006 Apr;273(7):1362-72.
- **The *Case of Bisphenol A*…** A good starting place for reading up the links between BPA and shape is the *Boston Globe* article *Is plastic making us fat?* (http://www.boston.com/news/health/articles/2008/01/14/is_plastic_making_us_fat/). The toxicology profile of BPA is available as a PDF at the CDC website (www.atsdr.cdc.gov/toxprofiles/tp115-c5.pdf). Other sources for this case are:

- Graeme Stemp-Morlock. Chemical Exposures_Exploring Developmental Origins of Obesity. *Environ Health Perspect.* 2007 May; 115(5): A242.
- Hugo ER, Brandebourg TD, Woo JG, et al. Bisphenol A at environmentally relevant doses inhibits adiponectin release from human adipose tissue explants and adipocytes. *Environ Health Perspect.* 2008
- Miyawaki J, Sakayama K, Kato H, et al. Perinatal and postnatal exposure to bisphenol a increases adipose tissue mass and serum cholesterol level in mice. *J Atheroscler Thromb.* 2007 Oct;14(5):245-52.
- Nunez AA, Kannan K, Giesy JP, et al. Effects of bisphenol A on energy balance and accumulation in brown adipose tissue in rats. *Chemosphere.* 2001 Mar;42(8):917-22.
- Phrakonkham P, Viengchareun S, Belloir C, et al. Dietary xenoestrogens differentially impair 3T3-L1 preadipocyte differentiation and persistently affect leptin synthesis. *J Steroid Biochem Mol Biol.* 2008 May;110(1-2):95-103.
- Takeuchi T, Tsutsumi O, Ikezuki Y, et al. Positive relationship between androgen and the endocrine disruptor, bisphenol A, in normal women and women with ovarian dysfunction. *Endocr J.* 2004 Apr;51(2):165-9.
- vom Saal FS, Welshons WV. Large effects from small exposures. II. The importance of positive controls in low-dose research on bisphenol A. *Environ Res.* 2006 Jan;100(1):50-76.
- vom Saal FS, Hughes C. An extensive new literature concerning low-dose effects of bisphenol A shows the need for a new risk assessment. *Environ Health Perspect.* 2005 Aug;113(8):926-33.
- Welshons WV, Nagel SC, vom Saal FS. Large effects from small exposures. III. Endocrine mechanisms mediating effects of bisphenol A at levels of human exposure. *Endocrinology.* 2006 Jun;147(6 Suppl):S56-69.

- **According to Jerrold Heindel, of the National Institute of Environmental Health Sciences, a number of chemicals cause weight gain at low levels of exposure**… This was discussed in the article *Born to be Big: Early exposure to common chemicals may be programming kids to be fat*. This article was written by Sharon Begley and appeared in the September 11, 2009 issue of *Newsweek*.
- **The *Case of the New Car Smell*…** A good starting point for learning more about vinyl shower curtains is the article *New Car Smell: VOCs account for the characteristic 'newness'* by Steve Ritter (http://pubs.acs.org/cen/whatstuff/stuff/8020stuff.html).
- **The *Case of a New Vinyl Shower Curtain*…** A good starting point for learning more about vinyl shower curtains is the *Consumer Affairs* article *Shower Curtains May Be Hazardous to Your Health: That 'new shower curtain smell' is a shower of chemicals* (http://www.consumeraffairs.com/news04/2008/06/shower_curtain.html) and *An environmental organization finds high concentrations of dangerous chemicals in curtains sold at major stores* by Tami Abdollah (http://articles.latimes.com/2008/jun/13/local/me-showercurtain13).
- **The *Case of Fragrance Products*…** Sources for this case include:
  - *Air Fresheners Unregulated, Potentially Dangerous, Group Says* (http://www.enn.com/top_stories/article/23538)
  - Anderson RC, Anderson JH. Toxic effects of air freshener emissions. *Arch Environ Health.* 1997 Nov-Dec;52(6):433-41.
  - Berres CR, Vos KD, Thomson DB, Baretta ED. In-home measurement of background particles and particulates and propellants produced by an air freshener. *Am Ind Hyg Assoc J.* 1976 May;37(5):305-10.
  - Cone JE, Shusterman D. Health effects of indoor odorants. *Environ Health Perspect.* 1991 Nov;95:53-9.
  - Farrow A, Taylor H, Northstone K, Golding J. Symptoms of mothers and infants related to total volatile organic compounds in household products. *Arch Environ Health.* 2003 Oct;58(10):633-41.
  - Gaygen DE, Hedge A. Effect of acute exposure to a complex fragrance on lexical decision performance. *Chem Senses.* 2009 Jan;34(1):85-91.
  - Hickey. Symptoms of mothers and infants related to total volatile organic compounds in household products. *Arch Environ Health.* 2003 Oct;58(10):633-41;
  - How Products Are Made: Air Freshener (http://science.enotes.com/how-products-encyclopedia/air-freshener).
  - Medina-Ramón M, Zock JP, Kogevinas M, et al. Short-term respiratory effects of cleaning exposures in female domestic cleaners. *Eur Respir J.* 2006 Jun;27(6):1196-203.
  - Singer BC, Destaillats H, Hodgson AT, Nazaroff WW. Cleaning products and air fresheners: emissions and resulting concentrations of glycol ethers and terpenoids. *Indoor Air.* 2006 Jun;16(3):179-91.
  - Hannah Wallace L, Nelson W, Ziegenfus R, et al. The Los Angeles TEAM Study: personal exposures, indoor-outdoor air concentrations, and breath concentrations of 25 volatile organic compounds. *J Expo Anal Environ Epidemiol.* 1991 Apr;1(2):157-92.

- **The chemicals and chemical additives in plastics migrate into**… For further reading on chemical migration we suggest starting with the following sources.
  - Bendall JG. Food contamination with styrene dibromide via packaging migration of leachate from polystyrene cold-storage insulation. *J Food Prot.* 2007 Apr;70(4):1037-40.
  - Benfenati E, Natangelo M, Davoli E, Fanelli R. Migration of vinyl chloride into PVC-bottled drinking-water assessed by gas chromatography-mass spectrometry. *Food Chem Toxicol.* 1991 Feb;29(2):131-4.
  - Brede C, Fjeldal P, Skjevrak I, Herikstad H. Increased migration levels of bisphenol A from polycarbonate baby bottles after dishwashing, boiling and brushing. *Food Addit Contam.* 2003 Jul;20(7):684-9.
  - Darowska A, Borcz A, Nawrocki J. Aldehyde contamination of mineral water stored in PET bottles. *Food Addit Contam.* 2003 Dec;20(12):1170-7.
  - Gramshaw JW, Soto-Valdez H. Migration from polyamide 'microwave and roasting bags' into roast chicken. *Food Addit Contam.* 1998 Apr;15(3):329-35.
  - Le HH, Carlson EM, Chua JP, Belcher SM. Bisphenol A is released from polycarbonate drinking bottles and mimics the neurotoxic actions of estrogen in developing cerebellar neurons. *Toxicol Lett.* 2008 Jan 30;176(2):149-56.
  - Limm W, Hollifield HC. Effects of temperature and mixing on polymer adjuvant migration to corn oil and water. *Food Addit Contam.* 1995 Jul-Aug;12(4):609-24.
  - López-Cervantes J, Paseiro-Losada P. Determination of bisphenol A in, and its migration from, PVC stretch film used for food packaging. *Food Addit Contam.* 2003 Jun;20(6):596-606.
  - Maragou NC, Makri A, Lampi EN, et al. Migration of bisphenol A from polycarbonate baby bottles under real use conditions. *Food Addit Contam.* 2008 Mar;25(3):373-83.
  - Monarca S, De Fusco R, Biscardi D, et al. Studies of migration of potentially genotoxic compounds into water stored in pet bottles. *Food Chem Toxicol.* 1994 Sep;32(9):783-8.
  - Shotyk W, Krachler M. Contamination of bottled waters with antimony leaching from polyethylene terephthalate (PET) increases upon storage. *Environ Sci Technol.* 2007 Mar 1;41(5):1560-3.
  - Skjevrak I, Due A, Gjerstad KO, Herikstad H. Volatile organic components migrating from plastic pipes (HDPE, PEX and PVC) into drinking water. *Water Res.* 2003 Apr;37(8):1912-20.
  - Soto-Valdez H, Gramshaw JW, Vandenburg HJ. Determination of potential migrants present in Nylon 'microwave and roasting bags' and migration into olive oil. *Food Addit Contam.* 1997 Apr;14(3):309-18.
  - Tawfik MS, Huyghebaert A. Polystyrene cups and containers: styrene migration. *Food Addit Contam.* 1998 Jul;15(5):592-9.
- **This process is called *odor-associative learning*…** To learn more about this process we suggest starting with Rachel S. Herz. Odor-associative Learning and Emotion: Effects on Perception and Behavior. *Chem. Senses* 30 (suppl 1): i250–i251, 2005.
- **In 2007 the Natural Resources Defense Council released the results of a study of 14 common household air fresheners**… This is available at the NRDC website (http://www.nrdc.org/health/home/airfresheners.asp).
- **The *Case of Chloracne*…** A good starting place to learn more about chloracne is the wikipedia page dedicated to this topic (http://en.wikipedia.org/wiki/Chloracne).

- **The Solution: Avoidance, Elimination, and Systemic Detoxification**… There are many resources available to learn more about these issues. We recommend reading Dr. Walter Crinnion's book *Clean, Green, and Lean: Get Rid of the Toxins That Make You Fat* (ISBN-10: 0470409231) as a guide to this topic.

Chapter 16

- **Reasoning Backwards**… Good introductions into some of the issues in drug approval, side effects, and polypharmacy include the following books.
  - *Over Dose: The Case Against the Drug Companies: Prescription Drugs, Side Effects, and Your Health* by Jay Cohen (ISBN-10: 1422352129)
  - *Overdosed America: The Broken Promise of American Medicine (P.S.)* by John Abramson (ISBN-10: 0061344761)
  - *Side Effects: A Prosecutor, a Whistleblower, and a Bestselling Antidepressant on Trial* by Alison Bass (ISBN-10: 1565125533)
  - *Selling Sickness: How the World's Biggest Pharmaceutical Companies Are Turning Us All Into Patients* by Ray Moynihan and Alan Cassels (ISBN-10: 156025856X)
- **In the period between 1995-6 and 2002-3 medication usage in the United States increased an average of 46 percent**… Sources for these statistics are the Medical Expenditure Panel Survey April

2007 *Trends in Outpatient Prescription Drug Utilization and Expenditures, 1997 and 2004* report published by the Agency for Healthcare, and the *Healthcare Cost and Utilization Project (HCUP)* sponsored by the Agency for Healthcare Research and Quality (http://hcup.ahrq.gov/HCUPnet.asp).

- **Two patients were given Risperidone alone for three months**.... Source is Fukui H, Murai T. Severe weight gain induced by combination treatment with risperidone and paroxetine. *Clin Neuropharmacol.* 2002 Sep-Oct;25(5):269-71.

- **Protease Inhibitors are antiviral medications used in the treatment of HIV**... For further reading in this area we suggest:
    - Benson JO, McGhee K, Coplan P, et al. Fat redistribution in indinavir-treated patients with HIV infection: A review of postmarketing cases. *J Acquir Immune Defic Syndr.* 2000 Oct 1;25(2):130-9.
    - Bernasconi E. Metabolic effects of protease inhibitor therapy. *AIDS Read.* 1999 Jul;9(4):254-6, 259-60, 266-9.
    - Capaldini L. Protease inhibitors' metabolic side effects: cholesterol, triglycerides, blood sugar, and "Crix belly." Interview with Lisa Capaldini, M.D. Interview by John S. James. *AIDS Treat News.* 1997 Aug 15;(No 277):1-4.
    - McDermott AY, Shevitz A, Knox T, et al. Effect of highly active antiretroviral therapy on fat, lean, and bone mass in HIV-seropositive men and women. *Am J Clin Nutr* 2001 Nov;74(5):679-86
    - Moyle G. Metabolic issues associated with protease inhibitors. *J Acquir Immune Defic Syndr.* 2007 Jun 1;45 Suppl 1:S19-26.
    - Nolan D. Metabolic complications associated with HIV protease inhibitor therapy. *Drugs.* 2003;63(23):2555-74.
    - Stricker RB, Goldberg B. Weight gain associated with protease inhibitor therapy in HIV-infected patients. *Res Virol.* 1998 Mar-Apr;149(2):123-6.

- **Investigations into Medications and Shape**... Suggested reading to gain a general idea of the shape and medication side effect issue include:
    - Cheskin LJ, Bartlett SJ, Zayas R, et al. Prescription medications: a modifiable contributor to obesity. *South Med J.* 1999 Sep;92(9):898-904.
    - Leslie WS, Hankey CR, Lean ME. Weight gain as an adverse effect of some commonly prescribed drugs: a systematic review. *QJM.* 2007 Jul;100(7):395-404.
    - Malone M. Medications associated with weight gain. *Ann Pharmacother.* 2005 Dec;39(12):2046-54.

- The *Case of Risperidone*... Sources for this case include:
    - Cohen S, Glazewski R, Khan S, Khan A. Weight gain with risperidone among patients with mental retardation: effect of calorie restriction. *J Clin Psychiatry.* 2001 Feb;62(2):114-6.
    - Fleischhaker C, Heiser P, Hennighausen K, et al. Weight gain associated with clozapine, olanzapine and risperidone in children and adolescents. *J Neural Transm.* 2007 Feb;114(2):273-80.
    - Hellings JA, Zarcone JR, Crandall K, et al. Weight gain in a controlled study of risperidone in children, adolescents and adults with mental retardation and autism. *J Child Adolesc Psychopharmacol.* 2001 Fall;11(3):229-38.
    - Martin A, Landau J, Leebens P, et al. Risperidone-associated weight gain in children and adolescents: a retrospective chart review. *J Child Adolesc Psychopharmacol.* 2000 Winter;10(4):259-68.
    - Robinson DG, Woerner MG, Napolitano B, et al. Randomized comparison of olanzapine versus risperidone for the treatment of first-episode schizophrenia: 4-month outcomes. *Am J Psychiatry.* 2006 Dec;163(12):2096-102.
    - Safer DJ. A comparison of risperidone-induced weight gain across the age span. *J Clin Psychopharmacol.* 2004 Aug;24(4):429-36.
    - Theleritis CG, Papadimitriou GN, Papageorgiou CC, et al. Excessive weight gain after remission of depression in a schizophrenic patient treated with risperidone: case report. *BMC Psychiatry.* 2006 Sep 5;6:37.

- The *Case of Amitriptyline*... Sources for this case are:
    - Berilgen MS, Bulut S, Gonen M, et al. Comparison of the effects of amitriptyline and flunarizine on weight gain and serum leptin, C peptide and insulin levels when used as migraine preventive treatment. *Cephalalgia.* 2005 Nov;25(11):1048-53.
    - Berken GH, Weinstein DO, Stern WC. Weight gain. A side-effect of tricyclic antidepressants. *J Affect Disord.* 1984 Oct;7(2):133-8.
    - Fernstrom MH, Kupfer DJ. Antidepressant-induced weight gain: a comparison study of four medications. *Psychiatry Res.* 1988 Dec;26(3):265-71.
    - Montgomery SA, Reimitz PE, Zivkov M. Mirtazapine versus amitriptyline in the long-term treatment of depression: a double-blind placebo-controlled study. *Int Clin Psychopharmacol.* 1998 Mar;13(2):63-73.

- Noyes R Jr, Garvey MJ, Cook BL, Samuelson L. Problems with tricyclic antidepressant use in patients with panic disorder or agoraphobia: results of a naturalistic follow-up study. *J Clin Psychiatry*. 1989 May;50(5):163-9.
- van Ophoven A, Hertle L. Long-term results of amitriptyline treatment for interstitial cystitis. *J Urol*. 2005 Nov;174(5):1837-40.

- **The *Case of Beta Blockers*...** Sources for this case include:
  - Butler J, Khadim G, Belue R, Chomsky D, Dittus RS, Griffin M, Wilson JR. Tolerability to beta-blocker therapy among heart failure patients in clinical practice. *J Card Fail*. 2003 Jun;9(3):203-9.
  - Lainscak M, Keber I, Anker SD. Body composition changes in patients with systolic heart failure treated with beta blockers: a pilot study. *Int J Cardiol*. 2006 Jan 26;106(3):319-22.
  - Maggioni F, Ruffatti S, Dainese F, et al. Weight variations in the prophylactic therapy of primary headaches: 6-month follow-up. *J Headache Pain*. 2005 Sep;6(4):322-4.
  - Lamont LS. Beta-blockers and their effects on protein metabolism and resting energy expenditure. *J Cardiopulm Rehabil* 1995 May-Jun;15(3):183-5.
  - Lamont LS, Brown T, Riebe D, Caldwell M. The major components of human energy balance during chronic beta-adrenergic blockade. *J Cardiopulm Rehabil* 2000 Jul-Aug;20(4):247-50.
  - Martinez-Mir I, Navarro-Badenes J, Palop V, et al. Weight gain induced by long-term propranolol treatment. *Ann Pharmacother* 1993 Apr;27(4):512 [Letter].
  - Messerli FH, Bell DS, Fonseca V, et al. Use of beta-blockers in obesity hypertension: potential role of weight gain. *Obes Rev* 2001 Nov;2(4):275-80.
  - Rossner S, Taylor CL, Byington RP, Furberg CD. Long term propranolol treatment and changes in body weight after myocardial infarction. *BMJ* 1990 Apr 7;300(6729):902-3.
  - Sharma AM, Pischon T, Hardt S, et al. Hypothesis: Beta-adrenergic receptor blockers and weight gain: A systematic analysis. *Hypertension* 2001 Feb;37(2):250-4.
  - Wright JT Jr, Bangalore S, Holdbrook FK, et al. Body weight changes with beta-blocker use: results from GEMINI. *Am J Med*. 2007 Jul;120(7):610-5.
  - Zhang JL, Zheng X, Zou DJ, et al. Effect of metformin on weight gain during antihypertensive treatment with a beta-blocker in Chinese patients. *Am J Hypertens*. 2009 Aug;22(8):884-90.

- **This difference between the average response and the variance of response**... For further reading on this topic we recommend the book *Where Medicine Went Wrong: Rediscovering the Path to Complexity* by Bruce J West.

- **The *Case of the Four Yard Run* illustrates**... Source for this is the article *Two Yards at a Time* by Mike Tanier published by Football Outsiders.

- **During several months of Gabapentin use**... Source is DeToledo JC, Toledo C, DeCerce J, Ramsay RE. Changes in body weight with chronic, high-dose gabapentin therapy. *Ther Drug Monit*. 1997 Aug;19(4):394-6.

- **The *Case of SSRI*...** Sources for this case are:
  - Fava M, Judge R, Hoog SL, Nilsson ME, Koke SC. Fluoxetine versus sertraline and paroxetine in major depressive disorder: changes in weight with long-term treatment. *J Clin Psychiatry*. 2000 Nov;61(11):863-7.
  - Maina G, Albert U, Salvi V, Bogetto F. Weight gain during long-term treatment of obsessive-compulsive disorder: a prospective comparison between serotonin reuptake inhibitors. *J Clin Psychiatry*. 2004 Oct;65(10):1365-71.
  - Michelson D, Amsterdam JD, Quitkin FM, et al. Changes in weight during a 1-year trial of fluoxetine. *Am J Psychiatry*. 1999 Aug;156(8):1170-6.
  - Orzack MH, Friedman LM, Marby DW. Weight changes on fluoxetine as a function of baseline weight in depressed outpatients. *Psychopharmacol Bull*. 1990;26(3):327-30.
  - Sherman C. Writer Weight Gain Varies With Antidepressants. *Clinical Psychiatry News* 27(5):9, 1999.
  - Sussman N, Ginsberg DL, Bikoff J. Effects of nefazodone on body weight: a pooled analysis of selective serotonin reuptake inhibitor- and imipramine-controlled trials. *J Clin Psychiatry*. 2001 Apr;62(4):256-60.
  - Van Ameringen M, Mancini C, Pipe B, et al. Topiramate treatment for SSRI-induced weight gain in anxiety disorders. *J Clin Psychiatry*. 2002 Nov;63(11):981-4.
  - Ward AS, Comer SD, Haney M, et al. Fluoxetine-maintained obese humans: effect on food intake and body weight. *Physiol Behav*. 1999 Jul;66(5):815-21.
  - Wise TN, Perahia DG, Pangallo BA, et al. Effects of the antidepressant duloxetine on body weight: analyses of 10 clinical studies. *Prim Care Companion J Clin Psychiatry*. 2006;8(5):269-78.

- The *Case of Oral Hypoglycemic Agents*... Sources for this case are:
  - Basu A, Jensen MD, McCann F, et al. Effects of Pioglitazone Versus Glipizide on Body Fat Distribution, Body Water Content, and Hemodynamics in Type 2 Diabetes. *Diabetes Care* 2008:29:510 –514.
  - Purnell JQ, Weyer C. Weight effect of current and experimental drugs for diabetes mellitus: from promotion to alleviation of obesity. *Treat Endocrinol.* 2003;2(1):33-47.
- The *Case of Drugs in our Drinking Water*... The issue of drugs in drinking water has been written about several times. *Science News* published articles back on 3-21-98 and again on 4-1-2000 and 6-17-2000. Newer articles on this topic include *Low Levels of Drugs Found in Drinking Water* by Kathleen Doheny published by WebMD Health News in 2008 and *Even if you're careful, drugs can end up in water* by Clarke Canfield (Published by the A.P. on February 7, 2010).
- The precautionary principle... To read more about this principle we suggest the Wikipedia page dedicated to this topic.
- The *Case of Medications Possibly Preventing Weight Loss*... Source for this case is Malone M, Alger-Mayer SA, Anderson DA. Medication associated with weight gain may influence outcome in a weight management program. *Ann Pharmacother.* 2005 Jul-Aug;39(7-8):1204-8. Epub 2005 May 31.
- The *Case of Oral Contraceptives*... Source is Reuter's news article titled *Want to get buff, ladies? Switch contraceptives* published on April 2009, which reported on research by Chang-Woock Lee and Steven Riechman of Texas A&M University in College Station and Mark Newman of the University of Pittsburgh in Pennsylvania.
- The *Case of Lithium*... Source is Henry C. Lithium side-effects and predictors of hypothyroidism in patients with bipolar disorder: sex differences. *J Psychiatry Neurosci.* 2002 Mar;27(2):104-7.
- Depot contraceptives, on average, cause massive gains in weight and body fat... Source is Berenson AB, Rahman M. Changes in weight, total fat, percent body fat, and central-to-peripheral fat ratio associated with injectable and oral contraceptive use. *Am J Obstet Gynecol.* 2009 Mar;200(3):329.e1-8.

Chapter 17

- The Case of Remaining Sedentary... Source for this case is Slentz CA, Aiken LB, Houmard JA, et al. Inactivity, exercise and visceral fat. STRRIDE: a randomized, controlled study of exercise intensity and amount. J Appl Physiol. 2005 Jul 7.
- Fitness trumps fatness... A good starting place is the new articles *Fitness trumps fatness in longevity study* (www.reuters.com/article/idUSN0450613820071205).
  Examples of studies that suggest this inference are:
  - Farrell SW, Braun L, Barlow CE, et al. The relation of body mass index, cardiorespiratory fitness, and all-cause mortality in women. *Obes Res* 2002 Jun;10(6):417-23
  - Farrell SW, Cortese GM, LaMonte MJ, Blair SN. Cardiorespiratory fitness, different measures of adiposity, and cancer mortality in men. *Obesity (Silver Spring).* 2007 Dec;15(12):3140-9.
  - LaMonte MJ, Blair SN. Physical activity, cardiorespiratory fitness, and adiposity: contributions to disease risk. *Curr Opin Clin Nutr Metab Care.* 2006 Sep;9(5):540-6.
  - Lee CD, Blair SN, Jackson AS. Cardiorespiratory fitness, body composition, and all-cause and cardiovascular disease mortality in men. *Am J Clin Nutr.* 1999 Mar;69(3):373-80.
  - Nocon M, Hiemann T, Müller-Riemenschneider F, et al. Association of physical activity with all-cause and cardiovascular mortality: a systematic review and meta-analysis. *Eur J Cardiovasc Prev Rehabil.* 2008 Jun;15(3):239-46.
  - Pedersen BK. Body mass index-independent effect of fitness and physical activity for all-cause mortality. *Scand J Med Sci Sports.* 2007 Jun;17(3):196-204.
  - Sui X, LaMonte MJ, et al. Cardiorespiratory fitness and adiposity as mortality predictors in older adults. *JAMA.* 2007;298:2507-2516.
- Data from the National Weight Control Registry... Source is Klem ML, Wing RR, McGuire MT, et al. A descriptive study of individuals successful at long-term maintenance of substantial weight loss. *Am J Clin Nutr* 1997;66:239-46
- The Case of More Isn't Better... To read more about differences between volitional and forced exercise we suggest reading:
  - Moraska A, Deak T, Spencer RL, et al. Treadmill running produces both positive and negative physiological adaptations in Sprague-Dawley rats. *Am J Physiol Regul Integr Comp Physiol.* 2000 Oct;279(4):R1321-9.
  - Narath E, Skalicky M, Viidik A. Voluntary and forced exercise influence the survival and body composition of ageing male rats differently. *Exp Gerontol* 2001 Nov;36(10):1699-711

- Schultz RL, Swallow JG, Waters RP, et al. Effects of excessive long-term exercise on cardiac function and myocyte remodeling in hypertensive heart failure rats. *Hypertension.* 2007 Aug;50(2):410-6.
- Talan MI, Ingram DK. Effects of voluntary and forced exercise on thermoregulation and survival in aged C57BL/6J mice. *Mech Ageing Dev.* 1986 Nov 14;36(3):269-79.

- **One group of volunteers ate 25 percent fewer calories for six months...** Source is Redman LM, Heilbronn LK, Martin CK, et al. Metabolic and behavioral compensations in response to caloric restriction: implications for the maintenance of weight loss. *PLoS One.* 2009;4(2):e4377.

- **If it's only a matter of calories, why does the same caloric deficit, achieved in different ways, produce such different shape and metabolic responses?...** We suggest reading:
  - Blundell JE, Stubbs RJ, Hughes DA, et al. Cross talk between physical activity and appetite control: does physical activity stimulate appetite? *Proc Nutr Soc.* 2003 Aug;62(3):651-61.
  - Chomentowski P, Dubé JJ, Amati F, et al. Moderate exercise attenuates the loss of skeletal muscle mass that occurs with intentional caloric restriction-induced weight loss in older, overweight to obese adults. *J Gerontol A Biol Sci Med Sci.* 2009 May;64(5):575-80.
  - Grillo CM, Brownell KD, Stunkard AJ. The metabolic and psychological importance of exercise in weight control. In: *Obesity: Theory and therapy.* Ed. Stunkard AJ, Wadden TA. Raven Press, NY, 1993;258
  - Larson-Meyer DE, Redman L, Heilbronn LK, et al. Caloric Restriction With or Without Exercise: The Fitness versus Fatness Debate. *Medicine and Science in Sports and Exercise.* 2010;42(1):152-
  - Long SJ, Hart K, Morgan LM. The ability of habitual exercise to influence appetite and food intake in response to high- and low-energy preloads in man. *Br J Nutr* 2002 May;87(5):517-23
  - Nicklas BJ, Wang X, You T, et al. Effect of exercise intensity on abdominal fat loss during calorie restriction in overweight and obese postmenopausal women: a randomized, controlled trial. *Am J Clin Nutr.* 2009 Apr;89(4):1043-52.
  - Serresse O, Boulay MR, Fournier G. Long-term exercise training with constant energy intake. 1: Effect on body composition and selected metabolic variables. *Int J Obes.* 1990 Jan;14(1):57-73.
  - Tremblay A, Despres JP, Bouchard C. The effects of exercise-training on energy balance and adipose tissue morphology and metabolism. *Sports Med* 1985 May-Jun;2(3):223-33
  - Weiss EP, Villareal DT, Racette SB, et al. Caloric restriction but not exercise-induced reductions in fat mass decrease plasma triiodothyronine concentrations: a randomized controlled trial. *Rejuvenation Res.* 2008 Jun;11(3):605-9.
  - Weiss EP, Racette SB, Villareal DT, et al. Lower extremity muscle size and strength and aerobic capacity decrease with caloric restriction but not with exercise-induced weight loss. *J Appl Physiol.* 2007 Feb;102(2):634-40.
  - Woo R, Garrow JS, Pi-Sunyer FX. Voluntary food intake during prolonged exercise in obese women. *Am J Clin Nutr* 1982 Sep;36(3):478-84.

- **On Intensity and Frequency...** For further reading in this area we suggest:
  - Bond Brill J, Perry AC, Parker L, et al. Dose-response effect of walking exercise on weight loss. How much is enough? *Int J Obes Relat Metab Disord* 2002 Nov;26(11):1484-93
  - Brandon LJ, Elliott-Lloyd MB. Walking, body composition, and blood pressure dose-response in African American and white women. *Ethn Dis.* 2006 Summer;16(3):675-81.
  - Chambliss HO. Exercise duration and intensity in a weight-loss program. *Clin J Sport Med.* 2005 Mar;15(2):113-5.
  - Gwinup G. Weight loss without dietary restriction: efficacy of different forms of aerobic exercise. *Am J Sports Med.* 1987 May-Jun;15(3):275-9.
  - Gwinup G. Effect of exercise alone on the weight of obese women. *Arch Intern Med.* 1975 May;135(5):676-80.
  - Johnson JL, Slentz CA, Houmard JA, et al. Exercise training amount and intensity on metabolic syndrome (from Studies of a Targeted Risk Reduction Intervention through Defined Exercise). *Am J Cardiol* 2007; 100:1759-1766.
  - Leon AS, Conrad J, Hunninghake DB, Serfass R. Effects of a vigorous walking program on body composition, and carbohydrate and lipid metabolism of obese young men. *Am J Clin Nutr.* 1979 Sep;32(9):1776-87.
  - Mougios V, Kazaki M, Christoulas K, et al. Does the intensity of an exercise programme modulate body composition changes? *Int J Sports Med.* 2006 Mar;27(3):178-81.
  - Slentz CA, Duscha BD, Johnson JL, et al. Effects of the amount of exercise on body weight, body composition, and measures of central obesity: STRRIDE--a randomized controlled study. *Arch Intern Med.* 2004 Jan 12;164(1):31-9.
  - van Aggel-Leijssen DP, Saris WH, Wagenmakers AJ, et al. Effect of exercise training at different intensities on fat metabolism of obese men. *J Appl Physiol.* 2002 Mar;92(3):1300-9.

- ▪ Wilmore JH, Despres JP, Stanforth PR, et al. Alterations in body weight and composition consequent to 20 wk of endurance training: the HERITAGE Family Study. *Am J Clin Nutr.* 1999 Sep;70(3):346-52.

- **Volunteers wore devices for seven days that were designed to detect and measure all movement**... Source is Healy GN, Dunstan DW, Salmon J, et al. Breaks in sedentary time: beneficial associations with metabolic risk. *Diabetes Care.* 2008 Apr;31(4):661-6.

- **Two hundred and two previously sedentary men and women were divided into two groups and followed for one year**... This research was conducted at the Fred Hutchinson Cancer Research Center and was described in the *USA Today* article *Simple step toward better health* published in the Dec 3, 2008 paper.

- **Walkable environments have strong associations with leaner shapes**... Source is Smith KR, Brown BB, Yamada I, et al. Walkability and body mass index density, design, and new diversity measures. *Am J Prev Med.* 2008 Sep;35(3):237-44.

- **The Case of Gradually Increasing Walking Duration**... Source is Gwinup G. Effect of exercise alone on the weight of obese women. *Arch Intern Med.* 1975 May;135(5):676-80.

- **The Case of the Dog Walkers**... This research was described in the news article *Daily Dog Walks Work Off Weight for Owners* (http://www.newswise.com/articles/daily-dog-walks-work-off-weight-for-owners?ret=/articles/list&category=&page=2&search[status]=3&search[sort]=date+desc&search[channel_id]=47).

- **On varying Our pace**... A good starting point for reading more about naturalistic movement like that suggested in this section is the article *Why I Do All This Walking* by Nassim Taleb (www.fooledbyrandomness.com/whyIwalk.pdf).

- **The Case of Varying Our Pace**... Source is Nemoto KI, Gen-No H, Masuki S, et al. Effects of High-Intensity Interval Walking Training on Physical Fitness and Blood Pressure in Middle-Aged and Older People. *Mayo Clin Proc.* 2007;82(7):803-811.

- **A study involving nearly 1000 female twins**... Source is Samaras K, Kelly PJ, Chiano MN, Spector TD, Campbell LV. Genetic and environmental influences on total-body and central abdominal fat: The effect of physical activity in female twins. *Ann Intern Med* 1999;130:873-882.

- **The Case of Exercise and Fish Oil**... Source is Hill AM, Buckley JD, Murphy KJ, Howe PR. Combining fish-oil supplements with regular aerobic exercise improves body composition and cardiovascular disease risk factors. *Am J Clin Nutr.* 2007 May;85(5):1267-1274.

Chapter 18

- **This requires stimulus and recovery. Each bout of exercise is a challenge to our body**... The book *Body By Science: A Research Based Program to Get the Results You Want in 12 Minutes a Week*, by authors John Little and Doug McGuff, M.D., provides an excellent introduction to the way weight training serves as a stimuli for adaptation and why sufficient recovery time is needed. An article called *Exertion is only half of the equation* by Meg Jordan, which appeared in *American Fitness* in the Jan-Feb 2003 issue, is another good source of information.

- **A muscle is weaker after an intense workout than it was before the workout**... The book *Body By Science: A Research Based Program to Get the Results You Want in 12 Minutes a Week*, by authors John Little and Doug McGuff, M.D., provides an excellent explanation of how muscles progressively weaken during a resistance training session.

- **Intricate adaptations are also occurring inside muscles**... To read more about these adaptations, as well as the specificity of adaptations, we recommend reading:
    - ▪ Brentano MA, Cadore EL, Da Silva EM, et al. Physiological adaptations to strength and circuit training in postmenopausal women with bone loss. *J Strength Cond Res.* 2008 Nov;22(6):1816-25.
    - ▪ Campos GE, Luecke TJ, Wendelin HK, et al. Muscular adaptations in response to three different resistance-training regimens: specificity of repetition maximum training zones. *Eur J Appl Physiol.* 2002 Nov;88(1-2):50-60.
    - ▪ Coffey VG, Hawley JA. The molecular bases of training adaptation. *Sports Med.* 2007;37(9):737-63.
    - ▪ Folland JP, Williams AG. The adaptations to strength training: morphological and neurological contributions to increased strength. *Sports Med.* 2007;37(2):145-68.
    - ▪ Goto K, Nagasawa M, Yanagisawa O, et al. Muscular adaptations to combinations of high- and low-intensity resistance exercises. *J Strength Cond Res.* 2004 Nov;18(4):730-7.
    - ▪ Hagerman FC, Walsh SJ, Staron RS, et al. Effects of high-intensity resistance training on untrained older men. I. Strength, cardiovascular, and metabolic responses. *J Gerontol A Biol Sci Med Sci.* 2000 Jul;55(7):B336-46.
    - ▪ Harber MP, Fry AC, Rubin MR, et al. Skeletal muscle and hormonal adaptations to circuit weight training in untrained men. *Scand J Med Sci Sports.* 2004 Jun;14(3):176-85.

- Kraemer WJ, Nindl BC, Ratamess NA, et al. Changes in muscle hypertrophy in women with periodized resistance training. *Med Sci Sports Exerc.* 2004 Apr;36(4):697-708.
- Paddon-Jones D, Keech A, Lonergan A, Abernethy P. Differential expression of muscle damage in humans following acute fast and slow velocity eccentric exercise. *J Sci Med Sport.* 2005 Sep;8(3):255-63.
- Staron RS, Karapondo DL, Kraemer WJ, et al. Skeletal muscle adaptations during early phase of heavy-resistance training in men and women. *J Appl Physiol.* 1994 Mar;76(3):1247-55.
- Stepto NK, Coffey VG, Carey AL, et al. Global gene expression in skeletal muscle from well-trained strength and endurance athletes. *Med Sci Sports Exerc.* 2009 Mar;41(3):546-65.

- **The Case of Eccentric and Concentric Muscle Activity...** Sources for this case are:
  - Farthing JP, Chilibeck PD. The effects of eccentric and concentric training at different velocities on muscle hypertrophy. *Eur J Appl Physiol.* 2003 Aug;89(6):578-86.
  - Friedmann-Bette B, Bauer T, Kinscherf R, et al. Effects of strength training with eccentric overload on muscle adaptation in male athletes. *Eur J Appl Physiol.* 2009 Nov 25.
  - Hortobágyi T, Hill JP, Houmard JA, et al. Adaptive responses to muscle lengthening and shortening in humans. *J Appl Physiol.* 1996 Mar;80(3):765-72.
  - Mayhew TP, Rothstein JM, Finucane SD, Lamb RL. Muscular adaptation to concentric and eccentric exercise at equal power levels. *Med Sci Sports Exerc.* 1995 Jun;27(6):868-73.
  - Mueller M, Breil FA, Vogt M, et al. Different response to eccentric and concentric training in older men and women. *Eur J Appl Physiol.* 2009 Sep;107(2):145-53.
  - Reeves ND, Maganaris CN, Longo S, Narici MV. Differential adaptations to eccentric versus conventional resistance training in older humans. *Exp Physiol.* 2009 Jul;94(7):825-33.
  - Vissing K, Brink M, Lønbro S, et al. Muscle adaptations to plyometric vs. resistance training in untrained young men. *J Strength Cond Res.* 2008 Nov;22(6):1799-810.

- **Two groups of young women were placed on strength-training programs for nine weeks...** Source is Gillies EM, Putman CT, Bell GJ. The effect of varying the time of concentric and eccentric muscle actions during resistance training on skeletal muscle adaptations in women. *Eur J Appl Physiol.* 2006 Jul;97(4):443-53.

- **This specificity is in evidence in the Case of Disuse and Use...** Sources for this case are:
  - Adams GR, Hather BM, Dudley GA. Effect of short-term unweighting on human skeletal muscle strength and size. *Aviat Space Environ Med.* 1994 Dec;65(12):1116-21.
  - Berg HE, Larsson L, Tesch PA. Lower limb skeletal muscle function after 6 wk of bed rest. *J Appl Physiol.* 1997 Jan;82(1):182-8.
  - Berg HE, Eiken O, Miklavcic L, Mekjavic IB. Hip, thigh and calf muscle atrophy and bone loss after 5-week bedrest inactivity. *Eur J Appl Physiol.* 2007 Feb;99(3):283-9. de
  - Boer MD, Seynnes OR, di Prampero PE, et al. Effect of 5 weeks horizontal bed rest on human muscle thickness and architecture of weight bearing and non-weight bearing muscles. *Eur J Appl Physiol.* 2008 Sep;104(2):401-7.
  - Durheim MT, Slentz CA, Bateman LA, et al. Relationships between exercise-induced reductions in thigh intermuscular adipose tissue, changes in lipoprotein particle size, and visceral adiposity. *Am J Physiol Endocrinol Metab.* 2008 Aug;295(2):E407-12.
  - Edgerton VR, Zhou MY, Ohira Y, et al. Human fiber size and enzymatic properties after 5 and 11 days of spaceflight. *J Appl Physiol.* 1995 May;78(5):1733-9.
  - Giangregorio L, Blimkie CJ. Skeletal adaptations to alterations in weight-bearing activity: a comparison of models of disuse osteoporosis. *Sports Med.* 2002;32(7):459-76.
  - Manini TM, Clark BC, Nalls MA, et al. Reduced physical activity increases intermuscular adipose tissue in healthy young adults. *Am J Clin Nutr.* 2007 Feb;85(2):377-84.
  - Mueller M, Breil FA, Vogt M, et al. Different response to eccentric and concentric training in older men and women. *Eur J Appl Physiol.* 2009 Sep;107(2):145-53.
  - Pace N, Kodama AM, Price DC, et al. Body composition changes in men and women after 2-3 weeks of bed rest. *Life Sci Space Res.* 1976;14:269-74.
  - Song MY, Ruts E, Kim J, Janumala I, et al. Sarcopenia and increased adipose tissue infiltration of muscle in elderly African American women. *Am J Clin Nutr.* 2004 May;79(5):874-80.
  - Staron RS, Leonardi MJ, Karapondo DL, et al. Strength and skeletal muscle adaptations in heavy-resistance-trained women after detraining and retraining. *J Appl Physiol.* 1991 Feb;70(2):631-40.
  - Trappe SW, Trappe TA, Lee GA, et al. Comparison of a space shuttle flight (STS-78) and bed rest on human muscle function. *J Appl Physiol.* 2001 Jul;91(1):57-64.

- **Muscle memory...** Wikipedia has a page dedicated to this topic that provides a good introduction to the concept of muscle memory. The news article *Muscle Memory: Scientists May Have Unwittingly Uncovered Its Mystery* is also a good resource (http://www.thinkmuscle.com/articles/haycock/muscle-memory.htm). One of the studies that support the concept of muscle memory is Staron RS, Leonardi

MJ, Karapondo DL, et al. Strength and skeletal muscle adaptations in heavy-resistance-trained women after detraining and retraining. *J Appl Physiol.* 1991 Feb;70(2):631-40.

- **A Study in Resistance (Weight) Training**… Sources for this section include:
    - Chilibeck PD, Calder AW, Sale DG, Webber CE. A comparison of strength and muscle mass increases during resistance training in young women. *Eur J Appl Physiol Occup Physiol.* 1998;77(1-2):170-5.
    - Chilibeck PD, Calder A, Sale DG, Webber CE. Twenty weeks of weight training increases lean tissue mass but not bone mineral mass or density in healthy, active young women. *Can J Physiol Pharmacol.* 1996 Oct;74(10):1180-5.
    - Cullinen K, Caldwell M. Weight training increases fat-free mass and strength in untrained young women. J Am Diet Assoc 1998 Apr;98(4):414-8
    - Fenkci S, Sarsan A, Rota S, Ardic F. Effects of resistance or aerobic exercises on metabolic parameters in obese women who are not on a diet. *Adv Ther.* 2006 May-Jun;23(3):404-13.
    - Treuth MS, Hunter GR, Kekes-Szabo T, et al. Reduction in intra-abdominal adipose tissue after strength training in older women. *J Appl Physiol* 1995:78;1425-1431.
    - Tsuzuku S, Kajioka T, Endo H, et al. Favorable effects of non-instrumental resistance training on fat distribution and metabolic profiles in healthy elderly people. *Eur J Appl Physiol.* 2007 Mar;99(5):549-55.
    - Watts K, Beye P, Siafarikas A, et al. Exercise training normalizes vascular dysfunction and improves central adiposity in obese adolescents. *J Am Coll Cardiol.* 2004 May 19;43(10):1823-7.
- **The Cases of Body Image Satisfaction**… Sources for this case are:
    - Borg P, Kukkonen-Harjula K, Fogelholm M, Pasanen M. Effects of walking or resistance training on weight loss maintenance in obese, middle-aged men: a randomized trial. *Int J Obes Relat Metab Disord* 2002 May;26(5):676-83
    - Williams PA, Cash TF. Effects of a circuit weight training program on the body images of college students. *Int J Eat Disord.* 2001 Jul;30(1):75-82.
- **Whole body vibration uses**… Sources are:
    - Bogaerts A, Delecluse C, Claessens AL, et al. Impact of whole-body vibration training versus fitness training on muscle strength and muscle mass in older men: a 1-year randomized controlled trial. *J Gerontol A Biol Sci Med Sci.* 2007 Jun;62(6):630-5.
    - Lamont HS, Cramer JT, Bemben DA, et al. Effects of 6 weeks of periodized squat training with or without whole-body vibration on short-term adaptations in jump performance within recreationally resistance trained men. *J Strength Cond Res.* 2008 Nov;22(6):1882-93.
- **A Study in Start-Stop Exercise**… Sources for this section include:
    - June of 2005, *Science Daily* article *A Few 30 Second Sprints As Beneficial As Hour Long Jog.*
    - May 2007, The *New York Times* article *A Healthy Mix of Rest and Motion.*
    - Goldsmith, Rochelle L., et al. Implementation of a Novel Cyclic Exercise Protocol: Short-Term Impact on Healthy Women. *Amer. J. Med. Sports* 2002;4.
    - Helgerud J, Høydal K, Wang E, et al. Aerobic high-intensity intervals improve VO2max more than moderate training. *Med Sci Sports Exerc.* 2007 Apr;39(4):665-71.
    - Nemoto KI, Gen-No H, Masuki S, et al. Effects of High-Intensity Interval Walking Training on Physical Fitness and Blood Pressure in Middle-Aged and Older People. *Mayo Clin Proc.* 2007;82(7):803-811
    - Pipes TV. Physiological responses of fire fighting recruits to high intensity training. *J Occup Med.* 1977 Feb;19(2):129-32.
    - Ratel S, Lazaar N, Dore E, et al. High-intensity intermittent activities at school: controversies and facts. *J Sports Med Phys Fitness.* 2004 Sep;44(3):272-80.
    - Talanian JL, Galloway SD, Heigenhauser GJ, et al. Two weeks of high-intensity aerobic interval training increases the capacity for fat oxidation during exercise in women. *J Appl Physiol.* 2007 Apr;102(4):1439-47.
    - Tjønna AE, Lee SJ, Rognmo Ø, et al. Aerobic interval training versus continuous moderate exercise as a treatment for the metabolic syndrome. A pilot study. *Circulation.* 2008;
    - Trapp EG, Chisholm DJ, Freund J, Boutcher SH. The effects of high-intensity intermittent exercise training on fat loss and fasting insulin levels of young women. *Int J Obes (Lond).* 2008 Jan 15.
    - Tremblay A, Simoneau JA, Bouchard C. Impact of exercise intensity on body fatness and skeletal muscle metabolism. *Metabolism.* 1994 Jul;43(7):814-8.
- **A single bout of resistance exercise measurably increased metabolic rate for the next two days. Studies have show lasting increases in metabolic rate with consistent resistant exercise**… Sources are:
    - Kirk EP, Donnelly JE, Smith BK, et al. Minimal Resistance Training Improves Daily Energy Expenditure and Fat Oxidation. *Med Sci Sports Exerc.* 2009 Apr 3.

- Williamson DL, Kirwan JP. A single bout of concentric resistance exercise increases basal metabolic rate 48 hours after exercise in healthy 59-77-year-old men. *J Gerontol A Biol Sci Med Sci.* 1997 Nov;52(6):M352-5.
- Van Etten LM, Westerterp KR, Verstappen FT, et al. Effect of an 18-wk weight-training program on energy expenditure and physical activity. *J Appl Physiol* 1997 Jan;82(1):298-304

- **What to Do and How To Do It**... Sources for this section are:
    - Gillies EM, Putman CT, Bell GJ. The effect of varying the time of concentric and eccentric muscle actions during resistance training on skeletal muscle adaptations in women. *Eur J Appl Physiol.* 2006 Jul;97(4):443-53.
    - Marx JO, Ratamess NA, Nindl BC, et al. Low-volume circuit versus high-volume periodized resistance training in women. *Med Sci Sports Exerc.* 2001 Apr;33(4):635-43.
    - Paddon-Jones D, Keech A, Lonergan A, Abernethy P. Differential expression of muscle damage in humans following acute fast and slow velocity eccentric exercise. *J Sci Med Sport.* 2005 Sep;8(3):255-63.
    - Taaffe DR, Pruitt L, Pyka G, et al. Comparative effects of high- and low-intensity resistance training on thigh muscle strength, fiber area, and tissue composition in elderly women. *Clin Physiol.* 1996 Jul;16(4):381-92.
    - Tanimoto M, Sanada K, Yamamoto K, et al. Effects of whole-body low-intensity resistance training with slow movement and tonic force generation on muscular size and strength in young men. *J Strength Cond Res.* 2008 Nov;22(6):1926-38.
    - Westcott WL, Winett RA, Anderson ES, et al. Effects of regular and slow speed resistance training on muscle strength. *J Sports Med Phys Fitness.* 2001 Jun;41(2):154-8.

- **The Importance of Recovery**... For further reading we recommend the article *Exertion is only half of the equation* by Meg Jordan, which appeared in *American Fitness* in the Jan-Feb 2003 issue, is another good source of information on the importance of recovery. The book *Body By Science: A Research Based Program to Get the Results You Want in 12 Minutes a Week*, by authors John Little and Doug McGuff, M.D., provides an excellent introduction to the way weight training serves as a stimuli for adaptation and why sufficient recovery time is needed.

Chapter 19

- **Glycemic index**... The website glycemicindex.com is a good resource for discovering more about this concept and the ratings for various foods.
- **According to the satiety index**... Original work on the satiety index was done by Susan Holt and published in:
    - Holt SH, Miller JC, Petocz P, Farmakalidis E. A satiety index of common foods. *Eur J Clin Nutr.* 1995 Sep;49(9):675-90.
    - Holt SH, Brand Miller JC, Petocz P. Interrelationships among postprandial satiety, glucose and insulin responses and changes in subsequent food intake. *Eur J Clin Nutr.* 1996 Dec;50(12):788-97.
    - Holt SH, Brand-Miller JC, Stitt PA. The effects of equal-energy portions of different breads on blood glucose levels, feelings of fullness and subsequent food intake. *J Am Diet Assoc.* 2001 Jul;101(7):767-73.
- **In 1890, the principle fats we ate were**... Source is Mary Enig. *Know Your Fats: The Complete Primer for Understanding the Nutrition of Fats, Oils, and Cholesterol.* 2000.
- **Estimates suggest that an average person consumes 40 to 59 pounds of high fructose corn syrup each year**... Consumption data is taken from reports provided by the United States Department of Agriculture Economic Research Service.
- **The Case of Peck's Rats**... Sources for this case are:
  Peck JW. Active regulation to be lean by rats with ventromedial hypothalamic lesions. *J Comp Physiol Psychol.* 1979 Aug;93(4):695-707.
    - Peck JW. Rats defend different body weights depending on palatability and accessibility of their food. *J Comp Physiol Psychol.* 1978 Jun;92(3):555-70.
- **The Case of the Fat Sand Rat indicates**... Sources for this case are:
    - Adler JH, Lazarovici G, Marton M, Levy E. The diabetic response of weanling sand rats (Psammomys obesus) to diets containing different concentrations of salt bush (Atriplex halimus). *Diabetes Res* 1986 Mar;3(3):169-71
    - Aharonson Z, Shani J, Sulman FG. Hypoglycaemic effect of the salt bush (Atriplex halimus)--a feeding source of the sand rat (Psammomys Obesus). *Diabetologia* 1969 Dec;5(6):379-83
    - Bennani-Kabchi N, el Bouayadi F, Kehel L, et al. Effect of Suaeda fruticosa aqueous extract in the hypercholesterolaemic and insulin-resistant sand rat. *Therapie* 1999 Nov-Dec;54(6):725-30

- Degen AA. Energy requirements of the fat sand rat (Psammomys obesus) when consuming the saltbush, Atriplex halimus: a review. *J Basic Clin Physiol Pharmacol* 1993 Apr-Jun;4(1-2):13-28
- Frenkel G, Kraicer PF, Shani J. Diabetes in the sand-rat: diabetogenesis, responses to mannoheptulose and atriplex ash. *Diabetologia* 1972 Nov;8(5):313-8
- Palgi N, Vatnick I, Pinshow B. Oxalate, calcium and ash intake and excretion balances in fat sand rats (Psammomys obesus) feeding on two different diets. *Comp Biochem Physiol A Mol Integr Physiol.* 2005 May;141(1):48-53.

- **Are all fats and oils equal when it comes to the affects they have on shape?**... Some of the research that calls into question the linear relation ship between fat calories and shape include:

  - Bes-Rastrollo M, Sanchez-Villegas A, de la Fuente C, et al. Olive oil consumption and weight change: the SUN prospective cohort study. *Lipids.* 2006 Mar;41(3):249-56.
  - Buettner R, Parhofer KG, Woenckhaus M, et al. Defining high-fat-diet rat models: metabolic and molecular effects of different fat types. *J Mol Endocrinol.* 2006 Jun;36(3):485-501.
  - Hill AM, Buckley JD, Murphy KJ, Howe PR. Combining fish-oil supplements with regular aerobic exercise improves body composition and cardiovascular disease risk factors. *Am J Clin Nutr.* 2007 May;85(5):1267-1274.
  - Hill JO, Lin D, Yakubu F, Peters JC. Development of dietary obesity in rats: influence of amount and composition of dietary fat. *Int J Obes Relat Metab Disord.* 1992 May;16(5):321-33.
  - Jang IS, Hwang DY, Chae KR, et al. Role of dietary fat type in the development of adiposity from dietary obesity-susceptible Sprague-Dawley rats. *Br J Nutr.* 2003 Mar;89(3):429-38.
  - Rolland V, Roseau S, Fromentin G, et al. Body weight, body composition, and energy metabolism in lean and obese Zucker rats fed soybean oil or butter. *Am J Clin Nutr.* 2002 Jan;75(1):21-30.
  - Takeda M, Imaizumi M, Sawano S, et al. Long-term optional ingestion of corn oil induces excessive caloric intake and obesity in mice. *Nutrition.* 2001 Feb;17(2):117-20.
  - Wien MA, Sabate JM, Ikle DN, et al. Almonds vs complex carbohydrates in a weight reduction program. *Int J Obes Relat Metab Disord.* 2003 Nov;27(11):1365-72.

- **The Case of Trans-Fats**... Sources for this case are:

  - Bortolotto JW, Reis C, Ferreira A, et al. Higher content of trans fatty acids in abdominal visceral fat of morbidly obese individuals undergoing bariatric surgery compared to non-obese subjects. *Obes Surg.* 2005 Oct;15(9):1265-70.
  - Dorfman SE, Laurent D, Gounarides JS, et al. Metabolic implications of dietary trans-fatty acids. *Obesity (Silver Spring).* 2009 Jun;17(6):1200-7.
  - Elias SL, Innis SM. Bakery foods are the major dietary source of trans-fatty acids among pregnant women with diets providing 30 percent energy from fat. *J Am Diet Assoc.* 2002 Jan;102(1):46-51.
  - Field AE, Willett WC, Lissner L, Colditz GA. Dietary fat and weight gain among women in the Nurses' Health Study. *Obesity (Silver Spring).* 2007 Apr;15(4):967-76.
  - Harris RB, Jones WK. Physiological response of mature rats to replacement of dietary fat with a fat substitute. *J Nutr.* 1991 Jul;121(7):1109-16.
  - Harris RB, Zhou J, Youngblood BD, et al. Effect of repeated stress on body weight and body composition of rats fed low- and high-fat diets. *Am J Physiol.* 1998 Dec;275(6 Pt 2):R1928-38.
  - Javadi M, Geelen MJ, Everts H, et al. Body composition and heat expenditure in broiler chickens fed diets with or without trans fatty acids. *J Anim Physiol Anim Nutr (Berl).* 2008 Feb;92(1):99-104.
  - Koh-Banerjee P, Chu NF, Spiegelman D, et al. Prospective study of the association of changes in dietary intake, physical activity, alcohol consumption, and smoking with 9-y gain in waist circumference among 16 587 US men. *Am J Clin Nutr.* 2003 Oct;78(4):719-27.
  - Lee E, Lee S, Park Y. n-3 Polyunsaturated fatty acids and trans fatty acids in patients with the metabolic syndrome: a case-control study in Korea. *Br J Nutr.* 2008 Feb 28;:1-6.
  - Lucas F, Ackroff K, Sclafani A. Dietary fat-induced hyperphagia in rats as a function of fat type and physical form. *Physiol Behav.* 1989 May;45(5):937-46.
  - Martin CA, Milinsk MC, Visentainer JV, et al. Trans fatty acid-forming processes in foods: a review. *An Acad Bras Cienc.* 2007 Jun;79(2):343-50.
  - Tetri LH, Basaranoglu M, Brunt EM, et al. Severe NAFLD with hepatic necroinflammatory changes in mice fed trans fats and a high-fructose corn syrup equivalent. *Am J Physiol Gastrointest Liver Physiol.* 2008 Nov;295(5):G987-95.

- **The Case of the African Green Monkeys**... Sources for this case are:

  - Gosline, Anna. Why fast foods are bad, even in moderation. *New Scientist,* 2006-06-12.
  - Kavanagh K, Jones KL, Sawyer J, et al. Trans fat diet induces abdominal obesity and changes in insulin sensitivity in monkeys. *Obesity (Silver Spring).* 2007 Jul;15(7):1675-84.

- **The U.S. Department of Agriculture (USDA) estimated that per person in 1980**… Data in this section is from the Economic Research Service of the USDA, which tracks annual production and consumption data for a variety of foods including different sweeteners. Other sources are:
  - Bray GA, Nielsen SJ, Popkin BM. Consumption of high-fructose corn syrup in beverages may play a role in the epidemic of obesity. *Am J Clin Nutr.* 2004 Apr;79(4):537-43.
  - Popkin BM, Nielsen SJ. The sweetening of the world's diet. *Obes Res.* 2003 Nov;11(11):1325-32.
- **The Case of Liquid Sugar**… Sources for this case are:
  - Ackroff K, Sclafani A. Sucrose-induced hyperphagia and obesity in rats fed a macronutrient self-selection diet. *Physiol Behav.* 1988;44(2):181-7.
  - Albala C, Ebbeling CB, Cifuentes M, et al. Effects of replacing the habitual consumption of sugar-sweetened beverages with milk in Chilean children. *Am J Clin Nutr* 2008 Sep;88(3):605-11.
  - Assy N, Nasser G, Kamayse I, et al. Soft drink consumption linked with fatty liver in the absence of traditional risk factors. *Can J Gastroenterol.* 2008 Oct;22(10):811-6.
  - Chen L, Appel LJ, Loria C, et al. Reduction in consumption of sugar-sweetened beverages is associated with weight loss: the PREMIER trial. *Am J Clin Nutr.* 2009 May;89(5):1299-306.
  - Ebbeling CB, Feldman HA, Osganian SK, et al. Effects of decreasing sugar-sweetened beverage consumption on body weight in adolescents: a randomized, controlled pilot study. *Pediatrics.* 2006 Mar;117(3):673-80.
  - Hu FB, Malik VS. Sugar-sweetened beverages and risk of obesity and type 2 diabetes: Epidemiologic evidence. *Physiol Behav.* 2010 Feb 6.
  - Kanarek RB, Orthen-Gambill N. Differential effects of sucrose, fructose and glucose on carbohydrate-induced obesity in rats. *J Nutr.* 1982 Aug;112(8):1546-54.
  - Kanarek RB, Hirsch E. Dietary-induced overeating in experimental animals. *Fed Proc.* 1977 Feb;36(2):154-8.
  - Levine AS, Kotz CM, Gosnell BA. Sugars: hedonic aspects, neuroregulation, and energy balance. *Am J Clin Nutr.* 2003 Oct;78(4):834S-842S.
  - Ramirez I. Feeding a liquid diet increases energy intake, weight gain and body fat in rats. *J Nutr.* 1987 Dec;117(12):2127-34.
  - Rattigan S, Clark MG. Effect of sucrose solution drinking option on the development of obesity in rats. *J Nutr.* 1984 Oct;114(10):1971-7.
  - Reid M, Hammersley R, Hill AJ, Skidmore P. Long-term dietary compensation for added sugar: effects of supplementary sucrose drinks over a 4-week period. *Br J Nutr.* 2007 Jan;97(1):193-203.
  - Sclafani A. Carbohydrate-induced hyperphagia and obesity in the rat: effects of saccharide type, form, and taste. *Neurosci Biobehav Rev.* 1987 Summer;11(2):155-62.
  - Sclafani A. Carbohydrate taste, appetite, and obesity: an overview. *Neurosci Biobehav Rev.* 1987 Summer;11(2):131-53.
  - Sclafani A, Xenakis S. Sucrose and polysaccharide induced obesity in the rat. *Physiol Behav.* 1984 Feb;32(2):169-74.
  - Sichieri R, Paula Trotte A, de Souza RA, Veiga GV. School randomised trial on prevention of excessive weight gain by discouraging students from drinking sodas. *Public Health Nutr.* 2009 Feb;12(2):197-202.
  - Tordoff MG, Alleva AM. Effect of drinking soda sweetened with aspartame or high-fructose corn syrup on food intake and body weight. *Am J Clin Nutr* 1990 Jun;51(6):963-9
  - *Study: Drink more water, lose more weight*: Appeared in Oct 24, 2006 issue of USA TODAY (http://www.usatoday.com/news/health/2006-10-24-water-diet_x.htm)
  - *US Soft Drink Consumption Grew 135% Since 1977, Boosting Obesity*: Appeared in Sep 17, 2005 issue of Science Daily (http://www.sciencedaily.com/releases/2004/09/040917091452.htm).
- **Let's continue our investigation of sweet calories with the sweet molecule called fructose**… Sources for the information provided about fructose are:
  - Bantle JP. Dietary fructose and metabolic syndrome and diabetes. *J Nutr.* 2009 Jun;139(6):1263S-1268S.
  - Bantle JP, Raatz SK, Thomas W, Georgopoulos A. Effects of dietary fructose on plasma lipids in healthy subjects. *Am J Clin Nutr.* 2000 Nov;72(5):1128-34.
  - Bray GA, Nielsen SJ, Popkin BM. Consumption of high-fructose corn syrup in beverages may play a role in the epidemic of obesity. *Am J Clin Nutr.* 2004 Apr;79(4):537-43.
  - Cha SH, Wolfgang M, Tokutake Y, et al. Differential effects of central fructose and glucose on hypothalamic malonyl-CoA and food intake. *Proc Natl Acad Sci U S A.* 2008 Nov 4;105(44):16871-5.
  - Collison KS, Saleh SM, Bakheet RH, et al. Diabetes of the Liver: The Link Between Nonalcoholic Fatty Liver Disease and HFCS-55. *Obesity (Silver Spring).* 2009 Mar 12.

- Elliott SS, Keim NL, Stern JS, et al. Fructose, weight gain, and the insulin resistance syndrome. *Am J Clin Nutr* 2002 Nov;76(5):911-22
- Hofmann SM, Tschöp MH. Dietary sugars: a fat difference. *J Clin Invest.* 2009;119:1089–1092
- Lane MD, Cha SH. Effect of glucose and fructose on food intake via malonyl-CoA signaling in the brain. *Biochem Biophys Res Commun.* 2009 Apr 24;382(1):1-5.
- Le KA, Faeh D, Stettler R, et al. A 4-wk high-fructose diet alters lipid metabolism without affecting insulin sensitivity or ectopic lipids in healthy humans. *Am J Clin Nutr.* 2006 Dec;84(6):1374-9.
- Light HR, Tsanzi E, Gigliotti J, et al. The type of caloric sweetener added to water influences weight gain, fat mass, and reproduction in growing Sprague-Dawley female rats. *Exp Biol Med (Maywood).* 2009 Jun;234(6):651-61.
- Marriott BP, Cole N, Lee E. National estimates of dietary fructose intake increased from 1977 to 2004 in the United States. *J Nutr.* 2009 Jun;139(6):1228S-1235S.
- Shapiro A, Mu W, Roncal C, et al. Fructose-induced leptin resistance exacerbates weight gain in response to subsequent high-fat feeding. *Am J Physiol Regul Integr Comp Physiol.* 2008 Nov;295(5):R1370-5.
- Swarbrick MM, Stanhope KL, Elliott SS, et al. Consumption of fructose-sweetened beverages for 10 weeks increases postprandial triacylglycerol and apolipoprotein-B concentrations in overweight and obese women. *Br J Nutr.* 2008 Nov;100(5):947-52.
- Teff KL, Elliott SS, Tschöp M, et al. Dietary fructose reduces circulating insulin and leptin, attenuates postprandial suppression of ghrelin, and increases triglycerides in women. *J Clin Endocrinol Metab.* 2004 Jun;89(6):2963-72.
- Tetri LH, Basaranoglu M, Brunt EM, et al. Severe NAFLD with hepatic necroinflammatory changes in mice fed trans fats and a high-fructose corn syrup equivalent. *Am J Physiol Gastrointest Liver Physiol.* 2008 Nov;295(5):G987-95.
- Tordoff MG, Alleva AM. Effect of drinking soda sweetened with aspartame or high-fructose corn syrup on food intake and body weight. *Am J Clin Nutr* 1990 Jun;51(6):963-9.

- **The Case of Sugar-Sweetened and Fructose-Sweetened Beverages**… Source is Jurgens H, Haass W, Castaneda TR, et al. Consuming fructose-sweetened beverages increases body adiposity in mice. *Obes Res.* 2005 Jul;13(7):1146-56.
- **The Case of Glucose-Sweetened and Fructose-Sweetened beverages**… Source is Stanhope KL, Schwarz JM, Keim NL, et al. Consuming fructose-sweetened, not glucose-sweetened, beverages increases visceral adiposity and lipids and decreases insulin sensitivity in overweight/obese humans. *J Clin Invest.* 2009 May;119(5):1322-34.
- **Is processed fructose more fattening than fructose found in a complex food like honey?**… Sources are:

- Ahmad A, Azim MK, Mesaik MA, Khan RA. Natural honey modulates physiological glycemic response compared to simulated honey and D-glucose. *J Food Sci.* 2008 Sep;73(7):H165-7.
- Al-Waili NS. Natural honey lowers plasma glucose, C-reactive protein, homocysteine, and blood lipids in healthy, diabetic, and hyperlipidemic subjects: comparison with dextrose and sucrose. *J Med Food.* 2004 Spring;7(1):100-7.
- Bahrami M, Ataie-Jafari A, Hosseini S, et al Effects of natural honey consumption in diabetic patients: an 8-week randomized clinical trial. *Int J Food Sci Nutr.* 2008 Oct 2:1-9.
- Busserolles J, Gueux E, Rock E, et al. Substituting honey for refined carbohydrates protects rats from hypertriglyceridemic and prooxidative effects of fructose. *J Nutr.* 2002 Nov;132(11):3379-82.
- Chepulis L, Starkey N. The long-term effects of feeding honey compared with sucrose and a sugar-free diet on weight gain, lipid profiles, and DEXA measurements in rats. *J Food Sci.* 2008 Jan;73(1):H1-7.
- Chepulis LM. The effect of honey compared to sucrose, mixed sugars, and a sugar-free diet on weight gain in young rats. *J Food Sci.* 2007 Apr;72(3):S224-9.
- Chepulis LM, Starkey NJ, Waas JR, Molan PC. The effects of long-term honey, sucrose or sugar-free diets on memory and anxiety in rats. *Physiol Behav.* 2009 Jun 22;97(3-4):359-68.
- Samanta A, Burden AC, Jones GR. Plasma glucose responses to glucose, sucrose, and honey in patients with diabetes mellitus: an analysis of glycaemic and peak incremental indices. *Diabet Med.* 1985 Sep;2(5):371-3.
- Shambaugh P, Worthington V, Herbert JH. Differential effects of honey, sucrose, and fructose on blood sugar levels. *J Manipulative Physiol Ther.* 1990 Jul-Aug;13(6):322-5.
- Yaghoobi N, Al-Waili N, Ghayour-Mobarhan M, et al. Natural honey and cardiovascular risk factors; effects on blood glucose, cholesterol, triacylglycerole, CRP, and body weight compared with sucrose. *ScientificWorldJournal.* 2008 Apr 20;8:463-9.

- **The Case of Palatability**… For further reading about how processed food is produced, including things done to increase palatability, we recommend reading:

- *The End of Overeating* by David Kessler, M.D. (ISBN-10: 1605297852)
- *The End of Food* by Paul Roberts (ISBN-10: 0618606238)
- *Food Politics* by Marion Nestle (ISBN-10: 0520254031)
- *Fast Food Nation* by Eric Schlosser (ISBN-10: 006116139X)

- **Palatability is influenced by the degree to which a food interacts with our senses, including our sense of taste**... For further reading on this topic we recommend:
Unlocking the Secrets of your Sense of Smell by Luke Vorstermans (can be found by doing a google search)
  - Levine AS, Kotz CM, Gosnell BA. Sugars and fats: the neurobiology of preference. *J Nutr.* 2003 Mar;133(3):831S-834S.
  - Louis-Sylvestre J, Giachetti I, Le Magnen J. Sensory versus dietary factors in cafeteria-induced overweight. *Physiol Behav.* 1984 Jun;32(6):901-5.
  - Rolls ET. Taste and olfactory processing in the brain and its relation to the control of eating. *Crit Rev Neurobiol.* 1997;11(4):263-87.
  - Rolls ET Sensory processing in the brain related to the control of food intake. *Proc Nutr Soc.* 2007 Feb;66(1):96-112.
  - Yamamoto T. Brain mechanisms of sweetness and palatability of sugars. *Nutr Rev.* 2003 May;61(5 Pt 2):S5-9.

- **The increase in palatability caused by MSG is observed in several ways**... Sources for the information about MSG are:
  - Bellisle F, Monneuse MO, Chabert M, et al. Monosodium glutamate as a palatability enhancer in the European diet. *Physiol Behav.* 1991 May;49(5):869-73.
  - Bellisle F. Effects of monosodium glutamate on human food palatability. *Ann N Y Acad Sci.* 1998 Nov 30;855:438-41.
  - Collison KS, Maqbool Z, Saleh SM, et al. Effect of dietary monosodium glutamate on trans fat-induced nonalcoholic fatty liver disease. *J Lipid Res.* 2009 Aug;50(8):1521-37.
  - Fernandez-Tresguerres Hernández JA. Effect of monosodium glutamate given orally on appetite control (a new theory for the obesity epidemic) *An R Acad Nac Med (Madr).* 2005;122(2):341-55; discussion 355-60 [Article in Spanish]
  - Fernstrom MH, Patil V, Fernstrom JD. The effect of dietary carbohydrate on the rise in plasma glutamate concentrations following oral glutamate ingestion in rats. *J Nutr Biochem.* 2002 Dec;13(12):734-746.
  - He K, Zhao L, Daviglus ML, et al. Association of monosodium glutamate intake with overweight in Chinese adults: the INTERMAP Study. *Obesity (Silver Spring).* 2008 Aug;16(8):1875-80.
  - Hermanussen M, Garcia AP, Sunder M, et al. Obesity, voracity, and short stature: the impact of glutamate on the regulation of appetite. *Eur J Clin Nutr.* 2005 Aug 31.
  - Okiyama A, Beauchamp GK. Taste dimensions of monosodium glutamate (MSG) in a food system: role of glutamate in young American subjects. *Physiol Behav.* 1998 Aug;65(1):177-81.
  - Prescott J. Effects of added glutamate on liking for novel food flavors. *Appetite.* 2004 Apr;42(2):143-50.
  - Rogers PJ, Blundell JE. Umami and appetite: effects of monosodium glutamate on hunger and food intake in human subjects. *Physiol Behav.* 1990 Dec;48(6):801-4.
  - Sasaki Y, Suzuki W, Shimada T, et al. Dose dependent development of diabetes mellitus and non-alcoholic steatohepatitis in monosodium glutamate-induced obese mice. *Life Sci.* 2009 Sep 23;85(13-14):490-8.
  - Yu T, Zhao Y, Shi W, Ma R, Yu L. Effects of maternal oral administration of monosodium glutamate at a late stage of pregnancy on developing mouse fetal brain. *Brain Res.* 1997 Feb 7;747(2):195-206.

- **Palatability influences how much we eat. It also influences shape**... To read more about the appetite and shape effects of palatability we recommend reading:
  - Ausman LM, Rasmussen KM, Gallina DL. Spontaneous obesity in maturing squirrel monkeys fed semipurified diets. *Am J Physiol.* 1981 Nov;241(5):R316-21.
  - Erlanson-Albertsson C. How palatable food disrupts appetite regulation. *Basic Clin Pharmacol Toxicol.* 2005 Aug;97(2):61-73.
  - Gale SK, Van Itallie TB, Faust IM. Effects of palatable diets on body weight and adipose tissue cellularity in the adult obese female Zucker rat (fa/fa). *Metabolism.* 1981 Feb;30(2):105-10.
  - Kanarek RB, Hirsch E. Dietary-induced overeating in experimental animals. *Fed Proc.* 1977 Feb;36(2):154-8.
  - Levin BE, Dunn-Meynell AA. Defense of body weight depends on dietary composition and palatability in rats with diet-induced obesity. *Am. J. Physiol. Regul. Integr. Comp. Physiol.* 2002 Jan;282(1):R46-54.
  - Levine AS, Kotz CM, Gosnell BA. Sugars and fats: the neurobiology of preference. *J Nutr.* 2003 Mar;133(3):831S-834S.

- Lindqvist A, de la Cour CD, Stegmark A, et al. Overeating of palatable food is associated with blunted leptin and ghrelin responses. *Regul Pept.* 2005 Sep 15;130(3):123-32.
- Lucas F, Sclafani A. Hyperphagia in rats produced by a mixture of fat and sugar. *Physiol Behav.* 1990 Jan;47(1):51-5.
- Peck JW. Rats defend different body weights depending on palatability and accessibility of their food. *J Comp Physiol Psychol.* 1978 Jun;92(3):555-70.
- Sclafani A, Lucas F, Ackroff K. The importance of taste and palatability in carbohydrate-induced overeating in rats. *Am J Physiol.* 1996 Jun;270(6 Pt 2):R1197-202.
- Yeomans MR, Blundell JE, Leshem M. Palatability: response to nutritional need or need-free stimulation of appetite? *Br J Nutr.* 2004 Aug;92 Suppl 1:S3-14.

- **The Case of the Cafeteria Diet...** Sources for this case are:
  - Esteve M, Rafecas I, Fernández-López JA, et al. Effect of a cafeteria diet on energy intake and balance in Wistar rats. *Physiol Behav.* 1994 Jul;56(1):65-71.
  - Gianotti M, Roca P, Palou A. Body weight and tissue composition in rats made obese by a cafeteria diet. Effect of 24 hours starvation. *Horm Metab Res.* 1988 Apr;20(4):208-12.
  - Prats E, Monfar M, Castellà J, Iglesias R, Alemany M. Energy intake of rats fed a cafeteria diet. *Physiol Behav.* 1989 Feb;45(2):263-72.
  - Rogers PJ, Blundell JE. Meal patterns and food selection during the development of obesity in rats fed a cafeteria diet. *Neurosci Biobehav Rev.* 1984 Winter;8(4):441-53.
  - Sclafani A, Springer D. Dietary obesity in adult rats: similarities to hypothalamic and human obesity syndromes. *Physiol Behav.* 1976 Sep;17(3):461-71.
  - Segués T, Salvadó J, Arola L, Alemany M. Long-term effects of cafeteria diet feeding on young Wistar rats. *Biochem Mol Biol Int.* 1994 May;33(2):321-8.
  - Shafat A, Murray B, Rumsey D. Energy density in cafeteria diet induced hyperphagia in the rat. *Appetite.* 2009 Feb;52(1):34-8.
  - Tulp OL, Frink R, Danforth E Jr. Effect of cafeteria feeding on brown and white adipose tissue cellularity, thermogenesis, and body composition in rats. *J Nutr.* 1982 Dec;112(12):2250-60.
  - Winn P, Herberg LJ. Changes in actual versus defended body weight elicited by a varied, palatable ("supermarket") diet in rats. *Physiol Behav.* 1985 Nov;35(5):683-7.

- **The Case of the Vending Machine Experiment...** The source for this case is Larson DE, Rising R, Ferraro RT, Ravussin E. Spontaneous overfeeding with a 'cafeteria diet' in men: effects on 24-hour energy expenditure and substrate oxidation. *Int J Obes Relat Metab Disord.* 1995 May;19(5):331-7. Other vending machine experiments that have shown similar results include:
  - Larson DE, Tataranni PA, Ferraro RT, Ravussin E. Ad libitum food intake on a "cafeteria diet" in Native American women: relations with body composition and 24-h energy expenditure. *Am J Clin Nutr.* 1995 Nov;62(5):911-7.
  - Rising R, Alger S, Boyce V, et al. Food intake measured by an automated food-selection system: relationship to energy expenditure. *Am J Clin Nutr.* 1992 Feb;55(2):343-9.
  - Venti CA, Votruba SB, Franks PW, et al. Reproducibility of ad libitum energy intake with the use of a computerized vending machine system. *Am J Clin Nutr.* 2010 Feb;91(2):343-8.

- **The Case of Softer Food...** This case is based on Oka K, Sakuarae A, Fujise T, et al. Food texture differences affect energy metabolism in rats. *J Dent Res.* 2003 Jun;82(6):491-4.

- **The Case of Puréeing...** This case is based on Laboure H, Saux S, Nicolaidis S. Effects of food texture change on metabolic parameters: short- and long-term feeding patterns and body weight. *Am J Physiol Regul Integr Comp Physiol* 2001 Mar;280(3):R780-9

- **This effect is put to use in several medical situations, including low birth weight children and institutionalized elderly...** Sources are:
  - Germain I, Dufresne T, Gray-Donald K. A novel dysphagia diet improves the nutrient intake of institutionalized elders. *J Am Diet Assoc.* 2006 Oct;106(10):1614-23.
  - Patel MR, Piazza CC, Layer SA, et al. A systematic evaluation of food textures to decrease packing and increase oral intake in children with pediatric feeding disorders. *J Appl Behav Anal.* 2005 Spring;38(1):89-100.

- **Feeding of softer food causes more food to be eaten and more weight to be gained...** For further reading of the effects of texture on shape we recommend reading:
  - Davidson TL, Swithers SE. Food viscosity influences caloric intake compensation and body weight in rats. *Obes Res.* 2005 Mar;13(3):537-44.
  - Laboure H, Van Wymelbeke V, Fantino M, Nicolaidis S. Behavioral, plasma, and calorimetric changes related to food texture modification in men. *Am J Physiol Regul Integr Comp Physiol* 2002 May;282(5):R1501-11
  - Mars M, Hogenkamp PS, Gosses AM, et al. Effect of viscosity on learned satiation. *Physiol Behav.* 2009 Apr 24.

- Mattes RD, Campbell WW. Effects of food form and timing of ingestion on appetite and energy intake in lean young adults and in young adults with obesity. *J Am Diet Assoc.* 2009 Mar;109(3):430-7.
- Mok E, Thibault L. Effect of diet textural characteristics on the temporal rhythms of feeding in rats. *Physiol Behav.* 1999 Jan 1-15;65(4-5):893-9.
- Mourao DM, Bressan J, Campbell WW, Mattes RD. Effects of food form on appetite and energy intake in lean and obese young adults. *Int J Obes (Lond).* 2007 Nov;31(11):1688-95.
- Murakami K, Sasaki S, Takahashi Y, et al. Hardness (difficulty of chewing) of the habitual diet in relation to body mass index and waist circumference in free-living Japanese women aged 18–22 y. *Am J Clinical Nutrition,* 2007;86(1):206-213.
- Peracchi M, Santangelo A, Conte D, et al. The physical state of a meal affects hormone release and postprandial thermogenesis. *Br J Nutr* 2000 Jun;83(6):623-8
- Ramirez I. Diet texture, moisture and starch type in dietary obesity. Physiol Behav. 1987;41(2):149-54.
- Ramirez I. Feeding a liquid diet increases energy intake, weight gain and body fat in rats. *J Nutr.* 1987 Dec;117(12):2127-34.
- Tieken SM, Leidy HJ, Stull AJ, et al. Effects of Solid versus Liquid Meal-replacement Products of Similar Energy Content on Hunger, Satiety, and Appetite-regulating Hormones in Older Adults. *Horm Metab Res.* 2007 May;39(5):389-94.
- **The Case of Monotonous Food**... Source for this case is Cabanac M. Rabe EF. Influence of a monotonous food on body weight regulation in humans. *Physiol Behav.* 1976 Oct;17(4):675-8.
- **Cases of Adding or Omitting Snacks**... Sources for this case are:
  - Raynor HA, Niemeier HM, Wing RR. Effect of limiting snack food variety on long-term sensory-specific satiety and monotony during obesity treatment. *Eat Behav.* 2006 Jan;7(1):1-14.
  - Whybrow S, Mayer C, Kirk TR, et al. Effects of two weeks' mandatory snack consumption on energy intake and energy balance. *Obesity (Silver Spring).* 2007 Mar;15(3):673-85.
- **Overweight women were asked to eat either an apple or pear 3 times a day**... Source for this is Conceição de Oliveira M, Sichieri R, Sanchez Moura A. Weight loss associated with a daily intake of three apples or three pears among overweight women. *Nutrition.* 2003 Mar;19(3):253-6.
- **Obese men and women were asked to eat half of a grapefruit before meals**... Source for this is Fujioka K, Greenway F, Sheard J, Ying Y. The effects of grapefruit on weight and insulin resistance: relationship to the metabolic syndrome. *J Med Food.* 2006 Spring;9(1):49-54.
- **The Case of More or Less Variety**... Source for this case is Stubbs RJ, Johnstone AM, Mazlan N, et al. Effect of altering the variety of sensorially distinct foods, of the same macronutrient content, on food intake and body weight in men. *Eur J Clin Nutr* 2001 Jan;55(1):19-28
- **These cases suggest that eating a greater variety of processed foods is fattening**... For further reading in the shape effects of dietary variety we recommend reading:
  - Ackroff K, Bonacchi K, Magee M, et al. Obesity by choice revisited: Effects of food availability, flavor variety and nutrient composition on energy intake. *Physiol Behav.* 2007 Apr 24.
  - Brondel L, Lauraine G, Van Wymelbeke V, et al. Alternation between foods within a meal. Influence on satiation and consumption in humans. *Appetite.* 2009 Oct;53(2):203-9.
  - Hetherington MM, Foster R, Newman T, et al. Understanding variety: tasting different foods delays satiation. *Physiol Behav.* 2006 Feb 28;87(2):263-71.
  - Louis-Sylvestre J, Giachetti I, Le Magnen J. Sensory versus dietary factors in cafeteria-induced overweight. *Physiol Behav.* 1984 Jun;32(6):901-5.
  - Raynor HA, Epstein LH. Dietary variety, energy regulation, and obesity. *Psychol Bull.* 2001 May;127(3):325-41.
  - Rolls BJ, Van Duijvenvoorde PM, Rowe EA. Variety in the diet enhances intake in a meal and contributes to the development of obesity in the rat. *Physiol Behav.* 1983 Jul;31(1):21-7.
  - Treit D, Spetch ML, Deutsch JA. Variety in the flavor of food enhances eating in the rat: a controlled demonstration. *Physiol Behav.* 1983 Feb;30(2):207-11.
- **The Case of Increased Fruits and Vegetables**... Source for this case is Ello-Martin JA, Roe LS, Ledikwe JH, et al. Dietary energy density in the treatment of obesity: a year-long trial comparing 2 weight-loss diets. *Am J Clin Nutr.* 2007 Jun;85(6):1465-77.
- **Scientists refer to this as sensory-specific satiety**... Good sources to learn more about sensory-specific satiety are:
  - Guinard JX, Brun P. Sensory-specific satiety: comparison of taste and texture effects. *Appetite.* 1998 Oct;31(2):141-57.
  - Johnson J, Vickers Z. Effects of flavor and macronutrient composition of food servings on liking, hunger and subsequent intake. *Appetite.* 1993 Aug;21(1):25-39.
  - Johnson J, Vickers Z. Factors influencing sensory-specific satiety. *Appetite.* 1992 Aug;19(1):15-31.

- Rolls BJ, Van Duijvenvoorde PM, Rolls ET. Pleasantness changes and food intake in a varied four-course meal. *Appetite*. 1984 Dec;5(4):337-48.
  - Sørensen LB, Møller P, Flint A, et al. Effect of sensory perception of foods on appetite and food intake: a review of studies on humans. *Int J Obes Relat Metab Disord*. 2003 Oct;27(10):1152-66.
- **Fragrance chemicals are essential for the modern food industry**... Good starting places for learning more about the flavor industry and food are:
  - *Fast Food Nation* by Eric Schlosser (ISBN-10: 006116139X)
  - *The End of Food* by Paul Roberts (ISBN-10: 0618606238)
  - *The End of Overeating* by David Kessler, M.D. (ISBN-10: 1605297852)
- **The Case of Flavored Chow**... Source for this case is Wene JD, Barnwell GM, Mitchell DS. Flavor preferences, food intake, and weight gain in baboons (Papio sp.). *Physiol Behav*. 1982 Mar;28(3):569-73.
- **The Case of Natural Food Flavors**... Henry CJ, Woo J, Lightowler HJ, et al. Use of natural food flavours to increase food and nutrient intakes in hospitalized elderly in Hong Kong. *Int J Food Sci Nutr*. 2003 Jul;54(4):321-7.
- **There is still a great deal to learn about the role flavor variety**... For further reading on the impact of flavor on shape we recommend reading:
  - Cabanac M, Duclaux R, Spector NH. Sensory Feedback in Regulation of Body Weight: is there a Ponderostat? *Nature* 1971;229;125 – 127.
  - Louis-Sylvestre J, Giachetti I, Le Magnen J. Sensory versus dietary factors in cafeteria-induced overweight. *Physiol Behav*. 1984 Jun;32(6):901-5.
  - Naim M, Brand JG, Kare MR, Carpenter RG. Energy intake, weight gain and fat deposition in rats fed flavored, nutritionally controlled diets in a multichoice ("cafeteria") design. *J Nutr*. 1985 Nov;115(11):1447-58.
  - Sclafani A, Lucas F, Ackroff K. The importance of taste and palatability in carbohydrate-induced overeating in rats. *Am J Physiol*. 1996 Jun;270(6 Pt 2):R1197-202.
  - Schiffman SS, Warwick ZS. Effect of flavor enhancement of foods for the elderly on nutritional status: food intake, biochemical indices, and anthropometric measures. *Physiol Behav*. 1993 Feb;53(2):395-402.
- **Obese volunteers who took 1 to 2 tbsp of vinegar**... Sources for the shape benefits of vinegar are:
  - Johnston, CS, Kim, CM, Buller, AJ. 2004. Vinegar improves insulin sensitivity to a high-carbohydrate meal in subjects with insulin resistance or type 2 diabetes. *Diabetes Care* 27(January): 281-282.
  - Kondo T, Kishi M, Fushimi T, et al. Vinegar intake reduces body weight, body fat mass, and serum triglyceride levels in obese Japanese subjects. *Biosci Biotechnol Biochem*. 2009 Aug;73(8):1837-43.
- **We have more bacteria in our gut**... Sources for the shape benefits of gut bacteria include:
  - DiBaise JK, Zhang H, Crowell MD, et al. Gut microbiota and its possible relationship with obesity. *Mayo Clin Proc*. 2008 Apr;83(4):460-9.
  - Lee HY, Park JH, Seok SH, et al. Human originated bacteria, Lactobacillus rhamnosus PL60, produce conjugated linoleic acid and show anti-obesity effects in diet-induced obese mice. *Biochim Biophys Acta*. 2006 Jul;1761(7):736-44.
  - Tennyson CA, Friedman G. Microecology, obesity, and probiotics. *Curr Opin Endocrinol Diabetes Obes*. 2008 Oct;15(5):422-7.
  - Tsai F, Coyle WJ. The microbiome and obesity: is obesity linked to our gut flora? *Curr Gastroenterol Rep*. 2009 Aug;11(4):307-13.
  - Woodard GA, Encarnacion B, Downey JR, et al. Probiotics improve outcomes after Roux-en-Y gastric bypass surgery: a prospective randomized trial. *J Gastrointest Surg*. 2009 Jul;13(7):1198-204.

Chapter 20

- **These types of instincts are complicated processes, relying on aspects of the conscious and unconscious**... To gain a better understanding of what we are referring to as instincts we recommend reading the book *Gut Feelings: The Intelligence of the Unconscious* by Gerd Gigerenzer (ISBN-10: 0143113763).
- **In the 1920s and 1930s, Dr. Clara M. Davis performed an experiment**... For further reading on this research we recommend reading:
  - Davis CM. Results of the self-selection of diets by young children. *CMAJ* 1939;257-261.
  - Strauss S. Clara M. Davis and the wisdom of letting children choose their own diets. *CMAJ* 2006;175(10):1199–1201.
- **Leann Birch, Ph.D., Jennifer Fisher, Ph.D., and Susan Johnson, Ph.D. have done a series of experiments**... The findings of these researchers can be found in:

- Birch LL, Deysher M. Caloric compensation and sensory specific satiety: evidence for self regulation of food intake by young children. *Appetite* 1986 Dec;7(4):323-31
- Birch LL, Fisher JO. Food intake regulation in children. Fat and sugar substitutes and intake. *Ann N Y Acad Sci.* 1997 May 23;819:194-220.
- Birch LL, Fisher JO. Development of Eating Behaviors Among Children and Adolescents. *Pediatrics* 1998:101(3);539-549.
- Birch LL, Fisher JO. Food intake regulation in children. Fat and sugar substitutes and intake. *Ann N Y Acad Sci* 1997 May 23;819:194-220
- Birch LL, McPhee LS, Bryant JL, Johnson SL. Children's lunch intake: effects of midmorning snacks varying in energy density and fat content. *Appetite* 1993 Apr;20(2):83-94
- Birch LL, Fisher JO, Davison KK. Learning to overeat: maternal use of restrictive feeding practices promotes girls' eating in the absence of hunger. *Am J Clin Nutr.* 2003 Aug;78(2):215-20.
- Birch LL, Johnson SL, Jones MB, Peters JC. Effects of a nonenergy fat substitute on children's energy and macronutrient intake. *Am J Clin Nutr* 1993 Sep;58(3):326-33
- Birch LL, McPhee LS, Bryant JL, Johnson SL. Children's lunch intake: effects of midmorning snacks varying in energy density and fat content. *Appetite* 1993 Apr;20(2):83-94
- Birch LL, Johnson SL, Andresen G, et al. The variability of young children's energy intake. *N Engl J Med* 1991;324:232-5
- Fisher JO, Birch LL. Restricting access to palatable foods affects children's behavioral response, food selection, and intake. Am J Clin Nutr 1999;69:1264-72
- Fisher JO, Birch LL. Restricting Access to Foods and Children's Eating. *Appetite* 1999:Vol. 32;405-419.
- Fisher JO, Birch LL. Parents' restrictive feeding practices are associated with young girls' negative self-evaluation of eating. *J Am Diet Assoc* 2000 Nov;100(11):1341-6
- Galloway AT, Fiorito LM, Francis LA, Birch LL. 'Finish your soup': counterproductive effects of pressuring children to eat on intake and affect. *Appetite.* 2006 May;46(3):318-23.
- Johnson SL. Birch LL. Parents' and children's adiposity and eating style. *Pediatrics* 1994:94(5):653-61.
- Johnson SL. Improving Preschoolers' self-regulation of energy intake. *Pediatrics* 2000;106:1429-35
- Ventura AK, Birch LL. Does parenting affect children's eating and weight status? *Int J Behav Nutr Phys Act.* 2008 Mar 17;5:15.

- **Research published in the August 2006 issue of the medical journal Pediatrics**... Source is Farrow C, Blissett J. Does maternal control during feeding moderate early infant weight gain? *Pediatrics.* 2006 Aug;118(2):e293-8.

- **Humans can learn whether foods**... The work of Clara Davis, as well as Birch, Fischer, and Johnson, provides evidence for this inference. Further evidence will be presented as this chapter unfolds.

- **Scientists refer to the drive to eat things with a specific flavor, or other characteristics, as specific appetite**... A good introduction to this topic can be found on Wikipedia. Other good sources for gaining a general understanding of specific appetite include:

  - Markison S. The role of taste in the recovery from specific nutrient deficiencies in rats. *Nutr Neurosci.* 2001;4(1):1-14.
  - Rozin P, Kalat JW. Specific hungers and poison avoidance as adaptive specializations of learning. *Psychol Rev.* 1971 Nov;78(6):459-86.

- **The Case of the Thiamin Deficient Rat**... The sources for this case are:

  - Appledorf H, Tannenbaum SR. Specific hunger for thiamine in the rat: selection of low concentrations of thiamine in solution. *J Nutr.* 1967 Jun;92(2):267-73.
  - Maier SF, Zahorik DM, Albin RW. Relative novelty of solid and liquid diet during thiamine deficiency determines development of thiamine-specific hunger. *J Comp Physiol Psychol.* 1971 Feb;74(2):254-62.
  - Rozin P. Specific hunger for thiamine: Recovery from deficiency and thiamine preference. *J Com Physiol Psychol* 1965;59(1):98-101.

- **Specific appetites for other [nutrients]**... For further reading on research on specific appetites for nutrients we recommend:

  - Bertino M, Tordoff MG. Sodium depletion increases rats' preferences for salted food. *Behav Neurosci.* 1988 Aug;102(4):565-73.
  - Brommage R, DeLuca HF. Self-selection of a high calcium diet by vitamin D-deficient lactating rats increases food consumption and milk production. *J Nutr.* 1984 Aug;114(8):1377-85.

- Denton DA, Eichberg JW, Shade R, Weisinger RS. Sodium appetite in response to sodium deficiency in baboons. *Am J Physiol.* 1993 Mar;264(3 Pt 2):R539-43.
- Denton DA, Nelson JF, Tarjan E. The voluntary correction of sodium deficiency by the rabbit. *Physiol Behav.* 1985 Feb;34(2):181-7.
- Deutsch JA, Moore BO, Heinrichs SC. Unlearned specific appetite for protein. Physiol Behav. 1989 Oct;46(4):619-24.
- DiBattista D. Effects of time-restricted access to protein and to carbohydrate in adult mice and rats. *Physiol Behav.* 1991 Feb;49(2):263-9.
- Dunlap S, Heinrichs SC. Neuronal depletion of omega-3 fatty acids induces flax seed dietary self-selection in the rat. *Brain Res.* 2009 Jan 23;1250:113-9.
- Fromentin G, Nicolaidis S. Rebalancing essential amino acids intake by self-selection in the rat. *Br J Nutr.* 1996 May;75(5):669-82.
- Geurden I, Cuvier A, Gondouin E, et al. Rainbow trout can discriminate between feeds with different oil sources. *Physiol Behav.* 2005 Jun 2;85(2):107-14.
- Hawkins RL, Inoue M, Mori M, Torii K. Lysine deficient diet and lysine replacement affect food directed operant behavior. *Physiol Behav.* 1994 Nov;56(5):1061-8.
- Henry Y. Self-selection of lysine by growing pigs: choice combinations between deficient or suboptimal and adequate or superoptimal dietary levels according to sex. *Reprod Nutr Dev.* 1993;33(6):489-502.
- Hughes BO, Wood-Gush DG. A specific appetite for calcium in domestic chickens. *Anim Behav.* 1971 Aug;19(3):490-9.
- Leshem M, Langberg J, Epstein AN. Salt appetite consequent on sodium depletion in the suckling rat pup. *Dev Psychobiol.* 1993 Mar;26(2):97-114.
- Leshem M, Del Canho S, Schulkin J. Calcium hunger in the parathyroidectomized rat is specific. *Physiol Behav.* 1999 Oct;67(4):555-9.
- McCaughey SA, Tordoff MG. Magnesium appetite in the rat. *Appetite.* 2002 Feb;38(1):29-38.
- McCaughey SA, Forestell CA, Tordoff MG. Calcium deprivation increases the palatability of calcium solutions in rats. *Physiol Behav.* 2005 Feb 15;84(2):335-42.
- Muramatsu K, Ishida M. Regulation of amino acid intake in the rat: self-selection of methionine and lysine. *J Nutr Sci Vitaminol (Tokyo).* 1982 Apr;28(2):149-62.
- Nakashima Y, Tsukita Y, Yokoyama M. Preferential fat intake of pups nursed by dams fed low fat diet during pregnancy and lactation is higher than that of pups nursed by dams fed control diet and high fat diet. *J Nutr Sci Vitaminol (Tokyo).* 2008 Jun;54(3):215-22.
- Peretti PO, Baird M. Experimental studies of food selective behavior in squirrel monkeys fed on riboflavin deficient diet. *J Nutr Sci Vitaminol (Tokyo).* 1975;21(3):199-206.
- Reed DR, Friedman MI, Tordoff MG. Experience with a macronutrient source influences subsequent macronutrient selection. *Appetite.* 1992 Jun;18(3):223-32.
- Rutkoski NJ, Levenson CW. Self-selection of copper-containing diets by copper-deficient and overloaded rats. *Physiol Behav.* 2000 Oct 1-15;71(1-2):117-21.
- Siu GM, Hadley M, Agwu DE, Draper HH. Self-regulation of phosphate intake in the rat: the influence of age, vitamin D and parathyroid hormone. *J Nutr.* 1984 Jun;114(6):1097-105.
- Schulkin J, Leibman D, Ehrman RN, et al. Salt hunger in the rhesus monkey. *Behav Neurosci.* 1984 Aug;98(4):753-6.
- Villalba JJ, Provenza FD, Hall JO, Peterson C. Phosphorus appetite in sheep: dissociating taste from postingestive effects. *J Anim Sci.* 2006 Aug;84(8):2213-23.
- Woodside B, Millelire L. Self-selection of calcium during pregnancy and lactation in rats. *Physiol Behav.* 1987;39(3):291-5.
- Yamamoto Y, Muramatsu K. Self-selection of histidine and arginine intake and the requirements for these amino acids in growing rats. *J Nutr Sci Vitaminol (Tokyo).* 1987 Jun;33(3):245-53.
- Yamamoto Y, Makita K, Muramatsu K. Self-selection of phenylalanine in the rat. *Nutr Sci Vitaminol (Tokyo).* 1984 Jun;30(3):273-83.
- Zuberbuehler CA, Messikommer RE, Wenk C. Choice feeding of selenium-deficient laying hens affects diet selection, selenium intake and body weight. *J Nutr.* 2002 Nov;132(11):3411-7.

- **Carbohydrate cravings are an example…** Some of the evidence that suggests that carbohydrate cravings might be intelligent include:
  - Corsica JA, Spring BJ. Carbohydrate craving: a double-blind, placebo-controlled test of the self-medication hypothesis. *Eat Behav.* 2008 Dec;9(4):447-54.
  - Gendall KA, Joyce PR, Abbott RM. The effects of meal composition on subsequent craving and binge eating. *Addict Behav.* 1999 May-Jun;24(3):305-15.
  - Rogers PJ, Smit HJ. Food craving and food "addiction": a critical review of the evidence from a biopsychosocial perspective. *Pharmacol Biochem Behav.* 2000 May;66(1):3-14.

- Wurtman JJ. The involvement of brain serotonin in excessive carbohydrate snacking by obese carbohydrate cravers. *J Am Diet Assoc.* 1984 Sep;84(9):1004-7.

- **In investigations conducted on human volunteers, sleep deprivation increases overall appetite**... Sources for this include:
    - Koban M, Sita LV, Le WW, Hoffman GE. Sleep deprivation of rats: the hyperphagic response is real. *Sleep.* 2008 Jul 1;31(7):927-33.
    - Nedeltcheva AV, Kilkus JM, Imperial J, et al. Sleep curtailment is accompanied by increased intake of calories from snacks. *Am J Clin Nutr.* 2009 Jan;89(1):126-33.
    - Sorensen G. Association of sleep adequacy with more healthful food choices and positive workplace experiences among motor freight workers. *Am J Public Health.* 2009 Nov;99 Suppl 3:S636-43.
    - Spiegel K, Tasali E, Penev P, Van Cauter E. Brief communication: Sleep curtailment in healthy young men is associated with decreased leptin levels, elevated ghrelin levels, and increased hunger and appetite. *Ann Intern Med.* 2004 Dec 7;141(11):846-50.

- **The Case of the Sleep-deprived Rats**... Source for this case is Everson CA, Wehr TA. Nutritional and metabolic adaptations to prolonged sleep deprivation in the rat. *Am J Physiol* 1993 Feb;264(2 Pt 2):R376-87

- **Water-deprived rats crave carbohydrates**... Source is Corey DT, Walton A, Wiener NI. Development of carbohydrate preference during water rationing: a specific hunger? *Physiol Behav.* 1978 May;20(5):547-52.

- **We can crave a food, even if it is a food we might judge as a "bad" choice, because eating it is the intelligent thing to do under the circumstances**... In addition to references listed above, other studies that support this inference include:
    - Dallman MF, Pecoraro NC, la Fleur SE. Chronic stress and comfort foods: self-medication and abdominal obesity. *Brain Behav Immun.* 2005 Jul;19(4):275-80.
    - Gendall KA, Joyce PR, Abbott RM. The effects of meal composition on subsequent craving and binge eating. *Addict Behav.* 1999 May-Jun;24(3):305-15.
    - Maniam J, Morris MJ. Palatable cafeteria diet ameliorates anxiety and depression-like symptoms following an adverse early environment. *Psychoneuroendocrinology.* 2009 Nov 23.
    - Mason P, Foo H. Food consumption inhibits pain-related behaviors. *Ann N Y Acad Sci.* 2009 Jul;1170:399-402.

- **Specific appetites, including cravings, are learned**... The notion that specific appetites for most nutrients are learned is not new. It was hypothesized more than 40 years ago in Smith M, Pool R, Weinbergh. Evidence for a learning theory of specific hunger. *J Comp Physiol Psychol.* 1958 Dec;51(6):758-63. With the exception of a few nutrients, most notable salt, current consensus is that specific appetites are learned. On the Wikipedia page dedicated to specific appetites, the role of learned appetites is described.

- **Rats were placed on a diet that resulted in a deficiency in brain levels of omega-3 essential fats**... Source is Dunlap S, Heinrichs SC. Neuronal depletion of omega-3 fatty acids induces flax seed dietary self-selection in the rat. *Brain Res.* 2009 Jan 23;1250:113-9.

- **Scientists refer to this as flavor learning**... Sources for the information contained in this section are:
    - Ackroff K, Sclafani A. Energy density and macronutrient composition determine flavor preference conditioned by intragastric infusions of mixed diets. *Physiol Behav.* 2006 Sep 30;89(2):250-60.
    - Ackroff K, Lucas F, Sclafani A. Flavor preference conditioning as a function of fat source. *Physiol Behav.* 2005 Jul 21;85(4):448-60.
    - Ackroff A. Learned flavor preferences. The variable potency of post-oral nutrient reinforcers. *Appetite* 2008;51(3);743-746.
    - Addessi E, Galloway AT, Birch L, Visalberghi E. Taste perception and food choices in capuchin monkeys and human children. *Primatologie.* 2004;6:101-128.
    - Baeyens F, Crombez G, Hendrickx H, Eelen P. Parameters of human evaluative flavor-flavor conditioning. *Learning and Motivation* 1995:26 (2); 141-160
    - Brunstrom JM. Does dietary learning occur outside awareness? *Conscious Cogn.* 2004 Sep;13(3):453-70.
    - Brunstrom JM. Dietary learning in humans: directions for future research. *Physiol Behav.* 2005 May 19;85(1):57-65.
    - Brunstrom JM, Fletcher HZ. Flavour-flavour learning occurs automatically and only in hungry participants. *Physiol Behav.* 2008 Jan 28;93(1-2):13-9.
    - Brunstrom JM, Mitchell GL. Flavor-nutrient learning in restrained and unrestrained eaters. *Physiol Behav.* 2007 Jan 30;90(1):133-41.
    - Brunstrom JM. Associative learning and the control of human dietary behavior. *Appetite.* 2007 Jul;49(1):268-71.
    - Brunstrom JM, Shakeshaft NG, Scott-Samuel NE. Measuring 'expected satiety' in a range of common foods using a method of constant stimuli. *Appetite.* 2008 Nov;51(3):604-14.

- Brunstrom JM, Witcomb GL. Automatic and nonautomatic processes in dietary restraint: further evidence for a commonality between food and drug abstinence. *Eat Behav.* 2004 Nov;5(4):365-73.
- Brunstrom JM, Downes CR, Higgs S. Effects of dietary restraint on flavour-flavour learning. *Appetite.* 2001 Dec;37(3):197-206.
- De Jonghe BC, Hajnal A, Covasa M. Conditioned preference for sweet stimuli in OLETF rat: effects of food deprivation. *Am J Physiol Regul Integr Comp Physiol.* 2007 May;292(5):R1819-27.
- Havermans RC, Jansen A. Increasing children's liking of vegetables through flavour-flavour learning. *Appetite.* 2007 Mar;48(2):259-62.
- Higgs S. Memory and its role in appetite regulation. *Physiol Behav.* 2005 May 19;85(1):67-72.
- Mobini S, Chambers LC, Yeomans MR. Effects of hunger state on flavour pleasantness conditioning at home: flavour-nutrient learning vs. flavour-flavour learning. *Appetite.* 2007 Jan;48(1):20-8.
- Myers KP, Sclafani A. Development of learned flavor preferences. *Dev Psychobiol.* 2006 Jul;48(5):380-8.
- Pérez C, Fanizza LJ, Sclafani A. Flavor preferences conditioned by intragastric nutrient infusions in rats fed chow or a cafeteria diet. *Appetite.* 1999 Feb;32(1):155-70.
- Sclafani A. Oral and postoral determinants of food reward. *Physiol Behav.* 2004 Jul;81(5):773-9.
- Villalba JJ, Provenza FD. Nutrient-specific preferences by lambs conditioned with intraruminal infusions of starch, casein, and water. *J Anim Sci.* 1999 Feb;77(2):378-87.
- Warwick ZS, Weingarten HP. Flavor-postingestive consequence associations incorporate the behaviorally opposing effects of positive reinforcement and anticipated satiety: implications for interpreting two-bottle tests. *Physiol Behav.* 1996 Sep;60(3):711-5.
- Warwick ZS, Bowen KJ, Synowski SJ. Learned suppression of intake based on anticipated calories: cross-nutrient comparisons. *Physiol Behav.* 1997 Dec;62(6):1319-24.
- Wilkinson LL, Brunstrom JM. Conditioning 'fullness expectations' in a novel dessert. *Appetite.* 2009 Jun;52(3):780-3.
- Yeomans MR, Gould NJ, Leitch M, Mobini S. Effects of energy density and portion size on development of acquired flavour liking and learned satiety. *Appetite.* 2009 Apr;52(2):469-78.

- **Salt is an exemption to the generalized rule**... For more about salt specific appetite we recommend reading:
  - Denton DA, Eichberg JW, Shade R, Weisinger RS. Sodium appetite in response to sodium deficiency in baboons. *Am J Physiol.* 1993 Mar;264(3 Pt 2):R539-43.
  - Leshem M. Biobehavior of the human love of salt. *Neurosci Biobehav Rev.* 2009 Jan;33(1):1-17.
  - Leshem M. Salt preference in adolescence is predicted by common prenatal and infantile mineralofluid loss. *Physiol Behav.* 1998 Feb 15;63(4):699-704.
  - Leshem M, Maroun M, Del Canho S. Sodium depletion and maternal separation in the suckling rat increase its salt intake when adult. *Physiol Behav.* 1996 Jan;59(1):199-204.
  - Mattes RD. The taste for salt in humans. *Am J Clin Nutr.* 1997 Feb;65(2 Suppl):692S-697S.
  - Morris MJ, Na ES, Johnson AK. Salt craving: the psychobiology of pathogenic sodium intake. *Physiol Behav.* 2008 Aug 6;94(5):709-21.
  - Sakai RR, Frankmann SP, Fine WB, Epstein AN. Prior episodes of sodium depletion increase the need-free sodium intake of the rat. *Behav Neurosci.* 1989 Feb;103(1):186-92.
  - Sakai RR, Fine WB, Epstein AN, Frankmann SP. Salt appetite is enhanced by one prior episode of sodium depletion in the rat. *Behav Neurosci.* 1987 Oct;101(5):724-31.

- **What we can detect is flavor and it is the flavor of the food with the substance, not the substance, that is remembered and for which there is a strong preference**... To better understand the role of taste and smell in specific appetite we recommend reading:
  - Heinrichs SC, Deutsch JA, Moore BO. Olfactory self-selection of protein-containing foods. *Physiol Behav.* 1990 Mar;47(3):409-13.
  - McCleary RA. Taste and post-ingestion factors in specific-hunger behavior. *J Comp Physiol Psychol.* 1953 Dec;46(6):411-21.
  - Miller MG, Teates JF. The role of taste in dietary self-selection in rats. *Behav Neurosci.* 1986 Jun;100(3):399-409.
  - Miller MG, Teates JF. Oral somatosensory factors in dietary self-selection after food deprivation and supplementation. *Behav Neurosci.* 1984 Jun;98(3):424-34.
  - Tordoff MG. Intragastric calcium infusions support flavor preference learning by calcium-deprived rats. *Physiol Behav.* 2002 Aug;76(4-5):521-9.

- **The Case of Sweet Taste and Calorie Prediction**... The source for this case is Swithers SE, Davidson TL. A role for sweet taste: calorie predictive relations in energy regulation by rats. *Behav Neurosci.* 2008 Feb;122(1):161-73.

- **The Case of Confusing the Tastes of Rat Pups…** The source for this case is Pierce WD, Heth CD, Owczarczyk JC, et al. Overeating by young obesity-prone and lean rats caused by tastes associated with low energy foods. *Obesity (Silver Spring)*. 2007 Aug;15(8):1969-79.
- **The Case of Consistency or Inconsistency…** The source for this case is Swithers SE, Doerflinger A, Davidson TL. Consistent relationships between sensory properties of savory snack foods and calories influence food intake in rats. *Int J Obes (Lond)*. 2006 Nov;30(11):1685-92.
  The Case of Uncoupling the Flavor-Calorie Relationship… The source for this case is Warwick ZS, Schiffmana SS. Flavor-calorie relationships: Effect on weight gain in rats. *Physiology & Behavior* 1991:50 (3);465-470.
- **Flavor-calorie confusion was fattening…** For further reading on the possible consequences of flavor learning confusion on appetite and shape we recommend reading:
  - Appleton KM, Rogers PJ, Blundell JE. Effects of a sweet and a nonsweet lunch on short-term appetite: differences in female high and low consumers of sweet/low-energy beverages. *J Hum Nutr Diet*. 2004 Oct;17(5):425-34.
  - Bauman RA, Raslear TG, Hursh SR, et al. Substitution and caloric regulation in a closed economy. *J Exp Anal Behav*. 1996 Mar;65(2):401-22.
  - Davidson TL, Swithers SE. A Pavlovian approach to the problem of obesity. *Int J Obes Relat Metab Disord*. 2004 Jul;28(7):933-5.
  - Epstein LH, Caggiula AR, Rodefer JS, et al. The effects of calories and taste on habituation of the human salivary response. *Addict Behav*. 1993 Mar-Apr;18(2):179-85.
  - Lavin JH, French SJ, Read NW. The effect of sucrose- and aspartame-sweetened drinks on energy intake, hunger and food choice of female, moderately restrained eaters. *Int J Obes Relat Metab Disord*. 1997 Jan;21(1):37-42.
  - Sclafani A, Weiss K, Cardieri C, Ackroff K. Feeding response of rats to no-fat and high-fat cakes. *Obes Res*. 1993 May;1(3):173-8.
  - Schiffman SS, Cahn H, Lindley MG. Multiple receptor sites mediate sweetness: evidence from cross adaptation. *Pharmacol Biochem Behav*. 1981 Sep;15(3):377-88.
  - Shaffer SE, Tepper BJ. Effects of learned flavor cues on single meal and daily food intake in humans. *Physiol Behav*. 1994 Jun;55(6):979-86.
  - Swithers SE, Baker CR, Davidson TL. General and persistent effects of high-intensity sweeteners on body weight gain and caloric compensation in rats. *Behav Neurosci*. 2009 Aug;123(4):772-80.
  - Warwick ZS, Synowski SJ, Coons V, Hendrickson A. Flavor-cued modulation of intake in rats: role of familiarity and impact on 24-h intake. *Physiol Behav* 1999 Oct;67(4):527-32.
- **Keep in mind that the human brain is biased against food novelty…** This is call neophobia. For more information on this topic we recommend reading:
  - Addessi E, Galloway AT, Visalberghi E, Birch LL. Specific social influences on the acceptance of novel foods in 2-5-year-old children. *Appetite*. 2005 Dec;45(3):264-71.
  - Addessi E, Galloway AT, Birch L, Visalberghi E. Taste perception and food choices in capuchin monkeys and human children. *Primatologie*. 2004;6:101-128.
  - Galloway AT, Lee Y, Birch LL. Predictors and consequences of food neophobia and pickiness in young girls. *J Am Diet Assoc*. 2003 Jun;103(6):692-8.
  - McFarlane T, Pliner P. Increasing willingness to taste novel foods: effects of nutrition and taste information. *Appetite*. 1997 Jun;28(3):227-38.
- **The Case of Watered-down Fat…** The source for this case is Castonguay TW, Burdick SL, Guzman MA, Collier GH, Stern JS. Self-selection and the obese Zucker rat: the effect of dietary fat dilution. *Physiol Behav*. 1984 Jul;33(1):119-26.
- **Our body can learn to associate fatty foods with having more calories when the only foods we eat with a fatty taste contain fat. Once it learns this lesson, it can apply it to future meals and we can compensate with both appetite and metabolism…** An example of a study that shows this for butter in lab animals is Rolland V, Roseau S, Fromentin G, et al. Body weight, body composition, and energy metabolism in lean and obese Zucker rats fed soybean oil or butter. *Am J Clin Nutr*. 2002 Jan;75(1):21-30.
- **If you crave chocolate…** Sources for this information are:
  - Cartwright F, Stritzke WG. A multidimensional ambivalence model of chocolate craving: construct validity and associations with chocolate consumption and disordered eating. *Eat Behav*. 2008 Jan;9(1):1-12.
  - Fletcher BC, Pine KJ, Woodbridge Z, Nash A. How visual images of chocolate affect the craving and guilt of female dieters. *Appetite*. 2007 Mar;48(2):211-7.
  - Gibson EL, Desmond E. Chocolate craving and hunger state: implications for the acquisition and expression of appetite and food choice. *Appetite*. 1999 Apr;32(2):219-40.
  - Hill AJ, Heaton-Brown L. The experience of food craving: a prospective investigation in healthy women. *J Psychosom Res*. 1994 Nov;38(8):801-14.

- Macht M, Mueller J. Interactive effects of emotional and restrained eating on responses to chocolate and affect. *J Nerv Ment Dis.* 2007 Dec;195(12):1024-6.
- Parker G, Parker I, Brotchie H. Mood state effects of chocolate. *J Affect Disord.* 2006 Jun;92(2-3):149-59.

- **One approach to appetite, a common one in a weight-obsessed culture, is the control approach. Another approach—the opposite one in this case—is a trust approach…** In obesity research the control approach manifests as dieting or dietary restraint (restrained eating). A trust approach would be more akin to dietary self-selection. For further reading on the appetite and shape effects of restraint and self-selection we recommend beginning with the following:
  - Berner LA, Avena NM, Hoebel BG. Bingeing, self-restriction, and increased body weight in rats with limited access to a sweet-fat diet. *Obesity (Silver Spring).* 2008 Sep;16(9):1998-2002.
  - Birch LL, Fisher JO, Davison KK. Learning to overeat: maternal use of restrictive feeding practices promotes girls' eating in the absence of hunger. *Am J Clin Nutr.* 2003 Aug;78(2):215-20.
  - Cottone P, Sabino V, Steardo L, Zorrilla EP. Consummatory, anxiety-related and metabolic adaptations in female rats with alternating access to preferred food. *Psychoneuroendocrinology.* 2009 Jan;34(1):38-49.
  - Fisher JO, Birch LL. Restricting access to palatable foods affects children's behavioral response, food selection, and intake. *Am J Clin Nutr.* 1999 Jun;69(6):1264-72.
  - Hirsch E, Walsh M. Effect of limited access to sucrose on overeating and patterns of feeding. *Physiol Behav.* 1982 Jul;29(1):129-34.
  - Jansen E, Mulkens S, Emond Y, Jansen A. From the Garden of Eden to the land of plenty. Restriction of fruit and sweets intake leads to increased fruit and sweets consumption in children. *Appetite.* 2008 Nov;51(3):570-5.
  - Kremers SP, Brug J, de Vries H, Engels RC. Parenting style and adolescent fruit consumption. *Appetite.* 2003 Aug;41(1):43-50.
  - Lemmens SG, Schoffelen PF, Wouters L, et al. Eating what you like induces a stronger decrease of 'wanting' to eat. *Physiol Behav.* 2009 Sep 7;98(3):318-25.
  - Larue-Achagiotis C, Martin C, Verger P, Louis-Sylvestre J. Dietary self-selection vs. complete diet: body weight gain and meal pattern in rats. *Physiol Behav.* 1992 May;51(5):995-9.
  - Polivy J, Coleman J, Herman CP. The effect of deprivation on food cravings and eating behavior in restrained and unrestrained eaters. *Int J Eat Disord.* 2005 Dec;38(4):301-9.
  - Ricciardelli LA, Williams RJ, Finemore J. Restraint as misregulation in drinking and eating. *Addict Behav.* 2001 Sep-Oct;26(5):665-75.
  - Rieth N, Larue-Achagiotis C. Exercise training decreases body fat more in self-selecting than in chow-fed rats. *Physiol Behav.* 1997 Dec;62(6):1291-7.
  - Shiraev T, Chen H, Morris MJ. Differential effects of restricted versus unlimited high-fat feeding in rats on fat mass, plasma hormones and brain appetite regulators. *J Neuroendocrinol.* 2009 Jul;21(7):602-9.
  - Soetens B, Braet C, Van Vlierberghe L, Roets A. Resisting temptation: effects of exposure to a forbidden food on eating behaviour. *Appetite.* 2008 Jul;51(1):202-5.
  - Stirling LJ, Yeomans MR. Effect of exposure to a forbidden food on eating in restrained and unrestrained women. *Int J Eat Disord.* 2004 Jan;35(1):59-68.

Index